2010
YEAR BOOK OF
ENDOCRINOLOGY®

The 2010 Year Book Series

Year Book of Anesthesiology and Pain Management™: Drs Chestnut, Abram, Black, Gravlee, Lien, Mathru and Roizen

Year Book of Cardiology®: Drs Gersh, Cheitlin, Elliott, Gold, Graham, and Suri

Year Book of Critical Care Medicine®: Drs Dellinger, Parrillo, Balk, Dorman, Dries, and Zanotti-Cavazzoni

Year Book of Dermatology and Dermatologic Surgery™: Dr Del Rosso

Year Book of Diagnostic Radiology®: Drs Osborn, Abbara, Birdwell, Elster, Manaster, Oestreich, Offiah, Rosado de Christenson, and Walker

Year Book of Emergency Medicine®: Drs Hamilton, Bruno, Handly, Mullin, Quintana, and Ramoska

Year Book of Endocrinology®: Drs Schott, Apovian, Clarke, Eugster, Ludlam, Meikle, Ovalle, Schinner, Schteingart, and Toth

Year Book of Gastroenterology™: Drs Talley, Dempsey, Harnois, Lange, Pearson, Picco, Rombeau, and Scolapio

Year Book of Hand and Upper Limb Surgery®: Drs Yao and Steinmann

Year Book of Medicine®: Drs Barker, Berney, Garrick, Gersh, Khardori, LeRoith, Talley, and Thigpen

Year Book of Neonatal and Perinatal Medicine®: Drs Fanaroff, Benitz, Donn, Neu, and Papile

Year Book of Neurology and Neurosurgery®: Drs Klimo and Rabinstein

Year Book of Obstetrics, Gynecology, and Women's Health®: Drs Dungan and Shulman

Year Book of Oncology®: Drs Thigpen, Arceci, Bauer, Byhardt, Gordon, and Lawton

Year Book of Ophthalmology®: Drs Rapuano, Cohen, Flanders, Hammersmith, Milman, Myers, Nelson, Penne, Pyfer, Sergott, Shields, and Vander

Year Book of Orthopedics®: Drs Morrey, Beauchamp, Huddleston, Swiontkowski, and Trigg

Year Book of Otolaryngology-Head and Neck Surgery®: Drs Sindwani, Balough, Franco, Gapany, and Mitchell

Year Book of Pathology and Laboratory Medicine®: Drs Raab, Parwani, Bejarano, and Bissell

Year Book of Pediatrics®: Dr Stockman

Year Book of Plastic and Aesthetic Surgery™: Drs Miller, Gosain, Gurtner, Gutowski, Ruberg, Salisbury, and Smith

Year Book of Psychiatry and Applied Mental Health®: Drs Talbott, Ballenger, Buckley, Frances, Krupnick, and Mack

Year Book of Pulmonary Disease®: Drs Barker, Jones, Maurer, Raza, Tanoue, and Willsie

Year Book of Sports Medicine®: Drs Shephard, Cantu, Feldman, Jankowski, Khan, Lebrun, Nieman, Pierrynowski, and Rowland

Year Book of Surgery®: Drs Copeland, Behrns, Daly, Eberlein, Fahey, Huber, Jones, Mozingo, and Pruett

Year Book of Urology®: Drs Andriole and Coplen

Year Book of Vascular Surgery®: Drs Moneta, Gillespie, Starnes, and Watkins

2010

The Year Book of ENDOCRINOLOGY®

Editor-in-Chief

Matthias Schott, MD, PhD

Associate Professor, Deputy Director of the Department of Endocrinology, Diabetology and Rheumatology, University Hospital of Düsseldorf, Düsseldorf, Germany

ELSEVIER
MOSBY

ELSEVIER
MOSBY

Vice President, Continuity: John A. Schrefer
Developmental Editor: Patrick Manley
Production Supervisor: Donna M. Skelton
Electronic Article Manager: Emily Ogle
Senior Illustrations and Permissions Coordinator: Dawn Vohsen

2010 EDITION

Composition by TnQ Books and Journals Pvt Ltd, India

Editorial Office:
Elsevier
Suite 1800
1600 John F. Kennedy Blvd
Philadelphia, PA 19103-2899

International Standard Serial Number: 0084-3741
International Standard Book Number: 978-0-323-06830-7

Associate Editors

Caroline M. Apovian, MD, FACP, FACN
Associate Professor of Medicine and Pediatrics, Boston University School of Medicine; Director, Center for Nutrition and Weight Management, Boston Medical Center, Boston, Massachusetts

Bart L. Clarke, MD
Associate Professor of Medicine, Mayo Clinic College of Medicine; Consultant, St. Mary's Hospital; Consultant, Rochester Methodist Hospital, Rochester, Minnesota

Erica Eugster, MD
Professor of Pediatrics, Director, Section of Pediatric Endocrinology/Diabetology, Riley Hospital for Children, Indiana University School of Medicine, Indianapolis, Indiana

William H. Ludlam, MD, PhD
Director, Seattle Pituitary Center, Neuroscience Institute, Swedish Medical Center, Seattle, Washington

A. Wayne Meikle, MD
Professor of Medicine and Pathology, University of Utah School of Medicine; Director of Endocrine Testing, ARUP Laboratories, The University of Utah Hospitals, Salt Lake City, Utah

Fernando Ovalle, MD, FACE
Associate Professor of Medicine; Director, Fellowship Training Program; Director, Diabetes & Endocrine Clinical Research Unit; Director, Multidisciplinary Comprehensive Diabetes Clinic, Division of Endocrinology, Diabetes & Metabolism, University of Alabama at Birmingham School of Medicine, Birmingham, Alabama

Sven Schinner, MD, PhD
Associate Professor of Medicine, Department of Endocrinology, Diabetes and Rheumatology, University Hospital of Düsseldorf, Düsseldorf, Germany

David E. Schteingart, MD
Professor, Department of Internal Medicine, Division of Metabolism, Endocrinology and Diabetes, University of Michigan Health System, Ann Arbor, Michigan

Peter P. Toth, MD, PhD, FAAFP, FICA, FAHA, FCCP, FACC
Director of Preventive Cardiology, Sterling Rock Falls Clinic, Ltd; Clinical Professor, University of Illinois College of Medicine, Peoria, Illinois; Southern Illinois University School of Medicine, Springfield, Illinois

Contributing Editors

Rosane Ness-Abramof, MD

Meir Hospital, Kfar Saba, Israel, and Sackler School of Medicine, Tel Aviv, Israel

Ava M. Port, MD

Obesity Medicine and Nutrition Fellow, Department of Endocrinology, Boston University School of Medicine, Boston, Massachusetts

Megan Ruth, PhD

Post-doctoral Fellow, Endocrinology, Diabetes and Nutrition, Boston University School of Medicine, Boston, Massachusetts

Holger S. Willenberg, MD, PhD

Assistant Professor, University Hospital of Düsseldorf, Düsseldorf, Germany

Table of Contents

Journals Represented

Journals represented in this YEAR BOOK are listed below.

American Heart Journal
American Journal of Cardiology
American Journal of Clinical Nutrition
American Journal of Hypertension
American Journal of Kidney Diseases
American Journal of Perinatology
American Surgeon
Annals of Surgery
Annals of Surgical Oncology
Arthritis & Rheumatism
British Journal of Cancer
Cancer
Cancer Research
Circulation
Clinica Chimica Acta
Clinical Cancer Research
Clinical Endocrinology
Clinical Endocrinology (Oxford)
Clinical Radiology
Clinics in Endocrinology and Metabolism
Critical Care Medicine
Diabetes
Diabetes Care
Endocrine Practice
Endocrinology
European Heart Journal
European Journal of Endocrinology
European Journal of Nuclear Medicine and Molecular Imaging
Fertility and Sterility
Haematologica
Heart
Human Reproduction
Intensive Care Medicine
Journal of Biological Chemistry
Journal of Bone Mineral Research
Journal of Clinical Endocrinology & Metabolism Journal of Clinical Oncology
Journal of Neurosurgery
Journal of Pathology
Journal of Pediatric Surgery
Journal of Pediatrics
Journal of Surgical Research
Journal of the American College of Cardiology
Journal of the American Medical Association
Lancet
Mayo Clinic Proceedings
Metabolism
Molecular Cancer Research

Nature Medicine
New England Journal of Medicine
Obstetrics & Gynecology
Pediatrics
Proceedings of the National Academy of Sciences of the United States of America
Science
Thyroid

Standard Abbreviations

The following terms are abbreviated in this edition: adrenocorticotropin hormone (ACTH); acquired immunodeficiency syndrome (AIDS); cardiopulmonary resuscitation (CPR); central nervous system (CNS); cerebrospinal fluid (CSF); computed tomography (CT); corticotropin-releasing hormone (CRH); deoxyribonucleic acid (DNA); electrocardiography (ECG); follicle-stimulating hormone (FSH); gonadotropin-releasing hormone (GnRH); growth hormone (GH); health maintenance organization (HMO); high-density lipoprotein (HDL); human immunodeficiency virus (HIV); insulin-dependent diabetes mellitus (IDDM); insulin-like growth factor I (IGF-I); intensive care unit (ICU); intermediate-density lipoprotein (IDL); intramuscular (IM); intravenous (IV); low-density lipoprotein (LDL); luteinizing hormone (LH); magnetic resonance (MR) imaging (MRI); multiple endocrine neoplasia (MEN); non-insulin-dependent diabetes mellitus (NIDDM); parathyroid hormone (PTH); prolactin (PRL); releasing hormone (RH); ribonucleic acid (RNA); thyrotropin-releasing hormone (TRH); thyroid-stimulating hormone or thyrotropin (TSH); thyroxine (T_4); triiodothyronine (T_3); ultrasound (US); and very-low-density lipoprotein (VLDL).

Note

The Year Book of Endocrinology is a literature survey service providing abstracts of articles published in the professional literature. Every effort is made to assure the accuracy of the information presented in these pages. Neither the editor nor the publisher of the Year Book of Endocrinology can be responsible for errors in the original materials. The editors' comments are their own opinions. Mention of specific products within this publication does not constitute endorsement.

To facilitate the use of the Year Book of Endocrinology as a reference tool, all illustrations and tables included in this publication are now identified as they appear in the original article. This change is meant to help the reader recognize that any illustration or table appearing in the Year Book of Endocrinology may be only one of many in the original article. For this reason, figure and table numbers appear to be out of sequence within the Year Book of Endocrinology.

Introduction

Within the last year, the world community of endocrinologists and endocrine researchers produced an abundant crop of important publications. Just to give you an idea: by performing a PubMed search for the keyword "thyroid," almost 5000 articles show up; by using the keywords "diabetes mellitus," more than 15 000 articles burst onto the computer screen. As the number and, importantly, the quality of publications increase each year, the section editors have the daunting task to review a large number in each field. Of course, there is a high chance that the co-editors and I have missed to mention important research articles that will prove to be of high importance in the future. On the other hand, this chance is now minimalized since an online system has been established by Elsevier where articles undergo a process of preselection. This helps the editors to evaluate each research article and pick up the most important articles in the field. Of the selected articles, this year's Editor's Choice is the article by Schlumberger et al entitled "Phase II study of safety and efficacy of motesanib in patients with progressive or symptomatic, advanced or metastatic medullary thyroid cancer."[1] In this article, the authors investigated the use of motesanib diphosphate, an oral inhibitor of the tyrosine kinases of VEGF receptors, platelet-derived growth-factor receptor, and KIT in progressive metastasized medullary thyroid cancers. The authors reported on a high rate (81%) of stable disease in patients whose cancer was initially progressive. From the point of view of a clinical endocrinologist, these findings are of major importance, as they show that multikinase inhibitors are clinically effective in this patient cohort. I hope you enjoy reading this book, and I hope that you will find the editors' comments useful.

Matthias Schott, MD, PhD

Reference

1. Schlumberger MJ, Elisei R, Bastholt L, et al. Phase II study of safety and efficacy of motesanib in patients with progressive or symptomatic, advanced or metastatic medullary thyroid cancer. *J Clin Oncol.* 2009;27:3794-3801.

1 Diabetes

Section A

INTRODUCTION

Beta-cell function and failure has been an important focus of scientific work in 2009. In particular, this was influenced by the identification of TCF7L2 as the strongest candidate gene for type 2 diabetes. Although the cellular effects of genetic variants in TCF7L2 are still largely unknown, it is clear that the major effect is on beta-cell function. The incretin system, either at the preclinical level or in various clinical trials for novel therapies, has been another area of focus for diabetes researchers and clinicians. Glucagon—a target for GLP-1 based therapies—has attracted attention with the broader clinical use of incretin-based therapy strategies. Some of these studies, like the LEAD-6 study or other clinical investigations,[1] will be presented in detail in this chapter.

Moreover, an interesting concept from animal models has been translated into humans: The bone–beta-cell axis. Previously, it has been established in animal models that bone signals to beta-cells via osteocalcin. This interesting concept is currently being investigated in humans, and there are some data[2] suggesting that this concept is also true in humans.

Taken together, there are plenty of novel research approaches to diabetes that will generate more questions and might eventually be translated into clinical practice.

Sven Schinner, MD, PhD

References

1. Hare KJ, Knop FK, Asmar M, et al. Preserved inhibitory potency of GLP-1 on glucagon secretion in type 2 diabetes mellitus. *J Clin Endocrinol Metab.* 2009; 94:4679-4687.
2. Winhofer Y, Handisurya A, Tura A, et al. Osteocalcin is related to enhanced insulin secretion in gestational diabetes mellitus. *Diabetes Care.* 2010;33:139-143.

PATHOGENESIS

Adaptive β-Cell Proliferation Is Severely Restricted With Advanced Age

Rankin MM, Kushner JA (Univ of Pennsylvania School of Medicine, Philadelphia)

Diabetes 58:1365-1372, 2009

Objective.—Regeneration of the insulin-secreting β-cells is a fundamental research goal that could benefit patients with either type 1 or type 2 diabetes. β-Cell proliferation can be acutely stimulated by a variety of stimuli in young rodents. However, it is unknown whether this adaptive β-cell regeneration capacity is retained into old age.

Research Design and Methods.—We assessed adaptive β-cell proliferation capacity in adult mice across a wide range of ages with a variety of stimuli: partial pancreatectomy, low-dose administration of the β-cell toxin streptozotocin, and exendin-4, a glucagon-like peptide 1 (GLP-1) agonist. β-Cell proliferation was measured by administration of 5-bromo-2′-deoxyuridine (BrdU) in the drinking water.

Results.—Basal β-cell proliferation was severely decreased with advanced age. Partial pancreatectomy greatly stimulated β-cell proliferation in young mice but failed to increase β-cell replication in old mice. Streptozotocin stimulated β-cell replication in young mice but had little effect in old mice. Moreover, administration of GLP-1 agonist exendin-4 stimulated β-cell proliferation in young but not in old mice. Surprisingly, adaptive β-cell proliferation capacity was minimal after 12 months of age, which is early middle age for the adult mouse life span.

Conclusions.—Adaptive β-cell proliferation is severely restricted with advanced age in mice, whether stimulated by partial pancreatectomy, low-dose streptozotocin, or exendin-4. Thus, β-cells in middle-aged mice appear to be largely postmitotic. Young rodents may not faithfully model the regenerative capacity of β-cells in mature adult mice.

▶ Secondary β-cell failure is a major problem in diabetes mellitus type 2.[1-3] Data from the UKPDS studies clearly demonstrated the progressive nature of β-cell dysfunction in the course of type 2 diabetes. In principle, β-cells have an astonishing potential to adapt to changing metabolic demands: increased insulin demand in pregnancy is a well-characterized model for the fast and effective response of β-cell adaption. Similarly, most obese patients can compensate insulin resistance—at least for a certain period of time—by increasing β-cell mass and insulin secretion thereby maintaining normoglycaemia. However, in the long run β-cell failure is a common finding and diabetes mellitus becomes overt.

Why do certain individuals compensate insulin resistance better than others, and why do older individuals have a higher incidence of type 2 diabetes?

Rankin and Kushner investigated the latter in mice. They used mice of different age and challenged the β-cells by different stimuli: loss of β-cells by surgery or low dose streptozotocin, which is toxic to β-cells. The remaining β-cells need to adapt to the metabolic demands. In addition, they administered exendin-4, a GLP-1 receptor agonist, which is known to increase β-cell proliferation.

What were the major findings?

1. Basal β-cell proliferation was much lower in old than in young animals.
2. The proliferative response of β-cells to partial pancreatectomy was lost in old mice.
3. The proliferative effect of exendin-4 was lost in old mice.

Of note, the proliferative capacity of β-cells decreased even after 12 months of age, which is early middle age for mice.

Obviously, these data are not easily translated into humans. However, at least in an animal model, β-cells loose their capacity of proliferative adaption markedly with age. This occurs relatively early given the mouse life span.

It will be exciting to try to translate these observations into human disease and it might open new strategies to prevent β-cell loss.

S. Schinner, MD, PhD

References

1. Teta M, Long SY, Wartschow LM, Rankin MM, Kushner JA. Very slow turn over of β-cells in aged adult mice. *Diabetes.* 2005;54:2557-2567.
2. Bonner-Weir S. β-cell turnover: its assessment and implications. *Diabetes.* 2001; 50:S20-S24.
3. Rhodes CJ. Type 2 diabetes-a matter of beta-cell life and death? *Science.* 2005;307: 380-384.

Age-Dependent Decline in β-Cell Proliferation Restricts the Capacity of β-Cell Regeneration in Mice

Tschen S-I, Dhawan S, Gurlo T, et al (Univ of California, Los Angeles)

Diabetes 58:1312-1320, 2009

Objective.—The aim of this study was to elucidate whether age plays a role in the expansion or regeneration of β-cell mass.

Research Design and Methods.—We analyzed the capacity of β-cell expansion in 1.5- and 8-month-old mice in response to a high-fat diet, after short-term treatment with the glucagon-like peptide 1 (GLP-1) analog exendin-4, or after streptozotocin (STZ) administration.

Results.—Young mice responded to high-fat diet by increasing β-cell mass and β-cell proliferation and maintaining normoglycemia. Old mice, by contrast, did not display any increases in β-cell mass or β-cell proliferation in response to high-fat diet and became diabetic. To further assess the plasticity of β-cell mass with respect to age, young and old mice were injected with a single dose of STZ, and β-cell proliferation was analyzed to assess the regeneration of β-cells. We observed a fourfold increase in β-cell proliferation in young mice after STZ administration, whereas no changes in β-cell proliferation were observed in older mice. The capacity to expand β-cell mass in response to short-term treatment with the

GLP-1 analog exendin-4 also declined with age. The ability of β-cell mass to expand was correlated with higher levels of Bmi1, a polycomb group protein that is known to regulate the *Ink4a* locus, and decreased levels of p16Ink4a expression in the β-cells. Young *Bmi1*$^{-/-}$ mice that prematurely upregulate p16^{Ink4a} failed to expand β-cell mass in response to exendin-4, indicating that p16^{Ink4a} levels are a critical determinant of β-cell mass expansion.

Conclusions.—β-Cell proliferation and the capacity of β-cells to regenerate declines with age and is regulated by the Bmi1/p16^{Ink4a} pathway.

▶ The reactive increase in insulin secretion and β-cell mass is a crucial mechanism to respond to insulin resistance in order to maintain normoglycemia. Once this mechanism fails, relative insulin deficiency develops, resulting in hyperglycemia.

In real life, obesity is the major challenge for β-cells, as it induces insulin resistance.

This article by Tschen et al must be seen in parallel with the accompanying article by Rankin and Kushner. The question is similar: Is there a difference in adaptive mechanisms of β-cells to metabolic challenges in young versus old animals? In this study by Tschen et al the major metabolic challenge was obesity. Again, young mice adapted adequately to diet-induced obesity. However, old mice failed to do so, showed no increase in β-cell mass, and developed diabetes mellitus. How can this be explained?

The authors investigated 2 markers for β-cell aging that regulate the cell cycle: Bmi-1 and p16. p16 inhibits cyclins and thereby the cell cycle. p16 is increased in the β-cells of old animals. In turn, p16 is negatively regulated by bmi-1. With age, Bmi-1 expression decreases while p16 expression increases. The authors find bmi-1 levels correlate with the adaptive proliferative capacity of β-cells. In line with this, Bmi-1 knockout mice upregulate p16 prematurely and fail to respond to exendin-4 with proliferation.

These data are interesting, suggesting potential molecular mechanisms of β-cell aging and the age-dependent failure of β-cells to adapt to metabolic challenges. Bmi-1 and p16 might be crucial regulators of this process.

S. Schinner, MD, PhD

β-Cell-Mediated Signaling Predominates Over Direct α-Cell Signaling in the Regulation of Glucagon Secretion in Humans

Cooperberg BA, Cryer PE (Washington Univ School of Medicine, St Louis, MO)

Diabetes Care 32:2275-2280, 2009

Objective.—Given evidence of both indirect and direct signaling, we tested the hypothesis that increased β-cell–mediated signaling of α-cells negates direct α-cell signaling in the regulation of glucagon secretion in humans.

Research Design and Methods.—We measured plasma glucagon concentrations before and after ingestion of a formula mixed meal and, on a separate occasion, ingestion of the sulfonylurea glimepiride in 24 basal insulin-infused, demonstrably β-cell–deficient patients with type 1 diabetes and 20 nondiabetic, demonstrably β-cell–sufficient individuals; the latter were infused with glucose to prevent hypoglycemia after glimepiride.

Results.—After the mixed meal, plasma glucagon concentrations increased from 22 ± 1 pmol/l (78 ± 4 pg/ml) to 30 ± 2 pmol/l (103 ± 7 pg/ml) in the patients with type 1 diabetes but were unchanged from 27 ± 1 pmol/l (93 ± 3 pg/ml) to 26 ± 1 pmol/l (89 ± 3 pg/ml) in the nondiabetic individuals ($P < 0.0001$). After glimepiride, plasma glucagon concentrations increased from 24 ± 1 pmol/l (83 ± 4 pg/ml) to 26 ± 1 pmol/l (91 ± 4 pg/ml) in the patients with type 1 diabetes and decreased from 28 ± 1 pmol/l (97 ± 5 pg/ml) to 24 ± 1 pmol/l (82 ± 4 pg/ml) in the nondiabetic individuals ($P < 0.0001$). Thus, in the presence of both β-cell and α-cell secretory stimuli (increased amino acid and glucose levels, a sulfonylurea) glucagon secretion was prevented when β-cell secretion was sufficient but not when β-cell secretion was deficient.

Conclusions.—These data indicate that, among the array of signals, indirect reciprocal β-cell–mediated signaling predominates over direct α-cell signaling in the regulation of glucagon secretion in humans.

▶ Hyperglycemia in type 2 diabetes mellitus is caused by dysregulation of insulin and glucagon secretion. While the absolute or relative insulin deficiency is well established, the hyperglucagonemia in diabetes is less recognized. However, with the implementation of incretin-based therapies for type 2 diabetes mellitus that suppress glucagon in addition to increasing insulin levels, the dysfunction of the α cell has attracted more attention.

The regulation of glucagon release is poorly understood. It is tonically suppressed by islet hormones, most of all insulin, and by glucose. Other factors regulating glucagon release are not completely characterised. Insulin deficiency or insulin resistance of glucagon-producing α cells can lead to a disinhibition of glucagon release. The resulting hyperglucagonemia induces hepatic glucose output and hyperglycemia.[1-4]

Cooperberg and colleagues investigated the regulation of glucagon release by direct signals and β-cell-derived signals in humans. They found that a mixed meal increased glucagon release in type 1 diabetic patients while it had no effect on glucagon levels in healthy controls. This increase in glucagon levels in T1DM subjects was despite an increase in blood glucose.

From this data it can be concluded that β-cell derived factors suppress glucagon release in response to a mixed meal.

Furthermore, both groups of subjects were treated with the sulphonylurea glimepiride. Blood glucose increased in T1DM patients lacking β-cells and remained unchanged in the control subjects as they received glucose infusions to maintain euglycemia. However, both groups responded inversely with respect to glucagon levels; glucagon went up in T1DM patients while it decreased in control subjects. Of note, T1DM patients received continuous insulin infusion during the ingestion of the mixed meal or glimepiride.

These data show that β-cell derived factors other than insulin contribute to the regulation of glucagon release.

The study is important as it points out the complexity of the regulation of α-cell function and sheds light on the intra-islet regulation not involving insulin.

S. Schinner, MD, PhD

References

1. Schinner S, Barthel A, Dellas C, et al. Protein kinase B activity is sufficient to mimic the effect of insulin on glucagon gene transcription. *J Biol Chem*. 2005; 280:7369-7376.
2. Unger RH, Orci L. The essential role of glucagon in the pathogenesis of diabetes mellitus. *Lancet*. 1975;1:143.
3. Gromada J, Franklin I, Wollheim CB. α-cells of the endocrine pancreas: 35 years of research but the enigma remains. *Endocr Rev*. 2007;28:84-116.
4. Gonzalez M, Boer U, Dickel C, et al. Loss of insulin-induced inhibition of glucagon gene transcription in hamster pancreatic islet alpha cells by long-term insulin exposure. *Diabetologia*. 2008;51:2012-2021.

β-Cell-Specific Overexpression of Glutathione Peroxidase Preserves Intranuclear MafA and Reverses Diabetes in *db/db* Mice

Harmon JS, Bogdani M, Parazzoli SD, et al (Pacific Northwest Diabetes Res Inst, Seattle, WA; et al)

Endocrinology 150:4855-4862, 2009

Chronic hyperglycemia causes oxidative stress, which contributes todamagein various tissues and cells, including pancreatic β-cells. The expression levels of antioxidant enzymes in the islet are low compared with other tissues, rendering the β-cell more susceptible to damage caused by hyperglycemia. The aim of this study was to investigate whether increasing levels of endogenous glutathione peroxidase-1 (GPx-1), specifically in β-cells, can protect them against the adverse effects of chronic hyperglycemia and assess mechanisms that may be involved. C57BLKS/J mice overexpressing the antioxidant enzyme GPx-1 only in pancreatic β-cells were generated. The biological effectiveness of the overexpressed GPx-1 transgene was documented when β-cells of transgenic mice were protected from streptozotocin. The transgene was then introgressed into the β-cells of *db/db* mice. Without use of hypoglycemic agents, hyperglycemia in *db/db*-GPx(+) mice was initially ameliorated compared with *db/db*-GPx(−) animals and then substantially reversed by 20 wk of age. β-Cell volume and insulin granulation and immunostaining were greater in *db/db*-GPx(+) animals compared with *db/db*-GPx(−) animals. Importantly, the loss of intranuclear musculoaponeurotic fibrosarcoma oncogene homolog A (MafA) that was observed in nontransgenic *db/db* mice was prevented by GPx-1 overexpression, making this a likely mechanism for the improved glycemic control. These studies demonstrate that enhancement of intrinsic antioxidant defenses of the *β*-cell protects it against deterioration during hyperglycemia.

▶ Pancreatic β-cells have only a few options to protect themselves against oxidative stress. In contrast to other cells, they express only few antioxidative enzymes rendering them especially vulnerable for oxidative stress. These enzymes include superoxide dismutaseses (SOD), catalase, and glutathione peroxidase (GPx). There is evidence that chronic hyperglycaemia induces the generation of reactive oxygen species (ROS) which, if not adequately metabolized, can lead to cellular damage. In β-cells, damage by oxidative stress is not only a model for the generation of autoimmune diabetes but also for β-cell failure in type 2 diabetes.

In this study, Harmon et al challenged this hypothesis by overexpression of GPx in β-cells in mice prone to develop diabetes.

The authors found overexpression of GPx to protect β-cells against streptozotocin induced β-cell loss. In addition, GPx overexpression in db/db mice (a model fpr type 2 diabetes) showed improved hyperglycemia, improved islet size, and insulin secretion.

These findings are interesting as they not only improve our understanding of β-cell physiology, but might also open possibilities for future therapies. Secondary β-cell failure and loss is still a major issue in the course of type 2 diabetes. Given that these findings of GPx saving β-cell function and mass would also hold true for the human situation, the next interesting step would be to investigate regulators of the expression of these antioxidative enzymes. Future studies are needed to translate the concept of improved antioxidative capacity for β-cells into clinical medicine.

For further reading on this subject I suggest articles by Morgan et al,[1] Tang et al,[2] and Choi et al.[3]

S. Schinner, MD, PhD

References

1. Morgan D, Oliveira-Emilio HR, Keane D, et al. Glucose, palmitate and pro-inflammatory cytokines modulate production and activity of a phagocyte-like NADPH oxidase in rat pancreatic islets and a clonal beta cell line. *Diabetologia.* 2007;50:359-369.
2. Tang C, Han P, Oprescu AI, et al. Evidence for a role of superoxide generation in glucose-induced beta-cell dysfunction in vivo. *Diabetes.* 2007;56:2722-2731.
3. Choi SW, Benzie IF, Ma SW, Strain JJ, Hannigan BM. Acute hyperglycemia and oxidative stress: direct cause and effect? *Free Radic Biol Med.* 2008;44:1217-1231.

γ-Carboxylation of osteocalcin and insulin resistance in older men and women

Shea MK, Gundberg CM, Meigs JB, et al (USDA Human Nutrition Res Ctr on Aging at Tufts Univ, Boston, MA; Yale Univ School of Medicine, New Haven, CT; Massachusetts General Hosp and Harvard Med School, Boston)
Am J Clin Nutr 90:1230-1235, 2009

Background.—The skeletal protein osteocalcin is γ-carboxylated by vitamin K. High serum uncarboxylated osteocalcin reflects low vitamin K status. In vitro and animal studies indicate that high uncarboxylated osteocalcin is associated with reduced insulin resistance. However, associations between osteocalcin and measures of insulin resistance in humans are less clear.

Objective.—Our aim was to examine cross-sectional and longitudinal associations between circulating forms of osteocalcin (total, uncarboxylated, and carboxylated) and insulin resistance in older men and women.

Design.—Cross-sectional associations between serum measures of total osteocalcin, carboxylated osteocalcin, and uncarboxylated osteocalcin and insulin resistance were examined in 348 nondiabetic men and women (mean age: 68 y; 58% female) by using the homeostasis model assessment of insulin resistance (HOMA-IR). Associations between each form of osteocalcin at baseline and 3-y change in HOMA-IR were examined in 162 adults (mean age: 69 y; 63% female) who did not receive vitamin K supplementation.

Results.—Lower circulating uncarboxylated osteocalcin was not associated with higher HOMA-IR at baseline or at 3-y follow-up. Those in the lowest tertiles of total osteocalcin and carboxylated osteocalcin at baseline had higher baseline HOMA-IR ($P = 0.006$ and $P = 0.02$, respectively). The concentration of carboxylated osteocalcin at baseline was inversely associated with a 3-y change in HOMA-IR ($P = 0.002$).

Conclusions.—In older adults, circulating uncarboxylated osteocalcin was not associated with insulin resistance. In contrast, elevated carboxylated osteocalcin and total osteocalcin were associated with lower insulin resistance, which supports a potential link between skeletal physiology and insulin resistance in humans. The role of vitamin K status in this association remains unclear and merits further investigation. This trial is registered at clinicaltrials.gov as NCT00183001.

▶ Osteocalcin is a noncollagenous protein produced by osteoblasts. The post-translational vitamin K-dependent γ-carboxylation allows the protein to bind calcium. In addition to its abundant presence in bone, osteocalcin can also be detected in blood. Mouse models demonstrated a role of osteocalcin in regulating insulin expression and insulin sensitivity in mice.[1,2] Moreover, osteocalcin led to increased energy expenditure.[2] In humans, total serum osteocalcin is also associated with improved insulin sensitivity, lower fat mass, and higher adiponectin levels.[3] In addition, vitamin K supplementation protected against the progression of insulin resistance in older men.

Shea et al investigated the association between total, carboxylated, and uncarboxylated osteocalcin and insulin resistance in elderly. They performed a cross-sectional study involving 348 nondiabetic men and women and a longitudinal study involving 162 participants. The baseline characteristics of all participants were similar. The cross-sectional results revealed a lower insulin resistance as assessed by homeostasis model assessment of insulin resistance (HOMA-IR) across the higher tertiles of total and carboxylated serum osteocalcin. In line with this, the higher tertile of total and carboxylated osteocalcin had lower fasting glucose and higher adiponectin levels. None of these parameters were associated with uncarboxylated serum osteocalcin. When adjusted for adiponectin, the association between total serum osteocalcin and HOMA-IR remained statistically significant, whereas the association between carboxylated osteocalcin and HOMA-IR did not.

At the 3-year follow-up, HOMA-IR was increased by 14%. In line with the cross-sectional findings, total and carboxylated serum osteocalcin decreased by 10% and 13%, respectively. A higher baseline concentration of carboxylated osteocalcin was associated with a reduction of HOMA-IR, plasma insulin concentration, and plasma glucose concentration after 3 years. No significant changes were found for uncarboxylated osteocalcin.

In contrast to these findings, Lee et al demonstrated uncarboxylated osteocalcin to be responsible for improved insulin sensitivity and increased insulin secretion in mice, and reported no effect of carboxylated osteocalcin on adiponectin and insulin expression in a cell-based assay. However, one should keep in mind possible species differences. Another recent study might help to explain the seemingly opposing findings. Hwang et al reported an association between uncarboxylated osteocalcin and improved β-cell function, whereas the carboxylated form of osteocalcin was found to be associated with improved insulin sensitivity in middle-aged male subjects.[4] Taken together, there is evidence for the effect of osteocalcin on glucose metabolism. The exact mechanisms, especially the mode of action of osteocalcin, however, still needs to be elucidated.

S. Schinner, MD, PhD

References

1. Lee NK, Sowa H, Hinoi E, et al. Endocrine regulation of energy metabolism by the skeleton. *Cell.* 2007 Aug 10;130:456-469.
2. Ferron M, Hinoi E, Karsenty G, Ducy P. Osteocalcin differentially regulates beta cell and adipocyte gene expression and affects the development of metabolic diseases in wild-type mice. *Proc Natl Acad Sci U S A.* 2008;105:5266-5270.
3. Pittas AG, Harris SS, Eliades M, Stark P, Dawson-Hughes B. Association between serum osteocalcin and markers of metabolic phenotype. *J Clin Endocrinol Metab.* 2009;94:827-832.
4. Hwang YC, Jeong IK, Ahn KJ, Chung HY. The uncarboxylated form of osteocalcin is associated with improved glucose tolerance and enhanced beta-cell function in middle-aged male subjects. *Diabetes Metab Res Rev.* 2009 Nov;25:768-772.

A Role for the CHC22 Clathrin Heavy-Chain Isoform in Human Glucose Metabolism

Vassilopoulos S, Esk C, Hoshino S, et al (Univ of California, San Francisco)
Science 324:1192-1196, 2009

Intracellular trafficking of the glucose transporter GLUT4 from storage compartments to the plasma membrane is triggered in muscle and fat during the body's response to insulin. Clathrin is involved in intracellular trafficking, and in humans, the clathrin heavy-chain isoform CHC22 is highly expressed in skeletal muscle. We found a role for CHC22 in the formation of insulin-responsive GLUT4 compartments in human muscle and adipocytes. CHC22 also associated with expanded GLUT4 compartments in muscle from type 2 diabetic patients. Tissue-specific introduction of CHC22 in mice, which have only a pseudogene for this protein, caused aberrant localization of GLUT4 transport pathway components in their muscle, as well as features of diabetes. Thus, CHC22-dependent membrane trafficking constitutes a species-restricted pathway in human muscle and fat with potential implications for type 2 diabetes.

▶ Mechanisms causing type 2 diabetes mellitus can be divided grossly into 2 groups: defects in the production of insulin or the action of insulin. In adipose tissue and muscle, insulin signaling leads to translocation of glucose transporter type 4 (GLUT4) from intracellular storage compartments to the plasma membrane to facilitate the passive diffusion of circulating glucose down its concentration gradient. The clathrin protein complex forms a coat on membrane vesicles and is involved in their selective intracellular transport. In contrast to the clathrin heavy chain (CHC)17 isoform, CHC22 is mainly expressed in muscle in humans. However, in mice it is a pseudogene.

Vassilopoulos et al found a strong colocalization of CHC22 with GLUT4 in human skeletal muscle. In muscle sections from diabetic patients, the intracellular GLUT4 storage compartments were expanded and the colocalization of CHC22 with GLUT4 was increased. Treatment of a human myoblast cell line or primary human adipocytes with siRNA to downregulate CHC22 led to reduced GLUT4 staining and protein content and a visible loss of the GLUT4 storage compartments. Furthermore, after CHC22 depletion, the myoblast cell line showed no insulin-stimulated increase in glucose uptake. These in vitro findings were confirmed by a transgenic mouse model in which the human CHC22 gene was introduced so that these mice expressed CHC22 protein in adipocytes and muscle. Transgenic mice displayed features of diabetes, that is, mildly depressed fasting blood insulin levels in older mice and impaired clearance of excess blood glucose in response to insulin. In the transgenic mice, enlarged GLUT4 storage compartment-like structures were detected underneath the plasma membrane. The GLUT4 content of the plasma membrane was reduced as compared with wild-type mice. Of note, analyses showed increased phosphorylated AKT in transgenic mice, a key player of the insulin signaling cascade.

First of all, the work by Vassilopoulos et al recalls the given species differences between humans and mice, a popular model to assess (patho) physiological mechanisms and to carefully interpret gained knowledge from animal models.

The presented findings add an interesting aspect to the pathophysiological consideration for type 2 diabetes mellitus, as they neither involve the production or secretion nor the direct action of insulin. AKT is involved in translocation of GLUT4 to the cell membrane in response to insulin, and the higher levels of phosphorylated AKT in CHC22 transgenic mice might—but not necessarily must—reflect an increased activation of insulin signaling, which, however, is not able to integrate GLUT4 into the cell membrane.

The mechanisms underlying the interaction between CHC22 and GLUT4 are poorly understood, and it will be interesting to figure out the mechanisms of CHC22 regulation and action and why colocalization of CHC22 and GLUT4 is increased in diabetic patients. For further reading, please see Esk et al.[1]

S. Schinner, MD, PhD

Reference

1. Esk C, Chen CY, Johannes L, Brodsky FM. The clathrin heavy chain isoform CHC22 functions in a novel endosomal sorting step. *J Cell Biol.* 2010;188: 131-144.

Circulating Fibroblast Growth Factor 21 Is Induced by Peroxisome Proliferator-Activated Receptor Agonists But Not Ketosis in Man

Christodoulides C, Dyson P, Sprecher D, et al (Churchill Hosp, Oxford, UK; Cardiovascular and Urogenital Centre for Excellence in Drug Discovery, PA; et al)

J Clin Endocrinol Metab 94:3594-3601, 2009

Context.—Murine fibroblast growth factor (FGF) 21 is a nutritionally regulated hormone secreted by the liver principally in response to peroxisome proliferator-activated receptor-α (PPARα) activation, which plays a critical role in regulating metabolism during ketosis. FGF21 is also a PPARγ target gene in mouse adipose tissue. Little information is available on FGF21 functions in humans.

Objective.—The aim of the study was to measure plasma FGF21 during fasting, ketogenic diet, and PPAR agonist treatment in humans.

Design and Setting.—We conducted a prospective study involving three patient groups at two university hospitals.

Patients.—Eight healthy male volunteers underwent a 48-h period of starvation followed by 24-h refeeding (group 1); seven obese individuals were allocated to a low-carbohydrate diet for 3 months (group 2); and three groups of healthy, overweight or obese male volunteers received treatment with a PPARα (20 μg/d GW590735) (n = 6), PPARδ (10 mg/d GW501516) (n = 6), or PPARγ agonist (rosiglitazone) (n = 10) for 2 wk (group 3).

Main Outcome Measures.—Fasting plasma FGF21 and serum 3-hydroxybutyrate were measured.

Results.—There was no significant variation in human plasma FGF21 during fasting and refeeding. A 3-month ketogenic diet was associated with a 42% decline in plasma FGF21 levels. Circulating FGF21 increased significantly in response to treatment with PPARα (39%) and PPARδ (32%), but not PPARγ agonists.

Conclusion.—FGF21 does not play a major role in regulating the fasting response or ketosis in man. However, plasma FGF21 is elevated in response to pharmacological activation of PPARα and PPARδ and may contribute to the beneficial metabolic effects observed in response to pharmacotherapy with these compounds.

▶ With their work, Christodoulides et al investigated the association between circulating fibroblast growth factor 21 (FGF21) and (1) starvation, (2) ketogenic high-fat and low-carbohydrate diet, and (3) treatment with proliferator-activated receptor-α (PPARα), PPARβ, or PPARγ agonists in man. FGF21 belongs to the FGF19 subfamily of FGFs and has been shown to act in an endocrine manner. It is mainly expressed in the liver, adipose tissue, and the pancreas.[1] Formerly, in vitro exposure of murine adipocytes to FGF21 has been shown to increase insulin-independent glucose uptake by up-regulating glucose transporter 1 (GLUT1) mRNA and protein.[2] Expression of FGF21 in the liver was stimulated by PPARα in response to fasting or directly by PPARα agonists. The endocrine action of FGF21 was demonstrated in transgenic mice, which overexpressed FGF21, specifically in the liver. These animals were among others protected from diet-induced obesity and impairment of glucose tolerance. These findings demonstrate that FGF21 is a nutritionally regulated hormone of the liver that regulates metabolism during ketosis.

However, in contrast to mice, Christodoulides et al found no involvement of FGF21 in the metabolic adaptation in man. There was no significant variation in plasma FGF21 after 48 hours fasting and 24 hours re-feeding. Furthermore, they report a decline of circulating FGF21 after 3 months of ingestion of ketogenic diet in humans, in contrast to previous findings in mice. Treatment of patients with the PPARα agonist GW590735 or the PPARγ agonist GW501516 for 2 weeks significantly and uniformly increased plasma FGF21 level, whereas treatment with the PPARβ agonist rosiglitazone had no consistent effect, that is, an increase of plasma FGF21 levels in 7 subjects, unchanged levels in 2 subjects, and a decline by 50% in 1 subject.

This study reminds us to carefully adopt findings gained in mouse models to the human system. It will have to be elucidated whether an increase in plasma FGF21 levels has the same favorable metabolic effect in humans like in mice. If so, this might help explaining some effects of drugs targeting PPAR's, which increase circulating FGF21 levels.

S. Schinner, MD, PhD

References

1. Wente W, Efanov AM, Brenner M, et al. Fibroblast growth factor-21 improves pancreatic beta-cell function and survival by activation of extracellular signal-regulated kinase 1/2 and Akt signaling pathways. *Diabetes*. 2006;55:2470-2478.
2. Kharitonenkov A, Shiyanova TL, Koester A, et al. FGF-21 as a novel metabolic regulator. *J Clin Invest*. 2005;115:1627-1635.

Osteocalcin Is Related to Enhanced Insulin Secretion in Gestational Diabetes Mellitus

Winhofer Y, Handisurya A, Tura A, et al (Med Univ of Vienna, Austria; Inst of Biomed Engineering, Padova, Italy; et al)

Diabetes Care 33:139-143, 2010

Objective.—There is growing evidence that osteocalcin, an osteoblast-derived protein locally acting on bone formation, can increase insulin secretion as well as insulin sensitivity and thus prevent the development of obesity and diabetes in experimental animals. In humans, osteocalcin has been reported to be decreased in patients with type 2 diabetes. Because gestational diabetes mellitus (GDM) can serve as a model of pre–type 2 diabetes, the aim of this study was to investigate osteocalcin in GDM.

Research Design and Methods.—Osteocalcin measurement and an oral glucose tolerance test were performed in 78 pregnant women (26 women had GDM and 52 women had normal glucose tolerance [NGT] during pregnancy; women were matched for age and BMI) and in 34 women post-partum.

Results.—During pregnancy osteocalcin was significantly higher in the women with GDM than in the women with NGT (15.6 ± 6.4 vs. 12.6 ± 4.0 ng/ml; $P < 0.015$), whereas no difference was observed between the two groups at 12 weeks postpartum (36.2 ± 10.2 vs. 36.2 ± 13.0 ng/ml), when osteocalcin was found to be increased compared with the level in the pregnant state in all women (+145 ± 102% in GDM vs. +187 ± 119% in NGT; $P < 0.0001$). Moreover, osteocalcin showed a significant correlation with basal and total insulin secretion in the whole study group ($R = 0.3$, $P < 0.01$).

Conclusions.—In GDM osteocalcin was higher and thus less restrained than in women with NGT during pregnancy and furthermore correlated with insulin secretion parameters. Therefore, it could be hypothesized that osteocalcin can enhance insulin secretion in insulin-resistant states; alternatively an effect of hyperinsulinemia on osteocalcin secretion cannot be excluded.

► Osteocalcin is secreted by osteoblasts and acts on bone formation. However, in 2007 Lee and colleagues described effects of bone-derived osteocalcin on insulin secretion in mice. This work opened a new perspective on the interaction between bone and metabolic regulation. Since then, it has been known that insulin regulates bone formation, but also that the adipocyte-derived hormone leptin exerts effects on bone. The new concept, however, proposes interactions between bone and pancreatic islets in both directions. The current article by Winhofer et al therefore investigates the association between osteocalcin levels and glycemic status in women with gestational diabetes (GDM).

They found a significant correlation between osteocalcin serum levels and glucose tolerance with higher levels in women with gestational diabetes. This correlated further with insulin levels.

This is an association study, however it is interesting as it translates the concepts from animal models into clinical medicine. The data suggest that osteoalcin stimulates insulin secretion in the patients with GDM. A key feature of gestational diabetes is insulin resistance. Therefore, an important question within this concept is how the bone can sense insulin resistance and eventually lead to increased insulin release.

For further reading on this subject I suggest articles by Lee et al,[1] Kanazawa et al,[2] and Pittas et al.[3]

S. Schinner, MD, PhD

References

1. Lee NK, Sowa H, Hinoi E, et al. Endocrine regulation of energy metabolism by the skeleton. *Cell.* 2007;130:456-469.
2. Kanazawa I, Yamaguchi T, Yamamoto M, et al. Serum osteocalcin level is associated with glucose metabolism and atherosclerosis parameters in type 2 diabetes mellitus. *J Clin Endocrinol Metab.* 2009;94:45-49.
3. Pittas AG, Harris SS, Eliades M, Stark P, Dawson-Hughes B. Association between serum osteocalcin and markers of metabolic phenotype. *J Clin Endocrinol Metab.* 2009;94:827-832.

The cAMP Sensor Epac2 Is a Direct Target of Antidiabetic Sulfonylurea Drugs

Zhang C-L, Katoh M, Shibasaki T, et al (Kobe Univ Graduate School of Medicine, Japan)

Science 325:607-610, 2009

Epac2, a guanine nucleotide exchange factor for the small guanosine triphosphatase Rap1, is activated by adenosine 3′,5′-monophosphate. Fluorescence resonance energy transfer and binding experiments revealed that sulfonylureas, widely used antidiabetic drugs, interact directly with Epac2. Sulfonylureas activated Rap1 specifically through Epac2. Sulfonylurea-stimulated insulin secretion was reduced both in vitro and in vivo in mice lacking Epac2, and the glucose-lowering effect of the sulfonylurea tolbutamide was decreased in these mice. Epac2 thus contributes to the effect of sulfonylureas to promote insulin secretion. Because Epac2 is also required for the action of incretins, gut hormones crucial for potentiating insulin secretion, it may be a promising target for antidiabetic drug development.

▶ As a guanine nucleotide exchange factor (GEF) for the Ras-like GTP-binding proteins Rap1 and Rap2, Epac is activated by cyclic adenosine monophosphate (cAMP). Stimulatory G-protein-coupled receptors trigger the generation of cAMP, which activates the protein kinase A (PKA) by binding to its regulatory subunits. Two isoforms of Epac exist, Epac1 and Epac2. Former work suggests a role of Epac2 in the potentiation of insulin secretion by cAMP, but in a PKA-independent manner.

Zhang et al showed that besides the cAMP sensing function of Epac2, it can also directly be activated by sulfonylureas. They demonstrated the direct binding of [^{3}H]-labelled glibenclamide to Epac2 in mouse clonal pancreatic β-cells (MIN6) and COS cells, which was inhibited by unlabelled tolbutamide but not by 8-bromoadenosine 3′,5′-monophosphate (8-Br-cAMP) in COS cells, suggesting a binding site for sulfonylureas in Epac2 distinct from that for cAMP. While in isolated pancreatic islets of Epac2−/− mice the glucose- and potassium-stimulated insulin secretion was similar to the controls, both tolbutamide- and glibenclamide-stimulated insulin secretions were significantly reduced. Administration of glucose alone did not lead to the differences in either serum insulin or blood glucose between Epac2-/- and wild-type mice. However, administration of glucose with tolbutamide significantly reduced the insulin response in Epac2-/- mice.

This report extends our understanding of the mode of action of sulfonylureas, a commonly used group of drugs in the treatment of type 2 diabetes mellitus. In addition, it offers a new target for the development of target-directed agents for the type 2 diabetes mellitus treatment.

For further reading I recommend reviews by Hinke[1] and Gloerich and Bos.[2]

S. Schinner, MD, PhD

References

1. Hinke SA. Epac2: a molecular target for sulfonylurea-induced insulin release. *Sci Signal.* 2009;2:e54.
2. Gloerich M, Bos JL. Epac: defining a new mechanism for cAMP action. *Annu Rev Pharmacol Toxicol.* 2010;50:355-375.

Complications

Post-Challenge Hyperglycemia in Older Adults Is Associated with Increased Cardiovascular Risk Profile

Crandall JP, Shamoon H, Cohen HW, et al (Albert Einstein College of Medicine, Bronx, NY)

J Clin Endocrinol Metab 94:1595-1601, 2009

Context.—Post-challenge hyperglycemia (PCH) is common in older adults and is associated with increased cardiovascular disease (CVD) risk and total mortality. However, PCH is rarely recognized in clinical settings, and the glycemic exposure and CVD risk profile of elderly individuals with PCH has not been defined.

Objective.—The aim of the study was to characterize metabolic and CVD risk profile of elderly subjects with PCH and to determine the effect of acute postprandial metabolic changes on vascular biomarkers.

Design.—We conducted a cross-sectional study with a standard meal challenge protocol.

Participants.—Older adults with normal glucose tolerance (n = 30) or PCH (fasting glucose <126 mg/dl and 2-h glucose ≥170 mg/dl; n = 28) participated in the study.

Main Outcome Measures.—We assessed fasting and postprandial levels of glucose, insulin, lipids, high sensitivity C-reactive protein, plasminogen activator inhibitor-1, and adiponectin and endothelial function using reactive hyperemia peripheral arterial tonometry.

Results.—Normal glucose tolerance and PCH subjects were matched for age, sex, body mass index, and ethnicity. Fasting glucose (102 ± 3 *vs.* 93 ± 2 mg/dl; $P < 0.001$) and glycosylated hemoglobin (5.7 vs. 5.4%; $P = 0.01$) were modestly higher in the PCH group, which was also more insulin resistant (homeostasis model assessment for insulin resistance, 7.0 ± 1.3 *vs.* 4.1 ± 0.6; $P = 0.03$). Fasting high sensitivity C-reactive protein was higher (2.6 ± 0.5 *vs.* 1.3 ± 0.2 mg/dl; $P = 0.05$), and adiponectin was lower (11.6 ± 1.6 *vs.* 14.0 ± 1.3 μg/ml; $P = 0.03$) in subjects with PCH. Peak and 6-h postprandial area under the curve glucose, insulin, and lipids were higher in PCH subjects, who also had higher fasting and postprandial levels of plasminogen activator inhibitor-1. Reactive hyperemia peripheral arterial tonometry declined postprandially only in PCH.

Conclusions.—Older adults with PCH experience significant fasting and postprandial metabolic dysregulation, which is accompanied by a proatherosclerotic and prothrombotic vascular profile.

▶ While it is clear that diabetes mellitus is a major risk factor for cardiovascular disease, there is ongoing debate on the contribution of impaired glucose tolerance (IGT) and impaired fasting glucose (IFG) to cardiovascular risk.

From a number of large-scale studies and meta-analyses there is evidence that IFG and IGT increase cardiovascular risk.[1-3] Probably the largest meta-analysis was performed by Coutinho and colleagues in 1999 and included a cumulative number of more than 100 000 patients.[1] The main outcome was an increased cardiovascular risk when the fasting plasma glucose was above 110 mg/dL.

In this study, Crandell and colleagues asked whether postchallenge hyperglycemia is associated with cardiovascular risk. They included patients with IGT and matched them to control subjects. Both groups were not diabetic by definition, but patients with IGT had a slightly higher glycosylated hemoglobin (HbA1c) (5.7% vs 5.4%) and fasting glucose (102 mg/dL vs 93 mg/dL). Patients with IGT had elevated, though subdiabetic, blood glucose values 2 hours after an oral glucose tolerance test (193 mg/dL). The patients in both groups were relatively old (71.4 years). The end point after a standard meal challenge was mainly reactive hyperemia peripheral arterial tonometry as a measure of endothelial function. As the main outcome, the authors found patients with IGT to have impaired endothelial function in response to a meal challenge.

The strengths of the study are the good clinical characterization of the patients and the physiologic stimulus (meal challenge). The end points are somehow indirect, but it is difficult to assess true clinical end points in that setting.

The article touches an interesting clinical topic and underlines the problem with defining cutoff values to determine the diagnosis of diabetes mellitus. In that context, it is interesting to take into account that the current diagnostic thresholds for diabetes derive from data from microvascular end points (retinopathy and nephropathy). Still it is conceivable but not clear whether macrovascular damage begins at blood glucose levels below the current diagnostic cutoff for diabetes mellitus.

S. Schinner, MD, PhD

References

1. Coutinho M, Gerstein HC, Wang Y, Yusuf S. The relationship between glucose and incident cardiovascular events. A metaregression analysis of published data from 20 studies of 95 783 individuals followed for 12.4 years. *Diabetes Care.* 1999;22:233-240.
2. Sorkin JD, Muller DC, Fleg JL, Andres R. The relation of fasting and 2-h postchallenge plasma glucose concentrations to mortality: data from the Baltimore Longitudinal Study of Aging with a critical review of the literature. *Diabetes Care.* 2005; 28:2626-2632.
3. Levitzky YS, Pencina MJ, D'Agostino RB, et al. Impact of impaired fasting glucose on cardiovascular disease: the Framingham Heart Study. *J Am Coll Cardiol.* 2008; 51:264-270.

Treatments

Liraglutide once a day versus exenatide twice a day for type 2 diabetes: a 26-week randomised, parallel-group, multinational, open-label trial (LEAD-6)

Buse JB, for the LEAD-6 Study Group (Univ of North Carolina School of Medicine, Chapel Hill; et al)

Lancet 347:39-47, 2009

Background.—Unlike most antihyperglycaemic drugs, glucagon-like peptide-1 (GLP-1) receptor agonists have a glucose-dependent action and promote weight loss. We compared the efficacy and safety of liraglutide, a human GLP-1 analogue, with exenatide, an exendin-based GLP-1 receptor agonist.

Methods.—Adults with inadequately controlled type 2 diabetes on maximally tolerated doses of metformin, sulphonylurea, or both, were stratified by previous oral antidiabetic therapy and randomly assigned to receive additional liraglutide 1·8 mg once a day (n = 233) or exenatide 10 μg twice a day (n = 231) in a 26-week open-label, parallel-group, multinational (15 countries) study. The primary outcome was change in glycosylated haemoglobin (HbA_{1c}). Efficacy analyses were by intention to treat. The trial is registered with ClinicalTrials.gov, number NCT00518882.

Findings.—Mean baseline HbA_{1c} for the study population was 8·2%. Liraglutide reduced mean HbA_{1c} significantly more than did exenatide (−1·12% [SE 0·08] *vs* −0·79% [0·08]; estimated treatment difference −0·33; 95% CI −0·47 to −0·18; p<0·0001) and more patients achieved a HbA_{1c} value of less than 7% (54% *vs* 43%, respectively; odds ratio 2·02; 95% CI 1·31 to 3·11; p = 0·0015). Liraglutide reduced mean fasting plasma glucose more than did exenatide (−1·61 mmol/L [SE 0·20] *vs* −0·60 mmol/L [0·20]; estimated treatment difference −1·01 mmol/L; 95% CI −1·37 to −0·65; p<0·0001) but postprandial glucose control was less effective after breakfast and dinner. Both drugs promoted similar weight losses (liraglutide −3·24 kg *vs* exenatide −2·87 kg). Both drugs were well tolerated, but nausea was less persistent (estimated treatment rate ratio 0·448, p<0·0001) and minor hypoglycaemia less frequent with liraglutide than with exenatide (1·93 *vs* 2·60 events per patient per year; rate ratio 0·55; 95% CI 0·34 to 0·88; p = 0·0131; 25·5% *vs* 33·6% had minor hypoglycaemia). Two patients taking both exenatide and a sulphonylurea had a major hypoglycaemic episode.

Interpretation.—Liraglutide once a day provided significantly greater improvements in glycaemic control than did exenatide twice a day, and was generally better tolerated. The results suggest that liraglutide might be a treatment option for type 2 diabetes, especially when weight loss and risk of hypoglycaemia are major considerations.

▶ The incretin hormone glucagon-like peptide-1 (GLP-1) is secreted by intestinal L-cells. It increases insulin secretion and inhibits glucagon release. In addition, GLP-1 inhibits gastric emptying thereby preventing postprandial glucose excursions and reducing food intake by acting on the central nervous system. These principles are used for the therapy of type 2 diabetes mellitus and, currently, there are 2 major different modes of pharmacological interventions to increase GLP-1 action. One is the inhibition of the enzyme Dipeptidyl-Peptidase-4 (DPP-4) that degrades not specifically GLP-1. Through this mechanism, endogenous GLP-1 levels are elevated. The other option is the exogenous administration of GLP-1 analogues. Exenatide is currently available; liraglutide was only made available recently. Exenatide is given twice daily, liraglutide once daily. In the past, a number of clinical studies (the LEAD) have proven the effect of liraglutide on glycemic control. This current study compared the effects of exenatide versus liraglutide on glycemic control.

Type 2 diabetic patients with inadequately controlled glycemic status (HbA1c 8.2%) under medication with metformin and/or sulfonylureas were assigned to receive either exenatide or liraglutide for 26 weeks. The primary end point was the change in HbA_{1c}.

Under this treatment regime, liraglutide led to a greater reduction in HbA1c levels than exenatide. Weight loss was comparable with both substances. Hypoglycemia is not a frequent problem with incretin-based drugs. However, as the patients received combinations with sulfonylureas hypoglycemia occurred. Liraglutide led to less (minor) hypoglycemia episodes than did exenatide.

These data demonstrate the effectiveness of liraglutide with respect to glycemic control. From the data obtained in this study one might assume a greater effectiveness and tolerability for liraglutide compared with exenatide. However, more trials are needed to eventually assess and compare the potency of these 2 drugs.

S. Schinner, MD, PhD

Preserved Inhibitory Potency of GLP-1 on Glucagon Secretion in Type 2 Diabetes Mellitus

Hare KJ, Knop FK, Asmar M, et al (Univ of Copenhagen, Denmark)
J Clin Endocrinol Metab 94:4679-4687, 2009

Objective.—Glucagon-like peptide-1 (GLP-1) is insulinotropic, but its effect on the α-cell is less clear. We investigated the dose-response relationship for GLP-1-induced glucagon suppression in patients with type 2 diabetes (T2DM) and healthy controls.

Design.—Ten patients with T2DM (duration of DM, 4 ± 1 yr; glycosylated hemoglobin, 7.1 ± 0.3%) were studied on 2 d, with stepwise increasing GLP-1 infusions (0.25, 0.5, 1.0, and 2.0 $pmol \cdot kg^{-1} \cdot min^{-1}$) (d 1) or saline (d 2) with plasma glucose (PG) clamped at fasting level. On d 3, patient PG was normalized overnight using a variable insulin infusion, followed by a 3-h GLP-1 infusion as on d 1. Ten healthy subjects were examined with the same protocol on d 1 and 2.

Results.—We observed similar dose-dependent stepwise suppression of glucagon secretion in both patients and controls. Significant suppression was observed at a GLP-1 infusion rate of 0.25 $pmol \cdot kg^{-1} \cdot min^{-1}$ (resulting in physiological plasma concentrations) as early as time 15 min in healthy controls and time 30 min in patients (d 1 and d 3). AUC for glucagon was significantly reduced on d 1 and 3 (1096 ± 109 and 1116 ± 108 3h·pmol/liter; $P = NS$) as compared to d 2 (1733 ± 193 3h·pmol/liter; $P < 0.01$) in patients with T2DM. A similar reduction in AUC for glucagon was observed in healthy controls [1122 ± 186 (d 1) *vs.* 1733 ± 312 3h·pmol/liter (d 2); $P < 0.001$].

Conclusions.—The diabetic α-cell appears to be highly sensitive to the inhibitory action of GLP-1 both during high and near-normalized PG levels, but responds with a short, nevertheless significant delay.

▶ Incretin based therapies for type 2 diabetes mellitus offer novel approaches for glucose control. It is well known that GLP-1 increases insulin secretion in response to glucose. Of note, GLP-1 also inhibits glucagon release, which is an additional mechanism to decrease blood glucose levels. In line with this, GLP-1 reduces blood glucose levels even in insulin deprived animal models and in patients with diabetes mellitus type1.[1,2] However, the effectiveness of GLP-1 in suppressing glucagon release in type 2 diabetic patients is not clear. In this study, Hare et al tested the response to GLP-1 with respect to glucagon suppression in healthy controls and 10 patients with type 2 diabetes mellitus. The diabetic patients were moderately obese (mean BMI 31.4 kg/m^2), their HbA1c was relatively good 7.1%, and they had a relatively short duration of diabetes (4 years). The controls and also the diabetic patients showed a strong increase in insulin release in response to GLP-1, indicating an early disease stage and a preserved beta-cell capacity. The authors found GLP-1 to inhibit glucagon levels in diabetic patients and controls to the same extent. This was independent of glucose that was clamped. It is also important to mention that controls and patients had comparable basal glucagon levels in this study. This observation and the preserved strong insulin response to GLP-1 are in contrast to previous findings indicating that the diabetic population investigated here is indeed particular with a very early disease stage. In patients affected more severely by diabetes, the GLP-1 responsiveness of the α-cells might differ.

In conclusion, this is an important study as it touches a clinically relevant and not well-understood topic. However, further studies in broader populations with diabetes are needed to fully unravel GLP-1 actions on α-cells under pathophysiological conditions.

S. Schinner, MD, PhD

References

1. Creutzfeldt WO, Kleine N, Willms B, Orskov C, Holst JJ, Nauck MA. Glucagonostatic actions and reduction of fasting hyperglycemia by exogenous glucagon-like peptide I(7-36) amide in type I diabetic patients. *Diabetes Care*. 1996;19:580-586.
2. Freyse EJ, Becher T, El-Hag O, Knospe S, Goke B, Fischer U. Blood glucose lowering and glucagonostatic effects of glucagon-like peptide I in insulin-deprived diabetic dogs. *Diabetes*. 1997;46:824-828.

Rosiglitazone evaluated for cardiovascular outcomes in oral agent combination therapy for type 2 diabetes (RECORD): a multicentre, randomised, open-label trial

Home PD, for the RECORD Study Team (Newcastle Diabetes Centre and Newcastle Univ, Newcastle upon Tyne, UK; et al)

Lancet 373:2125-2135, 2009

Background.—Rosiglitazone is an insulin sensitiser used in combination with metformin, a sulfonylurea, or both, for lowering blood glucose in people with type 2 diabetes. We assessed cardiovascular outcomes after addition of rosiglitazone to either metformin or sulfonylurea compared with the combination of the two over 5–7 years of follow-up. We also assessed comparative safety.

Methods.—In a multicentre, open-label trial, 4447 patients with type 2 diabetes on metformin or sulfonylurea monotherapy with mean haemoglobin A_{1c} (HbA_{1c}) of 7·9% were randomly assigned to addition of rosiglitazone (n = 2220) or to a combination of metformin and sulfonylurea (active control group, n = 2227). The primary endpoint was cardiovascular hospitalisation or cardiovascular death, with a hazard ratio (HR) non-inferiority margin of 1·20. Analysis was by intention to treat. This study is registered with ClinicalTrials.gov, number NCT00379769.

Findings.—321 people in the rosiglitazone group and 323 in the active control group experienced the primary outcome during a mean 5·5-year follow-up, meeting the criterion of non-inferiority (HR 0·99, 95% CI 0·85–1·16). HR was 0·84 (0·59–1·18) for cardiovascular death, 1·14 (0·80–1·63) for myocardial infarction, and 0·72 (0·49–1·06) for stroke. Heart failure causing admission to hospital or death occurred in 61 people in the rosiglitazone group and 29 in the active control group (HR 2·10, 1·35–3·27, risk difference per 1000 person-years 2·6, 1·1–4·1). Upper and distal lower limb fracture rates were increased mainly in women randomly assigned to rosiglitazone. Mean HbA_{1c} was lower in the rosiglitazone group than in the control group at 5 years.

Interpretation.—Addition of rosiglitazone to glucose-lowering therapy in people with type 2 diabetes is confirmed to increase the risk of heart failure and of some fractures, mainly in women. Although the data are inconclusive about any possible effect on myocardial infarction, rosiglitazone does not increase the risk of overall cardiovascular morbidity or mortality compared with standard glucose-lowering drugs.

▶ The thiazolidinediones (TZD) rosiglitazone and pioglitazone are in clinical use for lowering blood glucose levels in type 2 diabetes mellitus. Their modes of action are complex. The major target tissue seems to be the adipose tissue. TZDs lead to a redistribution of triglycerides from, for example, liver and muscle to the adipose tissue, thereby improving insulin sensitivity.[1]

However, fluid retention and heart failure have been issues with the use of rosiglitazone.[2] Therefore, the RECORD (Rosiglitazone Evaluated for Cardiac Outcomes and Regulation of Glycemia in Diabetes) trial aimed to investigate the cardiovascular tolerability of rosiglitazone. RECORD is a multicenter randomized prospective trial including over 4000 patients with type 2 diabetes mellitus. The mean follow-up was 5.5 years, and the primary end point was cardiovascular hospitalization or cardiovascular death. The patients received a combination of metformin and sulfonylurea or rosiglitazone in addition to either metformin or sulfonylurea. Of note, the mean HbA_{1c} was lower in the rosiglitazone group than in the control group after 5 years.

The incidence of cardiovascular death and cardiovascular hospitalization did not differ significantly between the 2 groups. However, significantly more patients in the rosiglitazone group developed heart failure causing admission to hospital or death (HR = 2.10; $P = .001$).

In addition, more patients under rosiglitazone experienced bone fractures. This is an established side effect of TZDs.

On one hand, these data demonstrate noninferiority of rosiglitazone to standard treatment with respect to the primary end points, namely cardiovascular hospitalization or cardiovascular death. On the other hand, it is worth mentioning that the risk for cardiovascular events was not significantly reduced under rosiglitazone despite better HBA_{1c} control. In addition, the RECORD trial confirms a higher risk for heart failure with rosiglitazone treatment.

S. Schinner, MD, PhD

References

1. Dormandy JA, Charbonnel B, Eckland DJ, et al. PROactive investigators. Secondary prevention of macrovascular events in patients with type 2 diabetes in the PROactive Study (PROspective pioglitAzone Clinical Trial In macroVascular Events): a randomised controlled trial. *Lancet.* 2005;366:1279-1289.
2. Nissen SE, Wolski K. Effect of rosiglitazone on the risk of myocardial infarction and death from cardiovascular causes. *N Engl J Med.* 2007;356:2457-2471.

Survival as a function of HbA_{1c} in people with type 2 diabetes: a retrospective cohort study

Currie CJ, Peters JR, Tynan A, et al (Cardiff Univ, UK; Univ Hosp of Wales, Cardiff, UK; Eli Lilly and Company, Indianapolis, IN; et al)
Lancet 375:481-489, 2010

Background.—Results of intervention studies in patients with type 2 diabetes have led to concerns about the safety of aiming for normal blood glucose concentrations. We assessed survival as a function of HbA_{1c} in people with type 2 diabetes.

Methods.—Two cohorts of patients aged 50 years and older with type 2 diabetes were generated from the UK General Practice Research Database from November 1986 to November 2008. We identified 27 965 patients whose treatment had been intensified from oral monotherapy to combination therapy with oral blood-glucose lowering agents, and 20 005 who had changed to regimens that included insulin. Those with diabetes secondary to other causes were excluded. All-cause mortality was the primary outcome. Age, sex, smoking status, cholesterol, cardiovascular risk, and general morbidity were identified as important confounding factors, and Cox survival models were adjusted for these factors accordingly.

Findings.—For combined cohorts, compared with the glycated haemoglobin (HbA_{1c}) decile with the lowest hazard (median HbA_{1c} 7·5%, IQR 7·5–7·6%), the adjusted hazard ratio (HR) of all-cause mortality in the lowest HbA_{1c} decile (6·4%, 6·1–6·6) was 1·52 (95% CI 1·32–1·76), and in the highest HbA_{1c} decile (median 10·5%, IQR 10·1-11·2%) was 1·79 (95% CI 1·56–2·06). Results showed a general U-shaped association, with the lowest HR at an HbA_{1c} of about 7·5%. HR for all-cause mortality in people given insulin-based regimens (2834 deaths) versus those given combination oral agents (2035) was 1·49 (95% CI 1·39–1·59).

Interpretation.—Low and high mean HbA_{1c} values were associated with increased all-cause mortality and cardiac events. If confirmed, diabetes guidelines might need revision to include a minimum HbA_{1c} value.

▶ There is ongoing debate about hemoglobin A1c (HbA1c) targets in type 2 diabetes. The ACCORD study published in 2008 raised questions on the safety of aggressive HbA1c lowering therapies especially in patients with a long duration of diabetes and cardiovascular comorbidities.

This study by Currie et al touches the same topic. However, the design of the study is different.

Currie and colleagues performed a retrospective study in patients with type 2 diabetes (mean age > 60 years; mean duration of diabetes approximately 5-8 years). The primary end point was survival as a function of the HbA1c. They followed 2 cohorts after these had an intensification of diabetes therapy (either adding an additional oral drug or adding insulin) for 4.5 years. Surprisingly, the authors found the lowest risk of death and large vessel events at an HbA1c level of 7.5%. HbA1c levels above and also below (!) 7.5% increased the mortality rate. This was true for oral-only treatment and insulin-based regimes.

What is new in this study?

The study underlines the tendency of the ACCORD study that—at least for some subgroups of patients—a less ambitious HbA1c target might be beneficial.

What are strengths and limitations of the study?

The study has been performed in a retrospective manner looking at data of patients who are treated by general practitioners. Therefore, the patients in this study did, of course, not have as tight follow-ups as in prospective study designs in specialized centers. However, in a way this is also a strength of the study as it reflects normal clinical practice.

Furthermore, one must mention that microvascular end points were not tested. The situation for these might be different from macrovascular end points. Also, the mean follow-up was 4.5 years. The UK Prospective Diabetes Study (UKPDS) follow-up study taught us that beneficial effects of glucose-lowering therapies for macrovascular end points take time.

This study is very interesting for clinicians treating patients with type 2 diabetes. It seems, however, premature to draw direct conclusions for HbA1c targets.

For further reading on this subject I suggest articles by the ADVANCE Collaborative Group,[1] the Action to Control Cardiovascular Risk in Diabetes Study Group,[2] and Holman et al.[3]

S. Schinner, MD, PhD

References

1. The ADVANCE Collaborative Group. Intensive blood glucose control and vascular outcomes in patients with type 2 diabetes. *N Engl J Med.* 2008;358: 2560-2572.

2. The Action to Control Cardiovascular Risk in Diabetes Study Group. Effects of intensive glucose-lowering in type 2 diabetes. *New Engl J Med.* 2008;358: 2545-2559.
3. Holman RR, Paul SK, Bethel A, Matthews DR, Neil AW. 10-year follow-up of intensive glucose control in type 2 diabetes. *N Engl J Med.* 2008;359: 1577-1589 (UKPDS 80).

Sustained Effects of Interleukin-1 Receptor Antagonist Treatment in Type 2 Diabetes

Larsen CM, Faulenbach M, Vaag A, et al (Hagedorn Res Inst and Steno Diabetes Ctr, Gentofte, Denmark; Univ Hosp Zurich, Switzerland; et al)
Diabetes Care 32:1663-1668, 2009

Objective.—Interleukin (IL)-1 impairs insulin secretion and induces β-cell apoptosis. Pancreatic β-cell IL-1 expression is increased and interleukin-1 receptor antagonist (IL-1Ra) expression reduced in patients with type 2 diabetes. Treatment with recombinant IL-1Ra improves glycemia and β-cell function and reduces inflammatory markers in patients with type 2 diabetes. Here we investigated the durability of these responses.

Research Design and Methods.—Among 70 ambulatory patients who had type 2 diabetes, A1C > 7.5%, and BMI > 27 kg/m^2 and were randomly assigned to receive 13 weeks of anakinra, a recombinant human IL-1Ra, or placebo, 67 completed treatment and were included in this double-blind 39-week follow-up study. Primary outcome was change in β-cell function after anakinra withdrawal. Analysis was done by intention to treat.

Results.—Thirty-nine weeks after anakinra withdrawal, the proinsulin-to-insulin (PI/I) ratio but not stimulated C-peptide remained improved (by −0.07 [95% CI −0.14 to −0.02], $P = 0.011$) compared with values in placebo-treated patients. Interestingly, a subgroup characterized by genetically determined low baseline IL-1Ra serum levels maintained the improved stimulated C-peptide obtained by 13 weeks of IL-1Ra treatment. Reductions in C-reactive protein (−3.2 mg/l [−6.2 to −1.1], $P = 0.014$) and in IL-6 (−1.4 ng/l [−2.6 to −0.3], $P = 0.036$) were maintained until the end of study.

Conclusions.—IL-1 blockade with anakinra induces improvement of the PI/I ratio and markers of systemic inflammation lasting 39 weeks after treatment withdrawal.

▶ Type 2 diabetes mellitus is characterised by subclinical inflammation. Interleukin-1 (IL-1), a proinflammatory cytokine, is produced in pancreatic islets in response to high glucose and to secretory products from adipocytes. In turn, IL-1 induces apoptosis of pancreatic β-cells and impairs their function. Apoptosis of β-cells and secondary β-cell failure is a major issue in type 2 diabetes and the cause for the progressive character of the disease. Therefore, inhibition of IL-1 action is a potential strategy to prevent or treat type 2 diabetes mellitus. This study is the follow-up observation of a previous trial, showing that IL-1 Ra treatment improves glycemic control and β-cell function. This follow-up aims to analyse sustained effects of IL-1 Ra treatment on A1c, β-cell function, and the inflammation status 39 weeks after withdrawal of IL-1 Ra. In this study, Larsen and colleagues treated 70 patients with type 2 diabetes mellitus over 13 weeks with a recombinant IL-1 receptor antagonist (IL-1 Ra). They used a placebo-controlled, double-blind randomized design to test the durability of glycemic control under IL-1 Ra treatment. After 13 weeks of treatment the IL-1 Ra was stopped, and after 39 weeks patients were analyzed with respect to glycemic control, surrogate parameters for β-cell function, and inflammation markers. The authors found no significant difference in A1C levels 39 weeks after withdrawal of IL-1 Ra versus placebo. However, the proinsulin/insulin ration as a surrogate parameter for β-cell function was improved in the IL-1 Ra group versus placebo group. However, c-peptide levels were not improved. In addition, IL-1 Ra treatment led to a sustained reduction in CRP (C-reactive protein) and IL-6 levels 39 weeks after withdrawal. In conclusion, it has been shown before that IL-1 Ra treatment improves glycemic control. However, the improvement of glycemic control is lost after 39 weeks of withdrawal of IL-1 Ra, but there is evidence for a potential prolonged effect on β-cell function.

For further reading on the subject I suggest articles by Larsen et al[1] and Maedler et al.[2,3]

S. Schinner, MD, PhD

References

1. Larsen CM, Faulenbach M, Vaag A, et al. Interleukin-1-receptor antagonist in type 2 diabetes mellitus. *N Engl J Med.* 2007;356:1517-1526.
2. Maedler K, Sergeev P, Ris F, et al. Glucose-induced β-cell production of IL-1 contributes to glucotoxicity in human pancreatic islets. *J Clin Invest.* 2002;110: 851-860.
3. Maedler K, Sergeev P, Ehses JA, et al. Leptin modulates β cell expression of IL-1 receptor antagonist and release of IL-1in human islets. *Proc Natl Acad Sci USA.* 2004;101:8138-8143.

Three-Year Efficacy of Complex Insulin Regimens in Type 2 Diabetes

Holman RR, Farmer AJ, Davies MJ, et al (Univ of Oxford, UK; Univ of Leicester, UK)

N Engl J Med 361:1736-1747, 2009

Background.—Evidence supporting the addition of specific insulin regimens to oral therapy in patients with type 2 diabetes mellitus is limited.

Methods.—In this 3-year open-label, multicenter trial, we evaluated 708 patients who had sub-optimal glycated hemoglobin levels while taking metformin and sulfonylurea therapy. Patients were randomly assigned to receive biphasic insulin aspart twice daily, prandial insulin aspart three times daily, or basal insulin detemir once daily (twice if required). Sulfonylurea therapy was replaced by a second type of insulin if hyperglycemia became unacceptable during the first year of the study or subsequently if glycated hemoglobin levels were more than 6.5%. Outcome measures were glycated hemoglobin levels, the proportion of patients with a glycated hemoglobin level of 6.5% or less, the rate of hypoglycemia, and weight gain.

Results.—Median glycated hemoglobin levels were similar for patients receiving biphasic (7.1%), prandial (6.8%), and basal (6.9%) insulin-based regimens ($P = 0.28$). However, fewer patients had a level of 6.5% or less in the biphasic group (31.9%) than in the prandial group (44.7%, $P = 0.006$) or in the basal group (43.2%, $P = 0.03$), with 67.7%, 73.6%, and 81.6%, respectively, taking a second type of insulin ($P = 0.002$). Median rates of hypoglycemia per patient per year were lowest in the basal group (1.7), higher in the biphasic group (3.0), and highest in the prandial group (5.7) ($P<0.001$ for the overall comparison). The mean weight gain was higher in the prandial group than in either the biphasic group or the basal group. Other adverse event rates were similar in the three groups.

Conclusions.—Patients who added a basal or prandial insulin-based regimen to oral therapy had better glycated hemoglobin control than patients who added a biphasic insulin-based regimen. Fewer hypoglycemic episodes and less weight gain occurred in patients adding basal insulin. (Current Controlled Trials number, ISRCTN51125379.)

▶ This article reports the results after 3 years of the 4-T (Treating to Target in Type 2 Diabetes) study. In this study, it is of particular importance to have a closer look at the study design. The study was performed to compare the effectiveness (glycemic control) and safety (hypoglycemia) of different insulin regimes in type 2 diabetes mellitus. Given the progressive nature of type 2 diabetes, most of the patients that start with oral antidiabetic drugs finally need insulin therapy to reach HbA1c targets.[1-4] In the 4-T study the patients receiving metformin and sulfonylureas were randomly assigned to either biphasic insulin twice daily or prandial insulin three times a day or basal insulin (detemir) at bedtime. After the beginning of the second year, however, sulfonylurea therapy was replaced by additional insulin if the HbA_{1c} was above 6.5%. This was necessary in most patients, namely in 68% to 82%. The standard for additional therapy was as follows: patients in the biphasic insulin group received additional prandial insulin (4-6 units); patients in the prandial group received additional basal insulin; and patients in the basal group received additional prandial insulin. The need for additional insulin was higher in the basal group (82% of the patients) than in the prandial group (74%) and in the biphasic group (68%). It is important to note that most patients ended up with complex insulin regimes (basal plus prandial) even though they started with a single insulin strategy.

The results after 3 years showed that the mean HbA1c reached did not differ significantly between the groups. However, the percentage of patients reaching a $HbA_{1c} \leq 6.5\%$ was higher in the prandial and basal group than in the biphasic group. However, weight gain and hypoglycemia were least when the therapy was started with basal insulin.

These data seem to be in favor of basal insulin as the starting strategy once oral drugs fail. It must, however, be mentioned and taken into consideration that the insulin doses and the dose of insulin per kg body weight were highest when basal insulin was used. This might—at least in part—explain the better glycemic control. Having this in mind, the advantages in safety (hypoglycemia) and weight gain appear, however, even more pronounced with basal insulin.

Furthermore, one must keep in mind that the resulting insulin therapy, for example between initial prandial insulin and initial basal insulin, had a large overlap. In conclusion, this is an important trial to study ideal insulin regimes in type 2 diabetes, but it seems premature to directly translate it into clinical practice.

S. Schinner, MD, PhD

References

1. Nathan DM, Buse JB, Davidson MB, et al. Medical management of hyperglycaemia in type 2 diabetes mellitus: a consensus algorithm for the initiation and adjustment of therapy: a consensus statement from the American Diabetes Association and the European Association for the Study of Diabetes. *Diabetologia.* 2009;52: 17-30.
2. Lasserson DS, Glasziou P, Perera R, Holman RR, Farmer AJ. Optimal insulin regimens in type 2 diabetes mellitus: systematic review and meta-analyses. *Diabetologia.* 2009;52:1990-2000.
3. Holman RR, Thorne KI, Farmer AJ, et al. Addition of biphasic, prandial, or basal insulin to oral therapy in type 2 diabetes. *N Engl J Med.* 2007;357:1716-1730.
4. Bretzel RG, Nuber U, Landgraf W, Owens DR, Bradley C, Linn T. Once-daily basal insulin glargine versus thrice-daily prandial insulin lispro in people with type 2 diabetes on oral hypoglycaemic agents (APOLLO): an open randomised controlled trial. *Lancet.* 2008;371:1073-1084 [erratum, Lancet 2008; 372:718].

Section B

Diabetic Complications

Intensive Glucose-Lowering Therapy Reduces Cardiovascular Disease Events in Veterans Affairs Diabetes Trial Participants With Lower Calcified Coronary Atherosclerosis

Reaven PD, for the Veterans Affairs Diabetes Trial (Phoenix Veterans Affairs Health Care System, AZ; et al)
Diabetes 58:2642-2648, 2009

Objective.—This study investigated the hypothesis that baseline calcified coronary atherosclerosis may determine cardiovascular disease events in response to intensive glycemic control within the Veterans Affairs Diabetes Trial (VADT).

Research Design and Methods.—At baseline, 301 type 2 diabetic participants in the VADT, a randomized trial comparing the effects of intensive versus standard glucose lowering on cardiovascular events, had baseline coronary atherosclerosis assessed by coronary artery calcium (CAC) measured by computed tomography. Participants were followed over the 7.5-year study for development of cardiovascular end points.

Results.—During a median follow-up duration of 5.2 years, 89 cardiovascular events occurred. Although intensive glucose-lowering therapy did not significantly reduce cardiovascular events in the substudy cohort as a whole, there was evidence that the response was modified by baseline CAC, as indicated by significant *P* values for treatment by log(CAC + 1) interaction terms in unadjusted and multivariable-adjusted models (0.01 and 0.03, respectively). Multivariable-adjusted hazard ratios (HRs) for the effect of treatment indicated a progressive diminution of benefit with increasing CAC. Subgroup analyses were also conducted for clinically relevant CAC categories: those above and below an Agatston score of 100. Among those randomized to intensive treatment, for the subgroup with CAC > 100, 11 of 62 individuals had events, while only 1 of 52 individuals with CAC ≤ 100 had an event. The multivariable HR for intensive treatment for those with CAC > 100 was 0.74 (95% CI 0.46–1.20; *P* = 0.21), while for the subgroup with CAC ≤ 100, the corresponding HR was 0.08 (0.008–0.77; *P* = 0.03), with event rates of 39 and 4 per 1,000 person-years, respectively.

Conclusions.—These data indicate that intensive glucose lowering reduces cardiovascular events in those with less extensive calcified coronary atherosclerosis.

▶ The data and results presented here are a part of an important sub study of the Veteran Affairs Diabetes Trial (VADT) and the Risk Factors, Atherosclerosis, and Clinical Events in Diabetes (RACED) trial. The VADT was a large (n = 1490) randomized trial comparing the effects of intensive versus standard glucose lowering on the cardiovascular event rates and outcomes of patients with type 2 diabetes and known coronary artery disease (CAD). After a little more than 5 years of follow-up, the group receiving intensive glycemic control experienced no significant reduction in cardiovascular events despite an average A1c 1.5% lower, throughout the trial.

The RACED sub study examined coronary artery calcium (CAC) in a subset (n = 301) of the VADT participants and tried to determine whether the effect of intensive glycemic control on cardiovascular disease (CVD) depended on the initial extent of underlying atherosclerosis as estimated by vascular calcium.

Although a relatively small study, the results of this study are very reassuring and give guidance to those who believe that controlling blood glucose intensively is important from a CVD perspective, despite the recent findings of the Action to Control Cardiovascular Risk in Diabetes (ACCORD), Action in Diabetes and Vascular Disease: Preterax and Diamicron Modified Release Controlled Evaluation (ADVANCE), and Bypass Angioplasty Revascularization Investigation 2 Diabetes (BARI-2D) studies. Furthermore, it gives guidance to those designing future studies in this area, supporting the concept that intensive glucose lowering therapy may be most effective in reducing CVD in those with less extensive coronary atherosclerosis.

F. Ovalle, MD

Metformin Associated With Lower Cancer Mortality in Type 2 Diabetes: ZODIAC-16

Landman GWD, Kleefstra N, van Hateren KJJ, et al (Isala Clinics, Zwolle, the Netherlands; et al)

Diabetes Care 33:322-326, 2010

Objective.—Several studies have suggested an association between specific diabetes treatment and cancer mortality. We studied the association between metformin use and cancer mortality in a prospectively followed cohort.

Research Design and Methods.—In 1998 and 1999, 1,353 patients with type 2 diabetes were enrolled in the Zwolle Outpatient Diabetes project Integrating Available Care (ZODIAC) study in the Netherlands. Vital status was assessed in January 2009. Cancer mortality rate was evaluated using standardized mortality ratios (SMRs), and the association between metformin use and cancer mortality was evaluated with a Cox proportional hazards model, taking possible confounders into account.

Results.—Median follow-up time was 9.6 years, average age at baseline was 68 years, and average A1C was 7.5%. Of the patients, 570 died, of which 122 died of malignancies. The SMR for cancer mortality was 1.47 (95% CI 1.22–1.76). In patients taking metformin compared with patients not taking metformin at baseline, the adjusted hazard ratio (HR) for cancer mortality was 0.43 (95% CI 0.23–0.80), and the HR with every increase of 1 g of metformin was 0.58 (95% CI 0.36–0.93).

Conclusions.—In general, patients with type 2 diabetes are at increased risk for cancer mortality. In our group, metformin use was associated with lower cancer mortality compared with nonuse of metformin. Although the design cannot provide a conclusion about causality, our results suggest a protective effect of metformin on cancer mortality.

▶ Diabetes is known to be associated with an increased risk of cancer, and most recently, the use of the insulin analog glargine was linked to an increased risk of cancer also, although this remains to be proven. A study designed to try to study further the association between insulin use and cancer concluded that it is possible that some of the apparent increased rates of cancer seen associated with insulin use in comparison with other drugs to treat diabetes was rather possibly, at least in part, the result of a decrease in the risk of cancer associated with metformin use in many of those patients not taking insulin.[1]

This study followed 1353 subjects with type 2 diabetes for approximately 10 years, and it is the first observational study with a prospective design to show an association between metformin use and lower cancer mortality risk. The group of subjects taking metformin in this study had, at the end, a cancer mortality risk comparable with that of the nondiabetic population. In other words, metformin seems to take away the excess risk of cancer mortality known to be associated with diabetes.

While the evidence for this association is growing stronger, a cause and effect relationship remains to be proven. Nonetheless, as the authors state, this finding further strengthens the position of metformin as the first-line therapy for type 2 diabetes.

F. Ovalle, MD

Reference

1. Currie CJ, Poole CD, Gale EA. The influence of glucose-lowering therapies on cancer risk in type 2 diabetes. *Diabetologia*. 2009;52:1766-1777.

Glycemic Control

A prospective randomised multi-centre controlled trial on tight glucose control by intensive insulin therapy in adult intensive care units: the Glucontrol study

Preiser J-C, Devos P, Ruiz-Santana S, et al (Univ Hosp, Liege, Belgium; Univ of Las Palmas de Gran Canaria, Spain; et al)
Intensive Care Med 35:1738-1748, 2009

Purpose.—An optimal target for glucose control in ICU patients remains unclear. This prospective randomized controlled trial compared the effects on ICU mortality of intensive insulin therapy (IIT) with an intermediate glucose control.

Methods.—Adult patients admitted to the 21 participating medico-surgical ICUs were randomized to group 1 (target BG 7.8–10.0 mmol/L) or to group 2 (target BG 4.4–6.1 mmol/L).

Results.—While the required sample size was 1,750 per group, the trial was stopped early due to a high rate of unintended protocol violations. From 1,101 admissions, the outcomes of 542 patients assigned to group 1 and 536 of group 2 were analysed. The groups were well balanced. BG levels averaged in group 1 8.0 mmol/L (IQR 7.1–9.0) (median of all values) and 7.7 mmol/L (IQR 6.7–8.8) (median of morning BG) versus 6.5 mmol/L (IQR 6.0–7.2) and 6.1 mmol/L (IQR 5.5–6.8) for group 2 ($p < 0.0001$ for both comparisons). The percentage of patients treated with insulin averaged 66.2 and 96.3%, respectively. Proportion of time spent in target BG was similar, averaging 39.5% and 45.1% (median (IQR) 34.3 (18.5–50.0) and 39.3 (26.2–53.6)%) in the groups 1 and 2, respectively. The rate of hypoglycaemia was higher in the group 2 (8.7%) than in group 1 (2.7%, $p < 0.0001$). ICU mortality was similar in the two groups (15.3 vs. 17.2%).

Conclusions.—In this prematurely stopped and therefore underpowered study, there was a lack of clinical benefit of intensive insulin therapy (target 4.4–6.1 mmol/L), associated with an increased incidence of hypoglycaemia, as compared to a 7.8–10.0 mmol/L target. (ClinicalTrials.gov # NCT00107601, EUDRA-CT Number: 200400391440).

▶ This multicenter randomized controlled trial attempted to determine what several others have tried lately: compare the effects on intensive care unit (ICU) mortality of intensive insulin therapy (IIT) with an intermediate glucose control. Unfortunately, the study data safety monitoring board (DSMB) decided to stop the study early because of a high rate of protocol violations. In other words, the proportion of blood glucose (BG) values in the assigned range was too low.

It is possible that the design of the study, assessing the quality of BG control in a much more detailed manner than most other studies (which used only the morning values), might have led to this high rate of protocol violations because the proportion of time in range calculated from the morning values was not lower than most of the other studies.

While we cannot draw any definite conclusions from this study, the available study data failed to show any clinically measurable benefit from tight (BG target 4.4-6.1 mmol/L) versus not so tight (BG target 7.8-10.0 mmol/L) control of glucose in the ICU. In addition, it showed an increased risk of hypoglycemia in the tight control group.

F. Ovalle, MD

Hyperglycemia-related mortality in critically ill patients varies with admission diagnosis

Falciglia M, Freyberg RW, Almenoff PL, et al (Univ of Cincinnati College of Medicine, OH)

Crit Care Med 37:3001-3009, 2009

Objective.—Hyperglycemia during critical illness is common and is associated with increased mortality. Intensive insulin therapy has improved outcomes in some, but not all, intervention trials. It is unclear whether the benefits of treatment differ among specific patient populations. The purpose of the study was to determine the association between hyperglycemia and risk-adjusted mortality in critically ill patients and in separate groups stratified by admission diagnosis. A secondary purpose was to determine whether mortality risk from hyperglycemia varies with intensive care unit type, length of stay, or diagnosed diabetes.

Design.—Retrospective cohort study.

Setting.—One hundred seventy-three U.S. medical, surgical, and cardiac intensive care units.

Patients.—Two hundred fifty-nine thousand and forty admissions from October 2002 to September 2005; unadjusted mortality rate, 11.2%.

Interventions.—None.

Measurements and Main Results.—A two-level logistic regression model determined the relationship between glycemia and mortality. Age, diagnosis, comorbidities, and laboratory variables were used to calculate a predicted mortality rate, which was then analyzed with mean glucose to determine the association of hyperglycemia with hospital mortality. Hyperglycemia was associated with increased mortality independent of illness severity. Compared with normoglycemic individuals (70–110 mg/dL), adjusted odds of mortality (odds ratio, [95% confidence interval]) for mean glucose 111–145, 146–199, 200–300, and >300 mg/dL was 1.31 (1.26–1.36), 1.82 (1.74–1.90), 2.13 (2.03–2.25), and 2.85 (2.58–3.14), respectively. Furthermore, the adjusted odds of mortality related to hyperglycemia varied with admission diagnosis, demonstrating a clear association in some patients (acute myocardial infarction, arrhythmia, unstable angina, pulmonary embolism) and little or no association in others. Hyperglycemia was associated with increased mortality independent of intensive care unit type, length of stay, and diabetes.

Conclusions.—The association between hyperglycemia and mortality implicates hyperglycemia as a potentially harmful and correctable abnormality in critically ill patients. The finding that hyperglycemia–related risk varied with admission diagnosis suggests differences in the interaction between specific medical conditions and injury from hyperglycemia. The design and interpretation of future trials should consider the primary disease states of patients and the balance of medical conditions in the intensive care unit studied.

▶ This is a massive retrospective cohort study designed to determine the association between hyperglycemia and mortality in critically ill patients. It was possible because of the integrated VA electronic medical record system throughout the United States.

If there was any doubt in anyone's mind about the association between hyperglycemia and mortality in the critically ill, this should put those questions to rest.

Most importantly, this large and powerful study helped identify several important trends in the strength of the association between hyperglycemia and mortality according to the admission diagnosis. Particularly interesting and thought-provoking is the magnitude of the association between cerebrovascular accidents (CVA) and hyperglycemia. Alternatively, the relatively weak associations between coronary artery bypass grafting (CABG), pulmonary veno-occlusive disease (PVOD), and amputations and hyperglycemia is interesting too.

This study should serve to help generate and support the hypothesis, and it should help guide the design of future studies. However, it clearly does not prove a cause and effect. So, whether we should treat our critically ill patients with hyperglycemia aggressively, with the goal of near-normoglycemia, remains an unanswered question.

F. Ovalle, MD

Hypoglycemia and Outcome in Critically Ill Patients

Egi M, Bellomo R, Stachowski E, et al (Okayama Univ Hosp, Japan; Austin Hosp, Melbourne, Victoria, Australia; Westmead Hosp, Sydney, New South Wales, Australia; et al)

Mayo Clin Proc 85:217-224, 2010

Objective.—To determine whether mild or moderate hypoglycemia that occurs in critically ill patients is independently associated with an increased risk of death.

Patients and Methods.—Of patients admitted to 2 hospital intensive care units (ICUs) in Melbourne and Sydney, Australia, from January 1, 2000, to October 14, 2004, we analyzed all those who had at least 1 episode of hypoglycemia (glucose concentration, <81 mg/dL). The independent association between hypoglycemia and outcome was statistically assessed.

Results.—Of 4946 patients admitted to the ICUs, a cohort of 1109 had at least 1 episode of hypoglycemia (blood glucose level, <81 mg/dL). Of these 1109 patients (22.4% of all admissions to the intensive care unit), hospital mortality was 36.6% compared with 19.7% in the 3837 nonhypoglycemic control patients (P<.001). Even patients with a minimum blood glucose concentration between 72 and 81 mg/dL had a greater unadjusted mortality rate than did control patients (25.9% vs 19.7%; unadjusted odds ratio, 1.42; 95% confidence interval, 1.12-1.80; P=.004.) Mortality increased significantly with increasing severity of hypoglycemia (P<.001). After adjustment for insulin therapy, hypoglycemia was independently associated with increased risk of death, cardiovascular death, and death due to infectious disease.

Conclusion.—In critically ill patients, an association exists between even mild or moderate hypoglycemia and mortality. Even after adjustment for insulin therapy or timing of hypoglycemic episode, the more severe the hypoglycemia, the greater the risk of death.

▶ This is a retrospective study conducted at 2 major teaching institutions in Australia. They enrolled 4946 patients admitted to their intensive care units (ICUs) over a period of 4 years and sought to determine whether mild to moderate hypoglycemia in the critically ill patient is associated with an increased risk of death. In summary, hypoglycemia was indeed independently associated with an increased risk of death, cardiovascular death, and death due to an infectious disease.

This study is another piece of the puzzle that has been rapidly progressing over the last few years. Not long ago, we all assumed that treating hyperglycemia intensively in the critically ill patient was a good idea, despite the well known increased risk of hypoglycemia, and many ICUs implemented protocols to achieve this. However, most recently, there have been several reports highlighting the increased risk of hypoglycemia with these protocols and the associated morbidity and mortality. It was not until the NICE-SUGAR study was published last year,[1] when all of a sudden the general attitude toward the treatment of hyperglycemia in the ICU suddenly changed. The NICE-SUGAR study found an increased 90-day mortality in the intensive insulin therapy group compared with the conventionally treated subjects.

At this point, further studies are needed to understand the pathophysiology of hypoglycemia in the critically ill individual and to find better ways to prevent it. As the authors point out, future studies will need to use continuous glucose monitoring systems (CGMS) to better document the glucose trends as well as the hyperglycemic and hypoglycemic events.

F. Ovalle, MD

Reference

1. NICE-SUGAR Study Investigators, Finfer S, Chittock DR, et al. Intensive versus conventional glucose control in critically ill patients. *N Engl J Med.* 2009;360: 1283-1297.

Prevention and Reversal of Diabetes

10-year follow-up of diabetes incidence and weight loss in the Diabetes Prevention Program Outcomes Study

Diabetes Prevention Program Research Group (Pennington Biomed Res Ctr, Baton Rouge, LA; et al)

Lancet 374:1677-1686, 2009

Background.—In the 2·8 years of the Diabetes Prevention Program (DPP) randomised clinical trial, diabetes incidence in high-risk adults was reduced by 58% with intensive lifestyle intervention and by 31% with metformin, compared with placebo. We investigated the persistence of these effects in the long term.

Methods.—All active DPP participants were eligible for continued follow-up. 2766 of 3150 (88%) enrolled for a median additional follow-up of 5·7 years (IQR 5·5–5·8). 910 participants were from the lifestyle, 924 from the metformin, and 932 were from the original placebo groups. On the basis of the benefits from the intensive lifestyle intervention in the DPP, all three groups were offered group-implemented lifestyle intervention. Metformin treatment was continued in the original metformin group (850 mg twice daily as tolerated), with participants unmasked to assignment, and the original lifestyle intervention group was offered additional lifestyle support. The primary outcome was development of diabetes according to American Diabetes Association criteria. Analysis was by intention-to-treat. This study is registered with ClinicalTrials.gov, number NCT00038727.

Findings.—During the 10·0-year (IQR 9·0–10·5) follow-up since randomisation to DPP, the original lifestyle group lost, then partly regained weight. The modest weight loss with metformin was maintained. Diabetes incidence rates during the DPP were 4·8 cases per 100 person-years (95% CI 4·1–5·7) in the intensive lifestyle intervention group, 7·8 (6·8–8·8) in the metformin group, and 11·0 (9·8–12·3) in the placebo group. Diabetes incidence rates in this follow-up study were similar between treatment groups: 5·9 per 100 person-years (5·1–6·8) for lifestyle, 4·9 (4·2–5·7) for metformin, and 5·6 (4·8–6·5) for placebo. Diabetes incidence in the 10 years since DPP randomisation was reduced by 34% (24–42) in the lifestyle group and 18% (7–28) in the metformin group compared with placebo.

Interpretation.—During follow-up after DPP, incidences in the former placebo and metformin groups fell to equal those in the former lifestyle group, but the cumulative incidence of diabetes remained lowest in the lifestyle group. Prevention or delay of diabetes with lifestyle intervention or metformin can persist for at least 10 years.

▶ This study, the Diabetes Prevention Program Outcomes Study (DPPOC), is the observational follow-up study of the participants in the Diabetes Prevention Program (DPP).

It was designed to determine whether the lower rates of diabetes observed in the lifestyle and metformin arms of the DPP were sustained. In other words, did the intervention help prevent, delay, or mask the onset of diabetes?

After an additional 5.7 years of follow-up (10 years after the randomization to DPP), those subjects who were originally assigned to the lifestyle intervention group gained back a good proportion of the weight they had lost during the DPP; those on the metformin arm maintained the weight they had lost; and those assigned to placebo maintained their original weight.

During the follow-up phase, the incidence rates of diabetes for the former placebo and metformin groups fell to levels similar to the former lifestyle group. However, the cumulative incidence of diabetes remained the lowest in the lifestyle group.

These results are consistent with those of most recent diabetes follow-up studies (eg, DCCT, EDIC, and UKPDS), demonstrating what some call a legacy effect or metabolic memory. This study demonstrates once again that early and aggressive treatment of diabetes and its comorbidities, pays off. Furthermore, it definitively shows that the lower rates of diabetes seen during the randomized phase of the DPP were not just the results of masking but rather represent evidence of true prevention of diabetes.

F. Ovalle, MD

2 Lipoproteins and Atherosclerosis

Introduction

Management of the many forms of dyslipidemia is an important part of practice in clinical endocrinology. Dyslipidemia is highly prevalent throughout the world. The reduction of atherogenic lipoprotein burden is a cornerstone in any attempt to decrease risk for cardiovascular disease in both the primary and secondary prevention settings. Our understanding of the role of lipoproteins and inflammation in atherosclerosis is burgeoning, and recent basic scientific and clinical trial investigations continue to reveal the enormous complexity intrinsic to the prevention and management of atherosclerotic disease.

In this edition of the YEAR BOOK OF ENDOCRINOLOGY, I have attempted to strike a balance among basic science, clinical studies, and large-scale intervention trials. In addition to covering post hoc analyses from statin trials, including AFCAPS/TexCAPS, TNT, and CORONA, an effort is made to present more recent insights from fibrate trials (FIELD and ACCORD) as well. New information about the role of statins and omega-3 fatty acids for arrhythmia prevention is covered. The efficacy of statins in the elderly and their acute impact on coronary plaque, the role of HDL elevation with statin therapy, the influence of proinflammatory HDL on atherosclerosis development and progression, the impact of ectopic pericardial fat on coronary disease, and at least part of the mechanistic basis for how vitamin D deficiency may induce atherosclerosis are also detailed. Studies exploring the potential role of trans fats in increasing risk for sudden cardiac death, paraoxonase polymorphisms and risk for cardiovascular events, the potential role of anthocyanins in lipid management, and the issue of how low you can take serum LDL-C in the setting of coronary disease, among other issues, are also addressed.

Lipoproteins offer up a vast platform from which to view the landscape of atherosclerosis. Atherosclerosis is a highly dynamic and plastic disease. Atherosclerotic plaque obviously progresses; but with aggressive management of dyslipidemia, it can also be made to regress and made less prone to rupture. While progress has been remarkable in the last year, obviously there is a long way to go. Many of the studies detailed in this chapter emphasize not only the complexity and the enormous number of molecular pathways that influence the development and progression of atherosclerosis, but also the many ways in which we can ever more intensively and beneficially impact the course and complications of this disease with interventions already at our disposal.

Peter P. Toth, MD, PhD

Clinical Trials of Drug Therapy

Effects of Increasing High-Density Lipoprotein Cholesterol and Decreasing Low-Density Lipoprotein Cholesterol on the Incidence of First Acute Coronary Events (from the Air Force/Texas Coronary Atherosclerosis Prevention Study)

Cui Y, Watson DJ, Girman CJ, et al (Merck & Compnay, Incorported, Whitehouse Station, NJ; et al)

Am J Cardiol 104:829-834, 2009

Reducing low-density lipoprotein (LDL) cholesterol with statins reduces cardiovascular risk, but the associations between increases in high-density lipoprotein (HDL) cholesterol and cardiovascular risk at different LDL levels have been less well characterized. To evaluate the associations between the 1-year changes in HDL cholesterol and LDL cholesterol with lovastatin and subsequent acute major coronary events (AMCEs), we studied 2,928 patients in the lovastatin arm who were followed for 5.2 years in a post-hoc analysis of the Air Force/Texas Coronary Atherosclerosis Prevention Study (AFCAPS/TexCAPS). The percentage of HDL cholesterol increase and apolipoproteins at year 1 and the incidence of AMCEs thereafter were assessed stratified by the LDL cholesterol levels. With lovastatin, LDL cholesterol was reduced by 25% on average to 115 mg/dl at year 1, and HDL cholesterol increased 6.0%. Patients with both an increase in HDL cholesterol of $\geq$7.5% and LDL cholesterol of <115 mg/dl at year 1 had the lowest event rate (3.53/1,000 person-years; $p = 0.028$). Similar results were found for an increase in HDL cholesterol of $\geq$7.5% and a decrease in LDL cholesterol of >25%, as well as for apolipoproteins A-I and B. The 1-year percent increase in HDL cholesterol appeared to be associated with a reduction in AMCEs in subsequent follow-up ($p = 0.07$ with the percentage of HDL cholesterol increase analyzed continuously). Patients with an HDL cholesterol increase of $\geq$7.5% had an AMCE rate of 5.18 compared with 7.66/1,000 person-years in patients with a lower HDL cholesterol increase ($p = 0.08$). In conclusion, lovastatin therapy was associated with a greater risk reduction of AMCEs when LDL cholesterol was substantially reduced and the HDL cholesterol increased by $\geq$7.5% (Fig 1).

▶ The Air Force/Texas Coronary Atherosclerosis Prevention Study (AFCAPS/TexCAPS) was the first clinical trial to demonstrate that treatment with a statin significantly reduced the risk for cardiovascular morbidity and mortality among

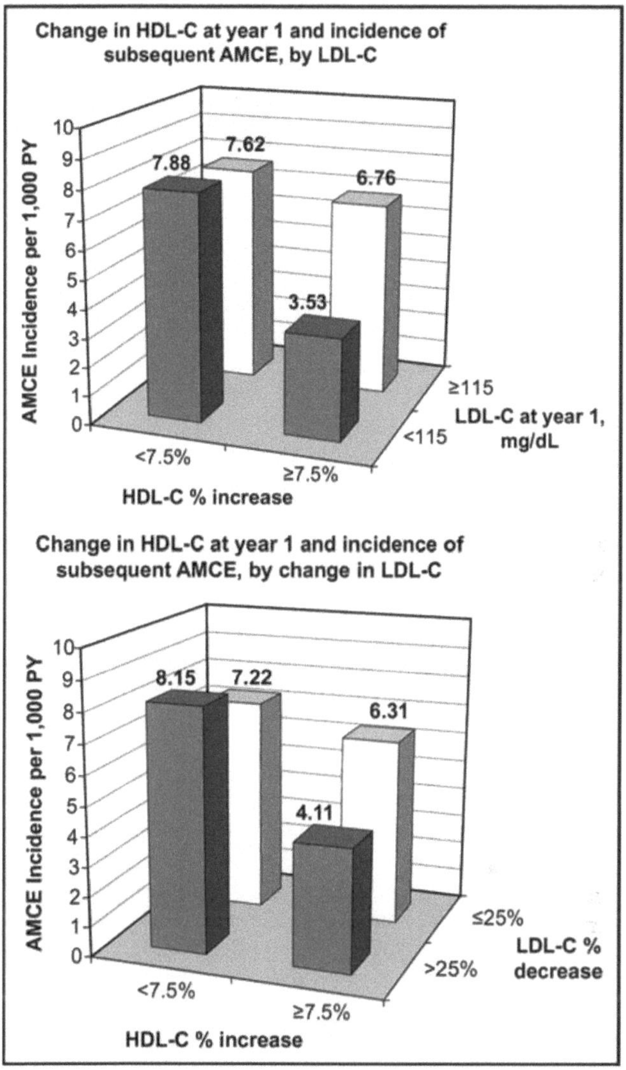

FIGURE 1.—HDL cholesterol percent change and incidence of AMCEs by LDL cholesterol. (*Top*) LDL cholesterol at year 1. (*Bottom*) LDL percent change. (Reprinted from Cui Y, Watson DJ, Girman CJ, et al. Effects of increasing high-density lipoprotein cholesterol and decreasing low-density lipoprotein cholesterol on the incidence of first acute coronary events (from the Air Force/Texas Coronary Atherosclerosis Prevention Study). *Am J Cardiol*. 2009;104:829-834, with permission from Elsevier Inc.)

men and women without a history of coronary artery disease. The subjects in this trial had average levels of low-density lipoprotein cholesterol (LDL-C) (155 mg/dL), triglycerides(165 mg/dL), and low levels of high-density lipoprotein cholesterol (HDL-C) (mean 37 mg/dL). In a previous analysis, it was shown that the patients with baseline HDL-C < 40 mg/dL derived 3 times more benefit in the primary composite end point of the trial than did those subjects with baseline HDL-C >40 mg/dL (45% vs 15%).[1] In this additional post hoc analysis, the investigators probe whether or not an HDL-C elevation on statin therapy >7.5% coupled with LDL-C reduction <115 mg/dL provides incremental risk reduction. Subjects with both an increase in HDL-C level of >7.5% and LDL-C level of <115 mg/dL at year 1 had the lowest event rate (3.53/1000 person-years; $P = .028$) compared to subjects with lower levels of HDL elevation or LDL-C reduction (Fig 1). Those subjects with HDL-C elevation >7.5% and a >25% reduction in LDL-C also did better compared with groups not achieving these changes in lipoprotein levels.

It has long been assumed that the primary benefit incurred by statin therapy is attributable to the reduction of atherogenic lipoprotein burden, especially LDL-C. Much skepticism surrounds the value of raising HDL-C and whether or not the modest increases in HDL-C stimulated by statin therapy contribute to overall risk reduction. This issue is complicated by the fact that, apart from using an infusible HDL mimetic, all currently available lipid-modifying therapies that increase HDL-C (statins, niacin, fibrates, and thiazolidinediones) impact serum levels of all components of the lipid profile, thereby necessitating multivariate regression analysis. A number of meta-analyses have shown that event rate reduction[2] and coronary atheromatous plaque regression based on intravascular ultrasonography[3] or quantitative coronary angiography[4] are a consequence of both aggressive LDL-C reduction and HDL-C elevation. This makes some sense on mechanistic grounds. Aggressive LDL-C reduction would be expected to provide less substrate for inducing endothelial cell dysfunction and promoting foam cell formation in the subendothelial space. Aggressive HDL raising may be associated with increased capacity for reverse cholesterol transport and other atheroprotective functions attributed to HDL particles.[5] Although a target for HDL-C elevation cannot be discerned from currently available clinical trials, this study provides important additional data supporting the importance of HDL-C elevation in patients with low baseline HDL-C levels. HDL-C elevation appears to contribute to cardiovascular risk reduction among patients with dyslipidemia treated with statin therapy. Consistent with other analyses, even a 2- to 3-mg/dL rise in HDL-C level appears to impact the risk for acute coronary events significantly.

P. P. Toth, MD, PhD

References

1. Downs JR, Clearfield M, Weis S, et al. Primary prevention of acute coronary events with lovastatin in men and women with average cholesterol levels: results of AFCAPS/TexCAPS. Air Force/Texas Coronary Atherosclerosis Prevention Study. *JAMA.* 1998;279:1615-1622.
2. Brown B, Zhao X, Cheung M. Should both HDL-C and LDL-C be targets for lipid therapy? A review of current evidence. *J Clin Lipidol.* 2007;1:88-94.
3. Nicholls SJ, Tuzcu EM, Sipahi I, et al. Statins, high-density lipoprotein cholesterol, and regression of coronary atherosclerosis. *JAMA.* 2007;297:499-508.
4. Ballantyne CM, Raichlen JS, Nicholls SJ, et al. for the ASTEROID Investigators. Effect of rosuvastatin therapy on coronary artery stenoses assessed by quantitative coronary angiography: a study to evaluate the effect of rosuvastatin on

intravascular ultrasound-derived coronary atheroma burden. *Circulation.* 2008; 117:2458-2466.
5. Toth PP. High-density lipoprotein: epidemiology, metabolism, and antiatherogenic effects. *Dis Mon.* 2001;47:365-416.

Paraoxonase Variants Relate to 10-Year Risk in Coronary Artery Disease: Impact of a High-Density Lipoprotein–Bound Antioxidant in Secondary Prevention

Regieli JJ, Jukema JW, Doevendans PA, et al (Univ Med Ctr Utrecht; Interuniversity Cardiology Inst of the Netherlands [ICIN/KNAW], Leiden; et al)
J Am Coll Cardiol 54:1238-1245, 2009

Objectives.—We investigated the effects of paraoxonase (PON)-1 variants on long-term clinical outcome in patients with coronary artery disease (CAD).

Background.—PON-1 is a potential therapeutic target to further reduce cardiovascular risk because it is a detoxifying esterase with antioxidant properties. The PON-1 knockout models result in higher susceptibility to atherosclerosis, and PON activity contributes to cardiovascular risk in humans. Human gene variants determine PON activity; however, the impact of these variants on recurrent cardiovascular events in vascular disease is as of yet unknown.

Methods.—We conducted a 10-year follow-up study of 793 CAD patients in the REGRESS (REgression GRowth Evaluation Statin Study) trial cohort, using nationwide registries. Genotypes were obtained of 2 PON-1 isotypes (L55M, rs854560, and Q192R, rs662), which were previously associated with PON activity. Absolute and relative risks by genotype were estimated using Kaplan-Meier and proportional hazards analyses.

Results.—Carriership of the PON-1 glutamine isotype at codon 192 and methionine at codon 55 was associated with a higher risk of death due to ischemic heart disease. Hazard ratios per allele copy were 1.71 (95% confidence interval: 1.0 to 2.8, $p = 0.03$) for the glutamine isotype at codon 192 and 1.56 (95% confidence interval: 1.1 to 2.3, $p = 0.03$) for methionine at codon 55. Both isotypes had previously been related to lower PON activity. No effect was observed on all-cause mortality.

Conclusions.—PON-1 gene variants influence the 10-year risk of fatal complications from CAD in male patients, despite no effect on all-cause mortality. These long-term findings confirm functional data on PON-1 activity, emphasize the relevance of this pathway in vascular disease, and enforce its putative role as a target to modify and estimate cardiovascular risk.

▶ Paraoxonase 1 (PON1) is synthesized by the liver and is carried by high-density lipoprotein (HDL) particles in serum. PON1, platelet activating factor acetylhydrolase, and redox-active methionine centers in apoprotein AI endow

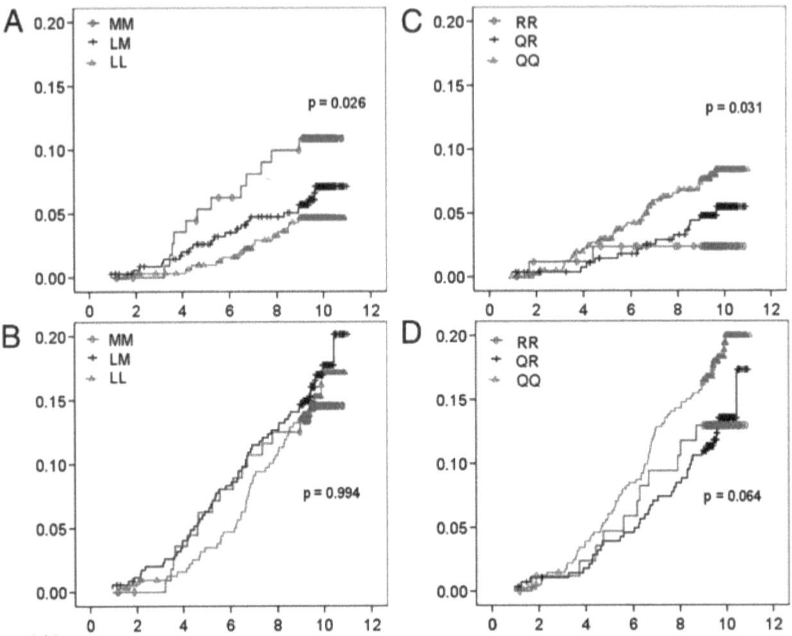

n at risk

LL	325	319	313	303	284	77
LM	352	344	334	319	304	103
MM	114	112	108	103	98	38

QQ	420	412	397	378	354	124
QR	287	282	278	270	259	78
RR	87	84	83	80	76	17

FIGURE 1.—Temporal patterns of 10-year risk by PON-1. Survival curves by paraoxonase-1 (PON-1) genotypes (A and B) methionine at codon 55 (M55L) and (C and D) glutamine at codon 192 (Q192R), vertically displaying cumulative absolute risk of death from (A and C) ischemic heart disease and (B and D) all-cause mortality. Follow-up time in years is displayed horizontally. (Reprinted from Regieli JJ, Jukema JW, Doevendans PA, et al. Paraoxonase variants relate to 10-year risk in coronary artery disease: impact of a high-density lipoprotein–bound antioxidant in secondary prevention. *J Am Coll Cardiol.* 2009;54:1238-1245, with permission from the American College of Cardiology Foundation.)

HDL with antioxidative capacity. These components of the HDL proteosome help to prevent the formation of oxidized low-density lipoprotein (LDL), the primary substrate for macrophage scavenging and foam cell formation. PON specifically hydrolyzes and inactivates bioactive oxidized phospholipids and cholesteryl esters.[1] Numerous polymorphisms in PON gene have been identified.[2] Loss-of-function mutations in PON are associated with increased risk for coronary artery disease (CAD) and stroke.[3]

Patients in this study were part of Regression Growth Evaluation Statin Study (REGRESS), which enrolled 884 men who were not diabetic but had symptomatic CAD. REGRESS was an angiographic trial that evaluated the effects of 24 months of pravastatin therapy on the evolution of atherosclerotic lesions. The impact of 2 loss-of-function polymorphisms in PON1 isotypes (L55M, rs854560, and Q192R, rs662) were studied in 793 men over a follow-up period of 10 years. Being homozygous for these polymorphisms was associated with a 1.71- and 1.56-fold increase in the risk for cardiovascular mortality, respectively. There was no significant association between these polymorphisms and risk for all-cause mortality. As seen in Fig 1, there is a clear gene-dose effect as patients progress from being homozygous for the wild-type allele to being heterozygous and then homozygous for the respective loss-of-function polymorphism.

These results from REGRESS suggest that the 192QR and 55LM loss-of-function polymorphisms represent an independent risk factor for coronary mortality in men with established CAD. It cannot be discerned from these data whether this also applies to women with CAD. Although statin therapy has been shown to increase PON expression in humans,[4] it is clear from this study that despite statin therapy, the 2 PON1 polymorphisms in this study still confer increased vulnerability for cardiovascular mortality. The presence of these polymorphisms could be potentially used to identify patients at particularly high risk for recurrent ischemic events. This study also shows that the relationship between HDL and risk for CAD-related events is highly complex, multifactorial, and strongly dependent on the activity and functionality of specific components of its proteosomic cargo.

P. P. Toth, MD, PhD

References

1. Mackness MI, Arrol S, Abbott C, Durrington PN. Protection of low-density lipoprotein against oxidative modification by high-density lipoprotein associated paraoxonase. *Atherosclerosis.* 1993;104:129-135.
2. Aviram M, Hardak E, Vaya J, et al. Human serum paraoxonases (PON1) Q and R selectively decrease lipid peroxides in human coronary and carotid atherosclerotic lesions: PON1 esterase and peroxidase-like activities. *Circulation.* 2000;101: 2510-2517.
3. Salonen JT, Malin R, Tuomainen TP, Nyyssonen K, Lakka TA, Lehtimaki T. Polymorphism in high density lipoprotein paraoxonase gene and risk of acute myocardial infarction in men: prospective nested case-control study. *BMJ.* 1999; 319:487-489. discussion 490.
4. Harangi M, Seres I, Varga Z, et al. Atorvastatin effect on high-density lipoprotein-associated paraoxonase activity and oxidative DNA damage. *Eur J Clin Pharmacol.* 2004;60:685-691.

Acute Effects of Statin Therapy on Coronary Atherosclerosis Following an Acute Coronary Syndrome

Rodés-Cabau J, Tardif J-C, Cossette M, et al (Quebec Heart and Lung Inst, Canada; Montreal Heart Inst, Quebec, Canada; Montreal Heart Inst Coordinating Ctr, Quebec, Canada)
Am J Cardiol 104:750-757, 2009

No data exist on the acute effects of statin therapy on human coronary atherosclerotic plaques. The objective of our study was to evaluate the early (<2 months) effects of newly initiated statin therapy on coronary atherosclerosis as evaluated by intravascular ultrasonography. The study population consisted of 74 patients (mean age 58 ± 8 years) who had

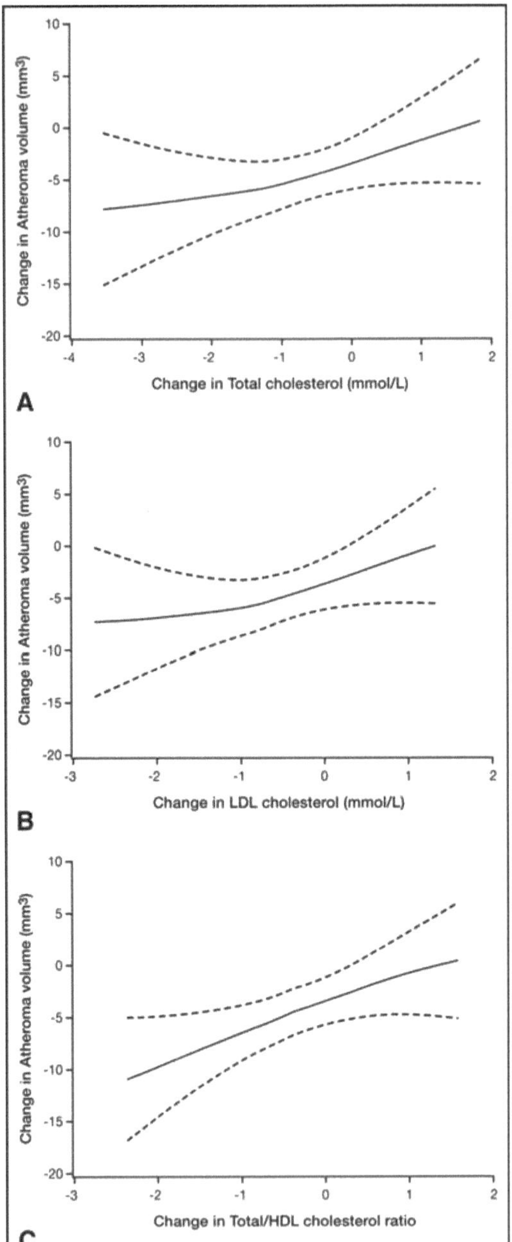

FIGURE 2.—Relations between changes in total cholesterol *(A)*, LDL cholesterol *(B)*, total to HDL cholesterol ratio *(C)* and change in atheroma volume on locally weighted smoothed scatterplots, with point estimates *(solid lines)* and upper and lower 95% confidence intervals *(dashed lines)*. (Reprinted from Rodés-Cabau J, Tardif J-C, Cossette M, et al. Acute effects of statin therapy on coronary atherosclerosis following an acute coronary syndrome. *Am J Cardiol.* 2009;104:750-757, with permission from Elsevier.)

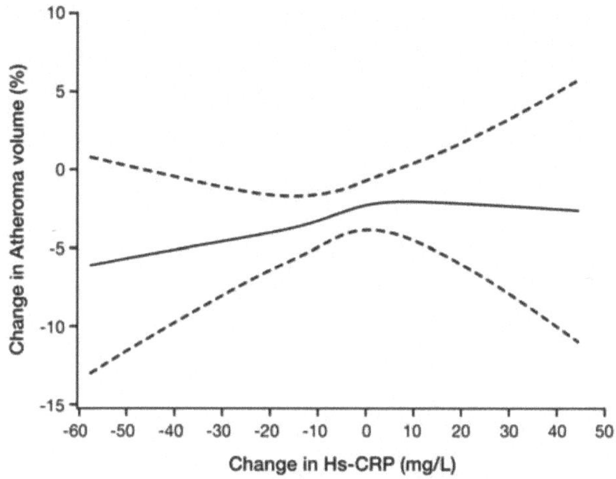

FIGURE 3.—Relation between change in hs-CRP level and percent change in atheroma volume, with point estimates *(solid lines)* and upper and lower 95% confidence intervals *(dashed lines)*. (Reprinted from Rodés-Cabau J, Tardif J-C, Cossette M, et al. Acute effects of statin therapy on coronary atherosclerosis following an acute coronary syndrome. *Am J Cardiol.* 2009;104:750-757, with permission from Elsevier.)

been included in the ERASE trial (evaluating the effects of reconstituted high-density lipoprotein infusions). All patients underwent serial intravascular ultrasonographic (IVUS) evaluation at baseline (3 ± 2 days after an acute coronary syndrome [ACS]) and after 6 ± 1 weeks of follow-up. Statin therapy was initiated after ACS in 36 patients who received ≤1 dose of statins before baseline IVUS examination (newly initiated statin therapy group), and 38 patients were already on a stable statin dose before the ACS (long-term statin therapy group). Atorvastatin at a dose of 40 mg/day was the most common regimen in the 2 groups. Percent changes in atheroma volume (prespecified primary efficacy parameter) were −4.71 ± 0.96% in the newly initiated statin therapy group ($p < 0.0001$) and −0.54 ± 0.89% in the long-term statin therapy group ($p = 0.546$; $p = 0.002$ for comparison between groups). Median nominal changes in atheroma volume were −9.10 mm^3 (interquartile range −12.56 to −3.73, $p < 0.0001$ vs baseline) and 1.21 mm^3 (interquartile range −6.41 to 3.76, $p = 0.429$ vs baseline) in the newly initiated and long-term statin therapy groups, respectively ($p = 0.003$ for comparison between groups). Greater decreases in total cholesterol ($r = 0.25$, $p = 0.035$), ratio of total to high-density lipoprotein cholesterol ($r = 0.28$, $p = 0.018$), and high-sensitivity C-reactive protein ($r = 0.31$, $p = 0.046$, for patients with high-sensitivity C-reactive protein measurements within 7 days after IVUS examination) were associated with larger percent changes in atheroma volume. In conclusion, newly initiated statin therapy is associated with rapid regression of coronary atherosclerosis within 2 months. This effect was in part associated with decreases in atherogenic lipid and inflammatory parameters. These results provide insight into the rapid clinical benefits of statin therapy after an ACS.

▶ Intravascular ultrasonography (IVUS) has emerged as an important means by which full thickness images of arterial walls are obtained. Importantly, IVUS is used to assess changes in atheromatous plaque volume and provides estimates of target lesion changes, such as stabilization, progression, or regression in response to therapeutic intervention. The Reversal of Atherosclerosis with Aggressive Lipid Lowering (REVERSAL)[1] and A Study To Evaluate the Effect of Rosuvastatin on Intravascular Ultrasound-Derived Coronary Atheroma Burden (ASTEROID)[2] used IVUS to evaluate the capacity of statin therapy to impact rates of atheromatous plaque progression over 18 and 24 months of follow-up, respectively. In this subgroup analysis of the Effect of Reconstituted High-Density Lipoprotein (rHDL) on Atherosclerosis Safety and Efficacy (ERASE) trial, serial IVUS is used to evaluate the impact of 2 months of statin therapy on atherosclerotic plaque volume in patients who sustain an acute coronary syndrome (ACS). The comparison groups comprised patients chronically treated with statins ($n = 38$) and patients naïve to statin therapy ($n = 36$).

Among statin naïve patients, statin therapy has significant and rapid impact on atheromatous plaque features with a 4.7% reduction in atheromatous plaque volume (PAV). These patients experienced a mean reduction in low-density lipoprotein cholesterol (LDL-C) from 100 to 63 mg/dL. Patients on chronic statin therapy experienced a more modest reduction in PAV of 0.54%. The reduction in PAV was highly correlated with magnitude of reduction in total cholesterol, LDL-C, total cholesterol to high-density lipoprotein cholesterol (HDL-C) ratio (Fig 2), and high-sensitivity C-reactive protein (hsCRP) (Fig 3). Within group, changes in HDL-C were not significant.

This study adds important information to our understanding of the role statins play in modulating atherosclerotic plaque burden. A nearly 5% regression in PAV is impressive after only 2 months of statin therapy. At least part of this regression is likely attributable to reductions in the volume of the lipid core of plaque. Studies such as the Myocardial Ischemia Reduction With Aggressive Cholesterol Lowering (MIRACL)[3] and Pravastatin or Atorvastatin Evaluation and Infection Therapy (PROVE-IT)[4] trials both demonstrated rapid event reductions (1-4 months) with statin therapy in patients who have sustained an ACS. This rapid time to event reduction has generally not been attributed to LDL-C reduction alone. Other explanations have included statin's ability to reduce systemic inflammatory tone (ie, reduce hsCRP) and a variety of pleiotropic effects, such as reversing endothelial dysfunction, improving endothelial nitric oxide production, decreasing endothelial adhesion molecule expression, and so forth. The ERASE trial certainly supports the conclusion that reducing atherogenic lipoprotein burden and serum levels of hsCRP beneficially impacts PAV in patients with an ACS. Although it is widely assumed that reducing PAV secondary to resorbing part of the lipid core of a plaque is beneficial, it remains to be seen whether magnitude of atherosclerotic plaque regression correlates with magnitude of reduction in risk for acute cardiovascular events.

P. P. Toth, MD, PhD

References

1. Nissen SE, Tuzcu EM, Schoenhagen P, et al. REVERSAL Investigators. Effect of intensive compared with moderate lipid-lowering therapy on progression of coronary atherosclerosis: a randomized controlled trial. *JAMA*. 2004;291:1071-1080.
2. Nissen SE, Nicholls SJ, Sipahi I, et al. ASTEROID Investigators. Effect of very high-intensity statin therapy on regression of coronary atherosclerosis: the ASTEROID trial. *JAMA*. 2006;295:1556-1565.
3. Schwartz GG, Olsson AG, Ezekowitz MD, et al. Myocardial Ischemia Reduction with Aggressive Cholesterol Lowering (MIRACL) Study Investigators. Effects of atorvastatin on early recurrent ischemic events in acute coronary syndromes: the MIRACL study: a randomized controlled trial. *JAMA*. 2001;285:1711-1718.
4. Cannon CP, Braunwald E, McCabe CH, et al. Intensive versus moderate lipid lowering with statins after acute coronary syndromes. *N Engl J Med*. 2004;350: 1495-1504.

Comparison of 80 versus 10 mg of *Atorvastatin* on Occurrence of Cardiovascular Events After the First Event (from the Treating to New Targets [TNT] Trial)

LaRosa JC, Deedwania PC, Shepherd J, et al (State Univ of New York, Brooklyn; VA Central California Healthcare System and UCSF School of Medicine, Fresno; Univ of Glasgow, UK; et al)

Am J Cardiol 105:283-287, 2010

Analyses of randomized clinical trials are usually restricted to examination of time to first event. However, because many patients have multiple events, this approach precludes much potentially useful clinical and economic data. To assess the effect on overall disease burden in the Treating to New Targets (TNT) study, we evaluated the effect of treatment with atorvastatin 80 versus 10 mg in the period after the occurrence of a first cardiovascular event. In TNT, 10,001 patients with stable coronary heart disease received double-blind therapy with atorvastatin 80 or 10 mg and were followed for 4.9 years. Post hoc time-to-event analysis was used to estimate separate hazard ratios for time to any first, second, third, fourth, and fifth recurrent cardiovascular events. During TNT, 3,082 patients had a first recurrent cardiovascular event, with 1,516, 698, 345, and 197 developing second, third, fourth, and fifth recurrent events, respectively. In patients receiving atorvastatin 80 mg, the relative risk of a first recurrent event was significantly decreased compared to those receiving atorvastatin 10 mg. Significant benefit with the 80-mg dose was also observed for second, third, fourth, and fifth recurrent events. Similar findings were recorded in 5,854 patients with type 2 diabetes mellitus and/or metabolic syndrome and in 3,809 patients ≥65 years of age compared to younger patients. In conclusion, treatment with atorvastatin 80 mg continued to significantly decrease the risk of any cardiovascular event over time compared to atorvastatin 10 mg in patients who had survived previous events. In TNT, analyses limited to the primary end point significantly underestimated the decrease in total cardiovascular

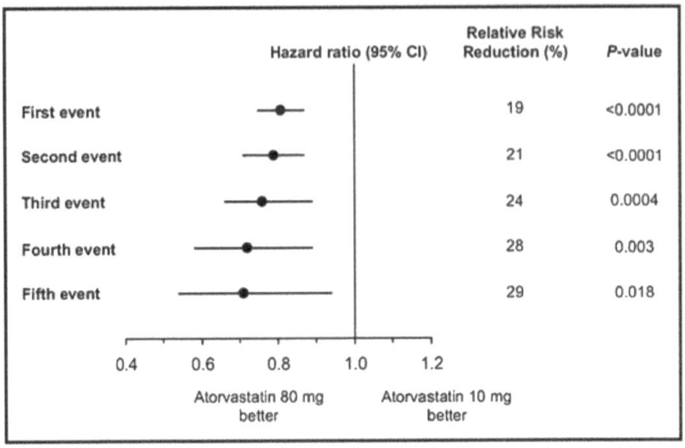

FIGURE 1.—Risk decrease in cardiovascular events. (Reprinted from LaRosa JC, Deedwania PC, Shepherd J, et al. Comparison of 80 versus 10 mg of atorvastatin on occurrence of cardiovascular events after the first event (from the Treating to New Targets [TNT] trial). *Am J Cardiol.* 2010;105:283-287, with permission from Elsevier.)

disease burden achieved by intensive low-density lipoprotein cholesterol lowering (Figs 1 and 2).

▶ In prospective randomized studies evaluating the effect of lipid-lowering therapy on cardiovascular events, it has been customary to evaluate time to first event. Patients with coronary artery disease (CAD) can sustain multiple events over the course of years. Consequently, traditional time to first event analyses can underestimate the full benefit of a given therapy, especially if recurrent events or events in different vascular beds occur in a significant percentage of patients enrolled in a clinical trial. In addition, because lipid-lowering therapies are intended to be continued in a lifelong manner in patients with established CAD, it is valuable to assess whether or not risk for multiple events in patients is reduced over time. In the Treating to New Targets trial, patients with stable CAD were randomized to treatment with either atorvastatin 80 or 10 mg daily. For the group as a whole, the primary composite end point of major cardiovascular events was reduced by 22% when comparing high- and low-dose atorvastatin therapies, respectively.[1]

This post hoc analysis of the Treating to New Targets Trial shows that second, third, fourth, and fifth major cardiovascular events (death, nonfatal myocardial infarction, fatal/nonfatal stroke, or resuscitated cardiac arrest) were all decreased in the study as a whole (Fig 1), and also in patients with type 2 diabetes mellitus/metabolic syndrome or patients ≥ 65 yrs of age (Fig 2), when comparing treatment with high- (80 mg) and low-dose atorvastatin (10 mg), respectively.

This analysis demonstrates statistically significant reductions in recurrent event rates. In this context, the benefit of sustained high-dose atorvastatin therapy is even greater than time to first event analysis would imply. In patients

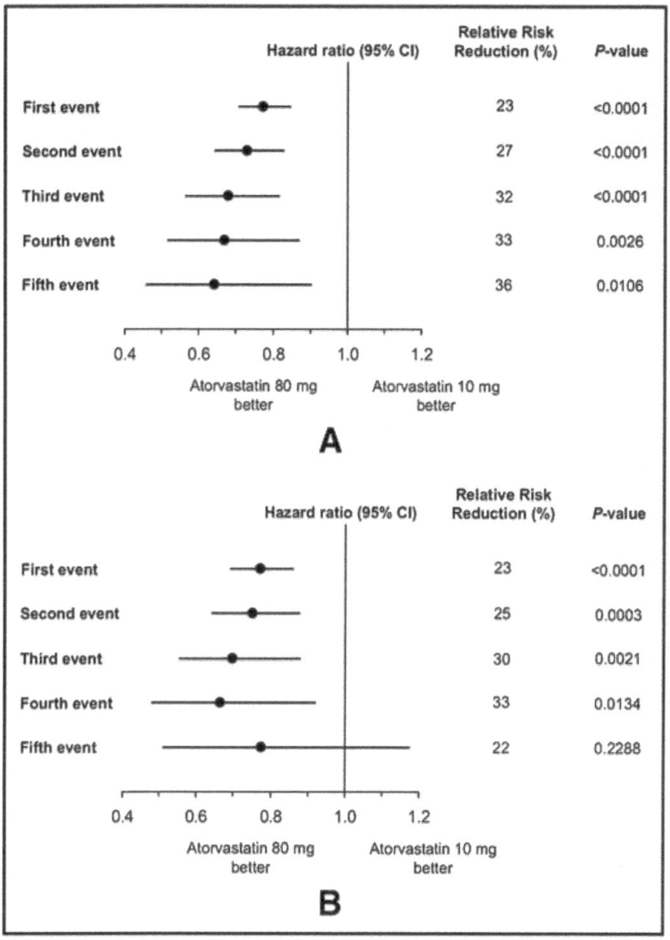

FIGURE 2.—Risk decrease in cardiovascular events in patients *(A)* with type 2 diabetes and/or metabolic syndrome and *(B)* ≥65 years of age. (Reprinted from LaRosa JC, Deedwania PC, Shepherd J, et al. Comparison of 80 versus 10 mg of atorvastatin on occurrence of cardiovascular events after the first event (from the Treating to New Targets [TNT] trial). *Am J Cardiol.* 2010;105:283-287, with permission from Elsevier.)

with established, stable CAD, these data support the use of high-dose statin therapy irrespective of the baseline lipid profile.

P. P. Toth, MD, PhD

Reference

1. LaRosa JC, Grundy SM, Waters DD, et al. Intensive lipid lowering with atorvastatin in patients with stable coronary disease. *N Engl J Med.* 2005;352:1425-1435.

Effects of Combination Lipid Therapy in Type 2 Diabetes Mellitus

The ACCORD Study Group (Columbia Univ College, NY)

N Engl J Med 362:1563-1574, 2010

Background.—We investigated whether combination therapy with a statin plus a fibrate, as compared with statin monotherapy, would reduce the risk of cardiovascular disease in patients with type 2 diabetes mellitus who were at high risk for cardiovascular disease.

Methods.—We randomly assigned 5518 patients with type 2 diabetes who were being treated with open-label simvastatin to receive either masked fenofibrate or placebo. The primary outcome was the first occurrence of nonfatal myocardial infarction, nonfatal stroke, or death from cardiovascular causes. The mean follow-up was 4.7 years.

Results.—The annual rate of the primary outcome was 2.2% in the fenofibrate group and 2.4% in the placebo group (hazard ratio in the fenofibrate group, 0.92; 95% confidence interval [CI], 0.79 to 1.08; P = 0.32). There were also no significant differences between the two study groups with respect to any secondary outcome. Annual rates of death were 1.5% in the fenofibrate group and 1.6% in the placebo group (hazard ratio, 0.91; 95% CI, 0.75 to 1.10; P = 0.33). Prespecified subgroup analyses suggested heterogeneity in treatment effect according to sex, with a benefit for men and possible harm for women (P = 0.01 for interaction), and a possible interaction according to lipid subgroup, with a possible benefit for patients with both a high baseline triglyceride level

TABLE 2.—Prespecified Primary and Secondary Outcomes

Outcome	Fenofibrate (N = 2765) No. of Events	Fenofibrate (N = 2765) Rate/Yr	Placebo (N = 2753) No. of Events	Placebo (N = 2753) Rate/Yr	Hazard Ratio (95% CI)	P Value
Primary outcome (major fatal or nonfatal cardiovascular event)	291	2.24	310	2.41	0.92 (0.79–1.08)	0.32*
Secondary outcomes						
Primary outcome plus revascularization or hospitalization for congestive heart failure	641	5.35	667	5.64	0.94 (0.85–1.05)	0.30
Major coronary disease event†	332	2.58	353	2.79	0.92 (0.79–1.07)	0.26
Nonfatal myocardial infarction	173	1.32	186	1.44	0.91 (0.74–1.12)	0.39
Stroke						
Any	51	0.38	48	0.36	1.05 (0.71–1.56)	0.80
Nonfatal	47	0.35	40	0.30	1.17 (0.76–1.78)	0.48
Death						
From any cause	203	1.47	221	1.61	0.91 (0.75–1.10)	0.33*
From cardiovascular cause	99	0.72	114	0.83	0.86 (0.66–1.12)	0.26
Fatal or nonfatal congestive heart failure	120	0.90	143	1.09	0.82 (0.65–1.05)	0.10

*P values were adjusted for interim monitoring.
†A major coronary disease event was defined as a fatal coronary event, nonfatal myocardial infarction, or unstable angina.

and a low baseline level of high-density lipoprotein cholesterol ($P = 0.057$ for interaction).

Conclusions.—The combination of fenofibrate and simvastatin did not reduce the rate of fatal cardiovascular events, nonfatal myocardial infarction, or nonfatal stroke, as compared with simvastatin alone. These results do not support the routine use of combination therapy with fenofibrate and simvastatin to reduce cardiovascular risk in the majority of high-risk patients with type 2 diabetes. (ClinicalTrials.gov number, NCT00000620.)

▶ The fibrates are an important class of lipid-lowering agent used to reduce serum levels of triglycerides, increase high-density lipoprotein cholesterol (HDL-C), and decrease low-density lipoprotein (LDL) particle number in patients with mixed forms of dyslipidemia. The fibrates activate lipoprotein lipase, stimulate hepatic apoA-I, and HDL secretion, and in experimental models have been shown to augment the reverse cholesterol transport. Gemfibrozil has been shown to reduce cardiovascular events in both the primary[1] and secondary[2] prevention settings and has also been shown to reduce the rate of progression of coronary artery disease (CAD).[3] Post hoc analyses of the Helsinki Heart Study (HHS), Bezafibrate Infarction Project (BIP), and the Fenofibrate Intervention and Event Lowering in Diabetes (FIELD) study demonstrated significant reductions in the primary composite end point of cardiovascular events in patients with elevated triglycerides and low serum HDL-C. Although the primary end point in both BIP and FIELD were negative for the studies as a whole (7.3% and 11% reductions, respectively), among patients with triglycerides >200 mg/dL in BIP[4] and those with triglycerides >204 mg/dL and HDL-C <42 mg/dL in FIELD,[5] risk reductions for the primary end point were 39.5% and 27%, respectively. Of interest in FIELD, microvascular end points, such as risk for proliferative retinopathy requiring laser photocoagulation, albuminuria, and lower extremity amputation, were also reduced significantly.[6]

The Action to Control Cardiovascular Risk in Diabetes (ACCORD) trial investigated whether combination therapy with a statin plus a fibrate would reduce the risk of cardiovascular events in patients with type 2 diabetes mellitus to a greater degree than statin monotherapy. At the time of randomization to either placebo or fenofibrate therapy, all patients were receiving open-label simvastatin therapy. Baseline lipid values at the time of assignment to study drug were as follows: LDL-C, 100 mg/dL; triglyceride, 160 mg/dL; and HDL-C, 38 mg/dL. There were no statistically significant differences between the groups—neither for the primary composite outcome nor for any of the secondary outcomes, including myocardial infarction, stroke, mortality, or heart failure (Table 2). However, for the prespecified subgroup with baseline triglycerides >204 mg/dL and HDL-C < 34 mg/dL, there was a 31% reduction in the primary composite end point of fatal and nonfatal cardiovascular events. There were no differences between treatment groups for risk of myalgia, myopathy, hepatotoxicity, gallstones, pulmonary embolism, or deep venous thrombosis. The incidence of micro- and macroalbuminuria was significantly lower in the group receiving combination simvastatin/fenofibrate therapy. This latter finding is consistent with the FIELD trial.

It is unfortunate that the ACCORD trial did not specifically randomize patients with baseline hypertriglyceridemia and low HDL-C. These are the groups that consistently derive benefit from fibrate therapy. With the high worldwide incidence of insulin resistance and metabolic syndrome, recruiting and randomizing such a population of subjects with diabetes mellitus would not have been difficult. Moreover, in clinical practice, physicians typically do not add a fibrate on to a statin as adjuvant therapy for triglycerides of 160 mg/dL and an HDL-C of 38 mg/dL. The ACCORD trial, however, affirms the benefit of fibrate adjuvant therapy in the setting of hypertriglyceridemia and low HDL-C. The ACCORD trial also affirms a signal for benefit on albuminuria with fenofibrate therapy. Moreover, combination therapy was safe and well tolerated compared with statin monotherapy. Because it is unlikely that another such combination trial exploring the value of combination statin-fibrate therapy compared with statin monotherapy will be undertaken, it is at least reassuring that the ACCORD trial demonstrated benefits in patients with hypertriglyceridemia and low HDL-C, with an effect size consistent with those observed in BIP and FIELD.

P. P. Toth, MD, PhD

References

1. Manninen V, Elo MO, Frick MH, et al. Lipid alterations and decline in the incidence of coronary heart disease in the Helsinki Heart Study. *JAMA*. 1988;260: 641-651.
2. Robins SJ, Collins D, Wittes JT, et al. Relation of gemfibrozil treatment and lipid levels with major coronary events: VA-HIT: a randomized controlled trial. *JAMA*. 2001;285:1585-1591.
3. Frick MH, Syvanne M, Nieminen MS, et al. Prevention of the angiographic progression of coronary and vein-graft atherosclerosis by gemfibrozil after coronary bypass surgery in men with low levels of HDL cholesterol. Lopid Coronary Angiography Trial (LOCAT) Study Group. *Circulation*. 1997;96:2137-2143.
4. Secondary prevention by raising HDL cholesterol and reducing triglycerides in patients with coronary artery disease: the Bezafibrate Infarction Prevention (BIP) study. *Circulation*. 2000;102:21-27.
5. Scott R, O'Brien R, Fulcher G, et al. Effects of fenofibrate treatment on cardiovascular disease risk in 9,795 individuals with type 2 diabetes and various components of the metabolic syndrome: the Fenofibrate Intervention and Event Lowering in Diabetes (FIELD) study. *Diabetes Care*. 2009;32:493-498.
6. Keech A, Simes RJ, Barter P, et al. Effects of long-term fenofibrate therapy on cardiovascular events in 9795 people with type 2 diabetes mellitus (the FIELD study): randomised controlled trial. *Lancet*. 2005;366:1849-1861.

Incidence and predictors of silent myocardial infarction in type 2 diabetes and the effect of fenofibrate: an analysis from the Fenofibrate Intervention and Event Lowering in Diabetes (FIELD) study

Burgess DC, Hunt D, Li L, et al (Univ of Sydney, Camperdown, Australia; Royal Melbourne Hosp, Victoria, Australia; et al)

Eur Heart J 31:92-99, 2010

Aims.—To determine the incidence and predictors of, and effects of fenofibrate on silent myocardial infarction (MI) in a large contemporary cohort of patients with type 2 diabetes in the Fenofibrate Intervention and Event Lowering in Diabetes (FIELD) study.

Methods and Results.—Routine electrocardiograms taken throughout the study were assessed by Minnesota-code criteria for the presence of new Q-waves without clinical presentation and analysed with blinding to treatment allocation and clinical outcome. Of all MIs, 36.8 were silent. Being male, older age, longer diabetes duration, prior cardiovascular disease (CVD), neuropathy, higher HbA_{1c}, albuminuria, high serum creatinine, and insulin use all significantly predicted risk of clinical or silent MI. Fenofibrate reduced MI (clinical or silent) by 19 [hazard ratio (HR) 0.81, 95 confidence interval (CI) 0.69–0.94; $P = 0.006$], non-fatal clinical MI by 24 ($P = 0.01$), and silent MI by 16 ($P = 0.16$). Among those having silent MI, fenofibrate reduced subsequent clinical CVD events by 78 (HR 0.22, 95 CI 0.08–0.65; $P = 0.003$).

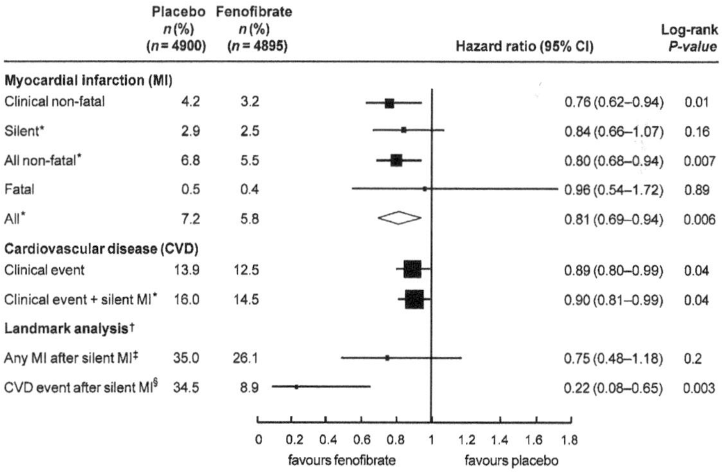

FIGURE 3.—Effects of fenofibrate treatment on myocardial infarction and cardiovascular events. *Interval-censored proportional-hazards methods were used. †Analyses were landmarked at 2 years (see methods for details). ‡Placebo group, 48 events, $n = 137$; fenofibrate group, 30 events, $n = 115$. §Placebo group, 20 events, $n = 58$; fenofibrate group, 4 events, $n = 45$. (Reprinted from Burgess DC, Hunt D, Li L, et al. Incidence and predictors of silent myocardial infarction in type 2 diabetes and the effect of fenofibrate: An analysis from the Fenofibrate Intervention and Event Lowering in Diabetes (FIELD) study. *Eur Heart J.* 2010;31:92-99, with permission from The European Society of Cardiology.)

Conclusion.—Silent and clinical MI have similar risk factors and increase the risk of future CVD events. Fenofibrate reduces the risk of a first MI and substantially reduces the risk of further clinical CVD events after silent MI, supporting its use in type 2 diabetes (Fig 3).

▶ Silent myocardial infarction (MI) is a serious complication of coronary artery disease (CAD). Patients with diabetes have increased risk for silent MI due to cardiac autonomic neuropathy stemming from chronic exposure to hyperglycemia. In this intriguing analysis of data from the Fenofibrate Intervention and Event Lowering in Diabetes (FIELD) study, the impact of fenofibrate therapy on risk for fatal/nonfatal and silent Q wave MI was explored. Despite a high drop-in rate of statin therapy in the placebo- and fenofibrate-treated groups, the investigators were able to show reductions in total, nonfatal, and silent MIs of 19%, 24%, and a statistically nonsignifcant 16%, respectively. However, among patients with silent MI by the end of year 2 (evaluated with sequential EKGs during the course of the trial), the risk for cardiovascular events was reduced significantly by 78% in the fenofibrate group relative to placebo (Fig 3). Thirty-seven percent of all MIs in this study were silent. This is a high incidence of MI that neither the patient nor the physician would have been aware of had the scheduled follow-up EKGs not been performed. The true incidence of MI may have been underestimated because non-Q wave MIs were not included in this analysis. This study emphasizes the importance of periodic screening for silent ischemia and perhaps stress testing in patients with diabetes mellitus, even if they have no perceptible symptoms of myocardial ischemia. This analysis also suggests that diabetic patients with a history of silent MI may benefit significantly from the addition of fenofibrate to their background pharmacologic therapy.

P. P. Toth, MD, PhD

Plasma Triglycerides and Cardiovascular Events in the Treating to New Targets and Incremental Decrease in End-Points Through Aggressive Lipid Lowering Trials of Statins in Patients With Coronary Artery Disease

Faergeman O, Holme I, Fayyad R, et al (Århus Univ Hosp, Denmark; Ullevål Univ Hosp, Oslo, Norway; Pfizer, Inc., NY; et al)

Am J Cardiol 104:459-463, 2009

We determined the ability of in-trial measurements of triglycerides (TGs) to predict new cardiovascular events (CVEs) using data from the Incremental Decrease in End Points through Aggressive Lipid Lowering (IDEAL) and Treating to New Targets (TNT) trials. The trials compared atorvastatin 80 mg/day with moderate-dose statin therapy (simvastatin 20 to 40 mg/day in IDEAL and atorvastatin 10 mg/day in TNT) in patients with clinically evident coronary heart disease or a history of myocardial infarction. The outcome measurement in the present research was CVE occurring after the first year of the trial. After adjusting for age, gender,

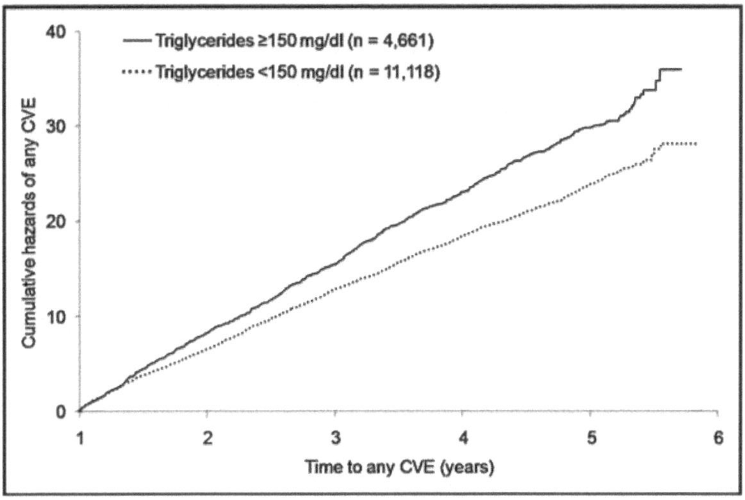

FIGURE 1.—Cumulative hazards of any CVE by on-treatment TGs in the IDEAL and TNT studies (HR 1.33, 95% CI 1.24 to 1.43, p <0.001). (Reprinted from Faergeman O, Holme I, Fayyad R, et al. Plasma triglycerides and cardiovascular events in the treating to new targets and incremental decrease in end-points through aggressive lipid lowering trials of statins in patients with coronary artery disease. *Am J Cardiol.* 2009;104:459-463, with permission from Elsevier.)

and study, risk of CVEs increased with increasing TGs (p <0.001 for trend across quintiles of TGs). Patients in the highest quintile had a 63% higher rate of CVEs than patients in the lowest quintile (hazard ratio 1.63, 95% confidence interval 1.46 to 1.81) and the relation of TGs to risk was apparent even within the normal range of TGs. The ability of TG measurements to predict risk decreased when high-density lipoprotein cholesterol and apolipoprotein B:apolipoprotein A-1 were included in the statistical analysis, and it was abolished with inclusion of further variables (diabetes, body mass index, glucose, hypertension, and smoking; (p = 0.044 and 0.621, respectively, for trend across quintiles of TGs). Similar results were obtained in patients in whom low-density lipoprotein cholesterol had been lowered to guideline-recommended levels. In conclusion, even slightly increased TG levels are associated with higher risk of recurrence of CVEs in statin-treated patients and should be considered a useful marker of risk (Figs 1-3).

▶ Hypertriglyceridemia is a defining feature of the metabolic syndrome, hyperchylomicronemia, and familial combined hyperlipidemia. It is associated with excess dietary fat intake, insulin resistance, and a large number of genetic polymorphisms in lipoprotein lipase and apoproteins CII and CIII, among other genetic loci. Prospective epidemiologic investigations have shown inconsistent relationships between serum triglyceride levels and risk for atherosclerotic disease. In general, multivariable analysis that controls standard risk factors, such as age, smoking status, hypertension, and serum high-density lipoprotein cholesterol (HDL-C) and low-density lipoprotein cholesterol (LDL-C),

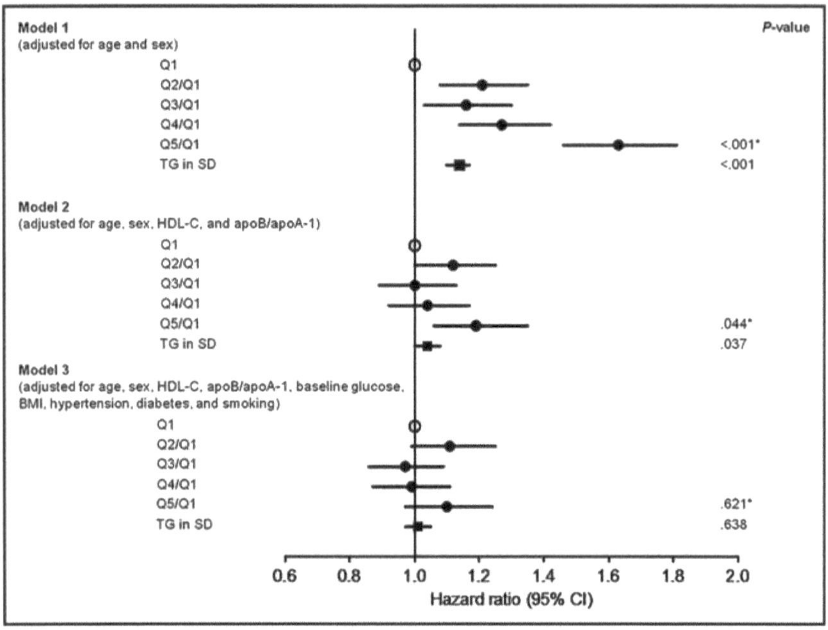

FIGURE 2.—Risk ratios for any CVE by quintiles (Q) of on-treatment TGs in the IDEAL and TNT studies (n = 15,779, *p values for trend across quintiles of TGs). BMI = body mass index; HDL-C = HDL cholesterol. (Reprinted from Faergeman O, Holme I, Fayyad R, et al. Plasma triglycerides and cardiovascular events in the treating to new targets and incremental decrease in end-points through aggressive lipid lowering trials of statins in patients with coronary artery disease. *Am J Cardiol.* 2009;104:459-463, with permission from Elsevier.)

frequently results in a nonsignifcant relationship between serum triglycerides and risk for coronary heart disease (CHD). A recent meta-analysis of 29 studies incorporating 262 565 subjects showed that when comparing risk in the first and third tertiles of serum triglycerides, hypertriglyceridemia is associated with an adjusted odds ratio of 1.72 for incident CHD.[1] The fibrate trials have done little to shed light on this issue, largely because the subjects enrolled in these trials for the most part have near normal fasting triglyceride levels. Hypertriglyceridemia alters lipoprotein metabolism and promotes HDL catabolism and increased production of small, dense LDL particles.

In this study, the impact of triglycerides on risk for cardiovascular events was evaluated in patients with stable CHD from the Incremental Decrease in End Points through Aggressive Lipid Lowering (IDEAL) and Treating to New Targets (TNT) trials.[2,3] When unadjusted for other risk factors, elevated triglycerides are associated with a 33% higher frequency of CHD-related events (Fig 1). Patients in the highest quintile had a 63% higher incidence of CHD events compared with those in the lowest quintile for triglycerides. However, whether evaluated in the cohorts as a whole or in patients who attained an LDL-C ≤100 mg/dL, once the analysis includes apoB, apoAI, body mass

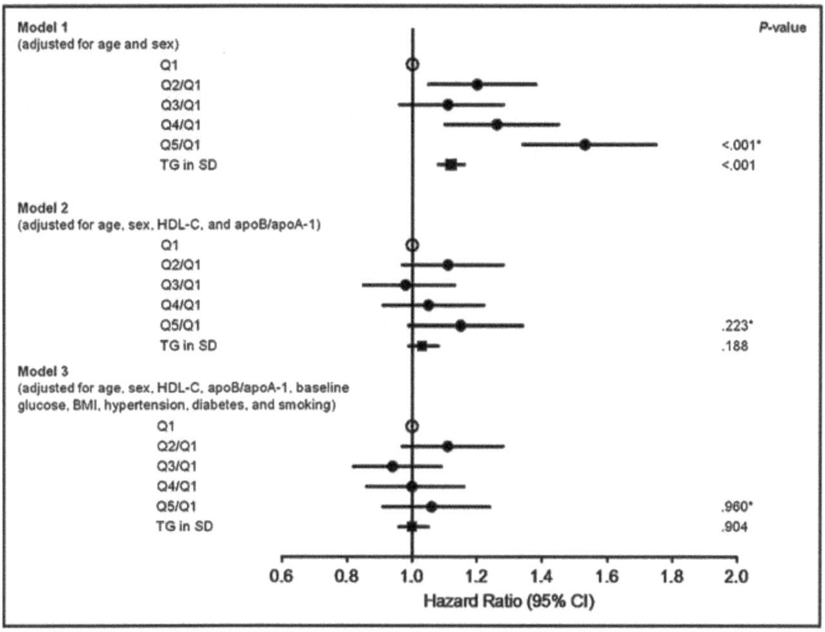

FIGURE 3.—Risk ratios for any CVE by quintiles of on-treatment TGs in patients treated to a LDL cholesterol concentration <100 mg/dl in the IDEAL and TNT studies (n = 10,801, *p values for trend across quintiles of TGs). Abbreviations as in Figure 2. (Reprinted from Faergeman O, Holme I, Fayyad R, et al. Plasma triglycerides and cardiovascular events in the treating to new targets and incremental decrease in end-points through aggressive lipid lowering trials of statins in patients with coronary artery disease. *Am J Cardiol.* 2009;104:459-463, with permission from Elsevier.)

index, diabetes status, and hypertension, the predictive significance of triglyceride levels is lost (Figs 2 and 3).

This analysis highlights the often-repeated observation that triglycerides are not an independent risk factor for CHD. They appear to be an effective marker of increased risk. Hypertriglyceridemia is associated with endothelial dysfunction and pancreatitis. Lowering serum triglycerides is therapeutically valuable, as this type of intervention is associated with improved vasoreactivity, reduced risk for pancreatitis, increases in serum HDL-C, and reductions in VLDL remnant particles and LDL particles. It is possible that the more optimal study to evaluate the role of triglycerides in risk will be to evaluate them in a postprandial setting. Designing such a study will have to control for insulin resistance, nutrient and fat compositions, intrinsic lipoprotein lipase activity, hepatic capacity to clear chylomicrons, and VLDL remnants, among other variables.

P. P. Toth, MD, PhD

References

1. Sarwar N, Danesh J, Eiriksdottir G, et al. Triglycerides and the risk of coronary heart disease: 10,158 incident cases among 262,525 participants in 29 Western prospective studies. *Circulation.* 2007;115:450-458.

2. Pedersen TR, Faergeman O, Kastelein JJ, et al. Incremental Decrease in End Points Through Aggressive Lipid Lowering (IDEAL) Study Group. Incremental decrease in end points through aggressive lipid lowering Study G. High-dose atorvastatin vs usual-dose simvastatin for secondary prevention after myocardial infarction: the IDEAL study: a randomized controlled trial. *JAMA*. 2005;294:2437-2445.
3. LaRosa JC, Grundy SM, Waters DD, et al. Treating to New Targets (TNT) Investigators. Intensive lipid lowering with atorvastatin in patients with stable coronary disease. *N Engl J Med*. 2005;352:1425-1435.

Safety and Efficacy of Achieving Very Low Low-Density Lipoprotein Cholesterol Levels With *Rosuvastatin* 40 mg Daily (from the ASTEROID Study)

Wiviott SD, Mohanavelu S, Raichlen JS, et al (Brigham and Women's Hosp and Harvard Med School, Boston, MA; AstraZeneca, Wilmington, Delaware; et al)
Am J Cardiol 104:29-35, 2009

Clinical trial evidence supports the use of intensive statin therapy for patients with coronary artery disease. High doses of potent statins have shown the greatest clinical benefit, but concerns persist regarding the efficacy and safety of achieving very low levels of low-density lipoprotein (LDL) cholesterol. We grouped patients treated with 40 mg of rosuvastatin daily by the LDL cholesterol achieved according to previous work (<40, 40 to <60, 60 to <80, 80 to <100, and ≥100 mg/dl) and by National Cholesterol Education Program targets (<70, 70 to <100, and ≥100 mg/dl) in A Study to Evaluate the Effect of Rosuvastatin on Intravascular Ultrasound-Derived Coronary Atheroma Burden (ASTEROID). The rates of key safety end points, including death, hemorrhagic stroke, and liver and muscle enzyme elevations, and key efficacy end points (atheroma burden) were compared using chi-square testing or Fisher's exact testing. The analysis included 471 patients who had had their LDL cholesterol measured at 3 months, of whom 340 (72.2%) had LDL cholesterol of <70 mg/dl, exhibiting excellent achievement of even the most stringent guideline-based goals. Of these 471 subjects, 192 (40.8%) had LDL cholesterol ≥40 mg/dl but <60 mg/dl, and 57 (12.1%) had LDL cholesterol <40 mg/dl. Adverse events occurred infrequently during the trial, and no pattern appeared relating the frequency of any adverse event to the achieved LDL cholesterol. Similarly, the on-treatment atheroma volume, change in atheroma volume, and high percentage of subjects with atheroma regression did not differ by the achieved LDL cholesterol. In conclusion, although the power to detect such changes was limited, these data showed no clear relation between the LDL cholesterol achieved by intensive statin therapy with rosuvastatin

TABLE 3.—Safety Outcomes by Low-Density Lipoprotein (LDL) Cholesterol Achieved (5 Groups)

Safety Outcome	LDL Cholesterol Achieved (mg/dl) <40 (n = 57)	40–<60 (n = 192)	60–<80 (n = 142)	80–<100 (n = 52)	≥100 (n = 28)	p Value*
Creatine kinase >5 × ULN	1 (2%)	2 (1%)	2 (1%)	1 (2%)	0 (0%)	0.88
Creatine kinase >10 × ULN	0 (0%)	0 (0%)	0 (0%)	0 (0%)	0 (0%)	1.0
Alanine aminotransferase >3 × ULN (2 occasions)	0 (0%)	1 (1%)	0 (0%)	0 (0%)	0 (0%)	1.0
Death	0 (0%)	0 (0%)	1 (1%)	0 (0%)	0 (0%)	0.59
Intracranial hemorrhage	0 (0%)	0 (0%)	1 (1%)	0 (0%)	0 (0%)	0.59
Withdrew owing to adverse event	4 (7%)	20 (10%)	15 (11%)	8 (15%)	3 (11%)	0.73
Myopathy	0 (0%)	0 (0%)	0 (0%)	0 (0%)	0 (0%)	1.0
Myositis	0 (0%)	0 (0%)	0 (0%)	0 (0%)	0 (0%)	1.0
Death/myocardial infarction/ stroke	0 (0%)	1 (1%)	3 (2%)	0 (0%)	0 (0%)	0.58

Data are presented as numbers (%).
ULN = upper limit of normal.
*For equality among cells (not-trend).

and adverse effects. Atheroma regression occurred in most patients and was not linked to the LDL cholesterol achieved (Table 3).

▶ For decades there has been a lingering suspicion that a low low-density lipoprotein cholesterol (LDL-C) could potentially be harmful. This is a fascinating issue. LDL particles are a by-product of very low-density lipoprotein (VLDL) catabolism. The VLDL particle is energy-rich by virtue of its triglyceride cargo. LDL-C is energy-poor and largely constitutes a spent particle for energy transport. Peripheral cells are incapable of catabolizing cholesterol. Hence, there is a dependence on reverse cholesterol transport by high-density lipoprotein (HDL) particles to mobilize and transport excess cholesterol back to the liver for elimination. Physiologically, mammals go to great lengths to try to remove LDL from blood, given the fact that it no longer appears to confer survival advantage. Hepatocytes express multiple LDL receptors (LDL receptor, LDL receptor-related protein). The macrophage has evolved families of scavenging receptors in an effort to clear LDL within the subendothelial space. Concern has also been expressed that if LDL-C falls to very low levels, perhaps steroidogenesis would somehow be impeded. This is incorrect, as HDL particles deliver cholesterol to steroidogenic organs, not LDL. Patients with lifelong very low levels of LDL-C (even in the teens and 20s) secondary to mutations in *PCSK9* have reduced risk for developing atherosclerosis but no readily characterizable increased risk for other diseases.[1,2] Despite these considerations, it is common for clinicians to ask, when it comes to LDL-C, how low is too low?"

In this post hoc evaluation of the A Study to Evaluate the Effect of Rosuvastatin on Intravascular Ultrasound-Derived Coronary Atheroma Burden (ASTEROID) trial, the authors probe the issue of whether or not adverse event rates increase as LDL-C is driven lower and lower (even to < 40 mg/dL) with rosuvastatin. There was no relationship between attained LDL-C and risk for myopathy, transaminitis, hepatotoxicity, intracranial hemorrhage, or acute cardiovascular events.

This data corroborates a post hoc evaluation of data from the Pravastatin or Atorvastatin Evaluation and Infection Therapy–Thrombolysis in Myocardial Infarction-22 (PROVE-IT TIMI22) trial. As LDL-C was driven lower and lower (to even <40 mg/dL), there was no increased risk for adverse events, and risk for cardiovascular events trended lower and lower.[3] Is it likely that when it comes to LDL, lower is better? Yes. Does risk for adverse events increase as LDL-C drops to even very low levels? Apparently not. Aggressive treatment of LDL-C is warranted in patients with established coronary artery disease. To date, the benefits certainly outweigh the risks.

P. P. Toth, MD, PhD

References

1. Cohen JC, Boerwinkle E, Mosley TH Jr, Hobbs HH. Sequence variations in PCSK9, low LDL, and protection against coronary heart disease. *N Engl J Med.* 2006;354:1264-1272.
2. Abifadel M, Varret M, Rabes JP, et al. Mutations in PCSK9 cause autosomal dominant hypercholesterolemia. *Nat Genet.* 2003;34:154-156.
3. Wiviott SD, Cannon CP, Morrow DA, Ray KK, Pfeffer MA, Braunwald E, PROVE IT-TIMI 22 Investigators. Can low-density lipoprotein be too low? The safety and efficacy of achieving very low low-density lipoprotein with intensive statin therapy: a PROVE IT-TIMI 22 substudy. *J Am Coll Cardiol.* 2005;46:1411-1416.

Epidemiology and Diagnosis

Low- and high-density lipoprotein cholesterol goal attainment in dyslipidemic women: The Lipid Treatment Assessment Project (L-TAP) 2

Santos RD, on behalf of the L-TAP 2 Investigators (Univ of São Paulo Hosp, Brazil; et al)

Am Heart J 158:860-866, 2009

Background.—Differences between women and men have been documented for both diagnostic testing and treatment in cardiology. This analysis evaluates whether low-density lipoprotein cholesterol (LDL-C) success rates according to current guidelines and high-density lipoprotein cholesterol (HDL-C) levels differ by gender in the L-TAP 2 population.

Methods.—Patients aged ≥20 years with dyslipidemia on stable lipid-lowering therapy were assessed in 9 countries between September 2006 and April 2007. Low-density lipoprotein cholesterol goal attainment by cardiovascular risk level and region and determinants of low HDL-C were compared between genders.

Results.—Of 9,955 patients (45.3% women) evaluated, women had a significantly lower overall LDL-C success rate than men (71.5% vs 73.7%, $P = .014$), due entirely to the difference in the high-risk/coronary heart disease (CHD) group (LDL-C goal <100 mg/dL, 62.6% vs 70.6%, $P < .0001$) Among CHD patients with ≥2 additional risk factors, only

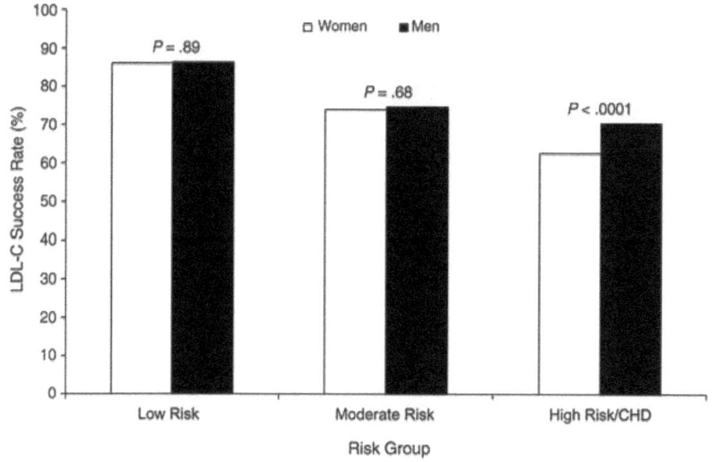

FIGURE 1.—Percentage of LDL-C success rate by gender and risk group. (Reprinted from Santos RD, on behalf of the L-TAP 2 Investigators. Low- and high-density lipoprotein cholesterol goal attainment in dyslipidemic women: the Lipid Treatment Assessment Project (L-TAP) 2. *Am Heart J*. 2009;158:860-866, with permission from Elsevier.)

26.7% of women and 31.5% of men (P =.021) attained the optional LDL-C goal of <70 mg/dL. High-density lipoprotein cholesterol was <50 mg/dL in 32.2% of women and <40 mg/dL in 26.8% of men (P < .0001), including 38.2% of women and 29.8% of men in the high risk/CHD group (P < .0001). Predictors of low HDL-C in women included diabetes, smoking, waist circumference, and hypertension.

Conclusions.—Cholesterol treatment has improved substantially since the original L-TAP a decade ago, when only 39% of women attained their LDL-C goal. However, high-risk women are undertreated compared to men, and a substantial opportunity remains to reduce their cardiovascular risk.

► Gender disparities for the diagnosis and management of cardiovascular disease have been identified and well characterized in recent years. Disparities in the management of cardiovascular risk factors, recognition of symptomatic coronary disease, and frequency of intervention in the setting of an acute coronary syndrome have all been quantified. In a consistent fashion, women were less aggressively treated than men. Fortunately, significant progress has been made in recent years in improving cardiovascular care for women. Progress is also being made in understanding how risk factors can incur differential levels of risk in men and women, and how women can specifically differ from men once symptomatic coronary disease develops.

In this evaluation by the Lipid Treatment Assessment Project (LTAP), it is apparent that significant progress is being made. There were no differences between genders in low-density lipoprotein cholesterol (LDL-C) goal attainment in the low- and moderate-risk groups (Fig 1). Among high-risk patients, the gap has narrowed. Achieving an LDL-C goal ≤100 mg/dL occurred in

62.6% and 70.6% of women and men, respectively. It cannot be discerned from these data what social, economic, or clinical barriers may have given rise to this difference. Among patients stratified to very high-risk status, whose optional LDL-C goal is ≤70 mg/dL, goal attainment was 31.5% and 26.7% for men and women, respectively. Approximately one-third and a quarter of women and men, respectively, had low levels of high-density lipoprotein (HDL).

Although this study points out a gender disparity in LDL-C goal attainment among high-risk patients, there are many positive findings. There were no differences for LDL-C goal attainment among lower risk patients. Moreover, compared with the previous LTAP evaluation, the percentage of high-risk women who attain an LDL-C ≤100 mg/dL has approximately doubled in 10 years.[1] This constitutes significant progress. Among very high-risk patients, it is likely that goal attainment would be improved for both men and women if the descriptor "optional goal" was dropped and the LDL-C target level hardened to ≤70 mg/dL. Much semantic ambiguity and clinical confusion would be removed. Characterizing low HDL-C is important, and this is not the first study to suggest a higher incidence of low HDL-C among women than men.[2] Treating low serum HDL-C will require more clinical trials to help determine whether there is, in fact, a therapeutic target for this lipid fraction. The target may actually depend upon gender, choice of therapeutic agent(s), risk factor burden, severity of coronary disease, and the resulting functionality of the HDL particles, among other considerations. This study stirs optimism. Goal attainment for both men and women is improving. But, as with all issues in medicine, there remains much room for improvement. It is important to continue to screen men and women for dyslipidemia, treat abnormal lipid profiles at all levels of risk, find better approaches for increasing compliance with lifestyle modification and pharmacologic intervention, and remain sensitive to socioeconomic and behavioral gender differences, which can influence treatment success rates.

P. P. Toth, MD, PhD

References

1. Pearson TA, Laurora I, Chu H, Kafonek S. The lipid treatment assessment project (L-TAP): a multicenter survey to evaluate the percentages of dyslipidemic patients receiving lipid-lowering therapy and achieving low-density lipoprotein cholesterol goals. *Arch Intern Med.* 2000;160:459-467.
2. Chapman MJ, Assmann G, Fruchart JC, Shepherd J, Sirtori C, European Consensus Panel on HDL-C. Raising high-density lipoprotein cholesterol with reduction of cardiovascular risk: the role of nicotinic acid – a position paper developed by the European Consensus Panel on HDL-C. *Curr Med Res Opin.* 2004;20:1253-1268.

Intake of total *trans*, *trans*-18:1, and *trans*-18:2 fatty acids and risk of sudden cardiac death in women

Chiuve SE, Rimm EB, Manson JE, et al (Harvard School of Public Health, Boston, MA; et al)

Am Heart J 158:761-767, 2009

Background.—Total intake of *trans* fat is associated with coronary heart disease (CHD), and recent reports in primarily male populations suggest that blood levels of specific *trans* isomers may have different effects on risk, particularly risk of sudden cardiac death (SCD).

Methods.—We prospectively examined the association between dietary intake of *trans* fat and SCD among 86,762 women from the Nurses' Health Study. Coronary heart disease risk factors, including diet and lifestyle factors, were updated via questionnaires every 2 to 4 years, beginning in 1980.

Results.—Over 26 years, we documented 317 SCD events. In the primary analysis, we found no significant association between intake of total *trans* fat, *trans*-18:1, or *trans*-18:2 isomers and risk of SCD. Compared to the lowest quintile of intake, the relative risk (95% CI) of SCD in the highest quintile was 1.28 (0.82-2.00) for total *trans*, 1.08 (0.64-1.83) for *trans*-18:1, and 1.19 (0.76-1.88) for *trans*-18:2. In a secondary prespecified analysis, total *trans* fat was significantly related to SCD among women who reported a diagnosis of CHD before SCD (relative risk 3.24, 95% CI 1.42-7.40 for the highest vs lowest quintile, P trend = .01); however, the test for interaction was not significant (P = .11).

Conclusions.—In this large prospective cohort of women, neither dietary intake of *trans* fat nor the individual *trans* isomers, *trans*-18:1 and *trans*-18:2, were significantly associated with risk of SCD. However, *trans* fat intake may be associated with SCD risk among women with CHD, suggesting that *trans* fat intake may play a greater role in SCD risk among those with clinically manifest atherosclerosis (Table 2).

▶ In contrast to the omega-3 fatty acids, trans fats are associated with an increased risk for coronary atherosclerosis[1,2] and sudden cardiac death (SCD).[3,4] Trans fats are derived from partially hydrogenated oils, and increased consumption is associated with increased serum levels of low-density lipoprotein cholesterol (LDL-C) and decreased levels of high-density lipoprotein cholesterol (HDL-C). There is an increased emphasis on the nutritional value of eliminating or at least minimizing the consumption of trans fats because of their adverse health consequences.

In this analysis from the Nurses' Health Study, investigators evaluated whether or not there is a relationship between the consumption of trans fat isomers (18:1, 18:2) or total trans fats and SCD. For the group as a whole, there was no significant relationship between trans fat consumption and risk after a variety of approaches to multivariate adjustment (Table 2). Among women with established CAD, however, there may be a relationship between

TABLE 2.—Relative Risks (95% CIs) of Sudden Cardiac Death According to Total *Trans*-Fat Intake

	Quintiles of Total *Trans* Fat (% Energy)					*P* Trend
Total *trans* (median intake, % energy)	0.77	1.12	1.43	1.83	2.55	
Cases	69	77	59	61	51	
Person-years	443 754	443 149	444 421	446 960	450 507	
Age and energy adjusted	1.0 (ref)	1.33 (0.96-1.85)	1.15 (0.81-1.63)	1.48 (1.03-2.12)	1.65 (1.11-2.45)	.01
Multivariate adjusted 1	1.0 (ref)	1.15 (0.83-1.60)	0.90 (0.63-1.28)	1.02 (0.71-1.48)	0.95 (0.63-1.43)	.95
Multivariate adjusted 2	1.0 (ref)	1.27 (0.91-1.79)	1.02 (0.70-1.48)	1.18 (0.80-1.74)	1.18 (0.76-1.83)	.64
Multivariate adjusted 3	1.0 (ref)	1.27 (0.90-1.79)	1.04 (0.72-1.52)	1.26 (0.85-1.87)	1.28 (0.82-2.00)	.36

Multivariate adjusted 1: adjusted for age, total energy intake, smoking, BMI, parental history of MI, menopausal status, use of postmenopausal hormones, aspirin use, multivitamin and vitamin E supplements, physical activity, and alcohol intake.

Multivariate adjusted 2: adjusted for multivariate 1 plus intake of ω-3 fatty acid, α-linolenic fatty acids, and ratio of polyunsaturated to saturated fatty acids.

Multivariate adjusted 3: adjusted for multivariate 2 plus diagnosis of CHD, stroke, diabetes, high blood pressure, or high cholesterol.

trans fat intake and SCD. When comparing the highest and lowest quintiles for women with CAD, the hazard ratio for SCD was 3.24, even after controlling for dietary factors and traditional CHD risk factors, but the interaction was not significant. The power of this study to detect a significant interaction was likely limited by the small numbers of women who developed CAD and sustained SCD. Moreover, during the course of this study, the enrichment of foodstuffs with trans fats had also decreased.

The finding of a possible relationship between trans fat intake and SCD is intriguing. This suggests that current recommendations to severely curtail food preparation with trans fat are valid and important, particularly in patients with established CAD. Any nutritional component with the capacity for augmenting the risk for sudden death should be looked upon as particularly toxic and contraindicated. The use of trans fats should be completely eliminated by food producers.

P. P. Toth, MD, PhD

References

1. Pietinen P, Ascherio A, Korhonen P, et al. Intake of fatty acids and risk of coronary heart disease in a cohort of Finnish men. The Alpha-Tocopherol, Beta-Carotene Cancer Prevention Study. *Am J Epidemiol.* 1997;145:876-887.
2. Oomen CM, Ocke MC, Feskens EJ, van Erp-Baart MA, Kok FJ, Kromhout D. Association between trans fatty acid intake and 10-year risk of coronary heart disease in the Zutphen Elderly Study: a prospective population-based study. *Lancet.* 2001;357:746-751.
3. Lemaitre RN, King IB, Mozaffarian D, et al. Plasma phospholipid trans fatty acids, fatal ischemic heart disease, and sudden cardiac death in older adults: the cardiovascular health study. *Circulation.* 2006;114:209-215.
4. Lemaitre RN, King IB, Raghunathan TE, et al. Cell membrane trans-fatty acids and the risk of primary cardiac arrest. *Circulation.* 2002;105:697-701.

Metabolic Syndrome

The association of pericardial fat with incident coronary heart disease: the Multi-Ethnic Study of Atherosclerosis (MESA)

Ding J, Hsu F-C, Harris TB, et al (Wake Forest Univ School of Medicine, Winston-Salem, NC; Natl Inst on Aging, Bethesda, MD; et al)
Am J Clin Nutr 90:499-504, 2009

Background.—Pericardial fat (ie, fat around the heart) may have a direct role in the atherosclerotic process in coronary arteries through local release of inflammation-related cytokines. Cross-sectional studies suggest that pericardial fat is positively associated with coronary artery disease independent of total body fat.

Objective.—We investigated whether pericardial fat predicts future coronary heart disease events.

Design.—We conducted a case-cohort study in 998 individuals, who were randomly selected from 6814 Multi-Ethnic Study of Atherosclerosis (MESA) participants and 147 MESA participants (26 from those 998 individuals) who developed incident coronary heart disease from 2000 to

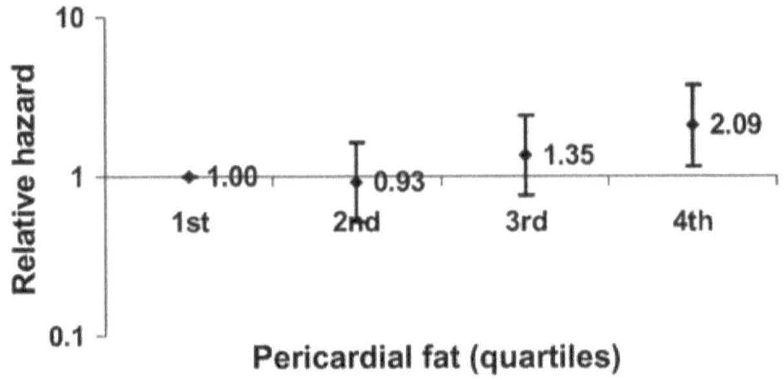

FIGURE 2.—Relative hazards (and 95% CIs) of coronary heart disease by quartiles of pericardial fat from a Cox proportional hazard model, adjusted for age, sex, ethnicity, and BMI in the Multi-Ethnic Study of Atherosclerosis (MESA) 1000 sample and in MESA participants who developed incident coronary heart disease, 2000–2005. (Reprinted from Ding J, Hsu F-C, Harris TB, et al. The association of pericardial fat with incident coronary heart disease: The Multi-Ethnic Study of Atherosclerosis (MESA). *Am J Clin Nutr.* 2009;90:499-504, with permission from the American Society for Nutrition.)

2005. The volume of pericardial fat was determined from cardiac computed tomography at baseline.

Results.—The age range of the subjects was 45–84 y (42% men, 45% white, 10% Asian American, 22% African American, and 23% Hispanic). Pericardial fat was positively correlated with both body mass index (correlation coefficient = 0.45, $P < 0.0001$) and waist circumference (correlation coefficient = 0.57, $P < 0.0001$). In unadjusted analyses, pericardial fat (relative hazard per 1-SD increment: 1.33; 95% CI: 1.15, 1.54), but not body mass index (1.00; 0.84, 1.18), was associated with the risk of coronary heart disease. Waist circumference (1.14; 0.97, 1.34; $P = 0.1$) was marginally associated with the risk of coronary heart disease. The relation between pericardial fat and coronary heart disease remained significant after further adjustment for body mass index and other cardiovascular disease risk factors (1.26; 1.01, 1.59). The relation did not differ by sex.

Conclusion.—Pericardial fat predicts incident coronary heart disease independent of conventional risk factors, including body mass index (Fig 1).

▶ Insulin resistance is associated with increased visceral adiposity. Insulin-resistant visceral adipose tissue undergoes multiple transformations, including an increased influx of macrophages secondary to elevated expression of monocyte chemoattractant protein-1.[1] Adipose tissue becomes an important source of adipocytokines, such as interleukin-1 and tumor necrosis factor-alpha, among others. As adipose tissue becomes more insulin resistant, hormone-sensitive lipase activity increases, resulting in augmented triglyceride hydrolysis and fatty acid release. With increased fatty acid availability, ectopic fat deposition increases. This results in hepatic steatosis, pericardial steatosis, and increase in both intra- and extramyocellular lipid deposition. All of these changes are associated with increased risk for diabetes mellitus and atherosclerotic disease. Pericardial fat mass is associated with increased secretion of inflammatory mediators[2] and coronary artery disease.[3,4]

The Multi-Ethnic Study of Atherosclerosis (MESA) is a community-based prospective cohort study designed primarily to investigate prevalence, correlates, and progression of subclinical cardiovascular disease in 6814 whites, blacks, Hispanics, and Asian Americans aged 45 to 84 years in Baltimore, Maryland; Chicago, Illinois; Forsyth County, North Carolina; Los Angeles, California; New York, New York; and St Paul, Minnesota. In this analysis, pericardial fat volume measured by computed tomography was correlated with risk for incident coronary artery disease (CAD). For each 1 standard deviation (SD) increase in pericardial fat, risk for incident CAD increased by 33%. Pericardial fat volume correlated with both body mass index (BMI) and waist circumference. There was no association between BMI and incident CAD. Risk for CAD increased as a function of pericardial fat quartile. When comparing the highest to lowest quartiles of pericardial fat volume, risk for CAD increased 2-fold even after controlling for other established CAD risk factors.

In recent years, much investigation has focused on the relationship among visceral adiposity, insulin resistance, and hepatic steatosis. Pericardial/epicardial adiposity is also adversely impacted by these changes. A number of studies now show that as pericardial adiposity increases, risk for CAD escalates. Considerable investigation will be required to more fully determine how ectopic pericardial fat deposition occurs, how metabolic derangements in it impact coronary atherogenesis, and whether or not these changes can be reversed and the fat resorbed with weight loss and relief of insulin resistance. All of a sudden, lipids in multiple forms appear to impact CAD development and progression: lipoproteins delivered into the subendothelial space via blood as well as lipid mass surrounding an artery, by either inducing inflammation or somehow serving as another source of atherogenic lipid (eg, it may expose the artery to a constant flux of fatty acids). Clearly, ectopic adipose tissue formation/deposition is toxic and further underscores the dramatic need to reduce the incidence of obesity and insulin resistance worldwide.

P. P. Toth, MD, PhD

References

1. Wellen KE, Hotamisligil GS. Obesity-induced inflammatory changes in adipose tissue. *J Clin Invest.* 2003;112:1785-1788.
2. Mazurek T, Zhang L, Zalewski A, et al. Human epicardial adipose tissue is a source of inflammatory mediators. *Circulation.* 2003;108:2460-2466.
3. de Vos AM, Prokop M, Roos CJ, et al. Peri-coronary epicardial adipose tissue is related to cardiovascular risk factors and coronary artery calcification in post-menopausal women. *Eur Heart J.* 2008;29:777-783.
4. Rosito GA, Massaro JM, Hoffmann U, et al. Pericardial fat, visceral abdominal fat, cardiovascular disease risk factors, and vascular calcification in a community-based sample: the Framingham Heart Study. *Circulation.* 2008;117:605-613.

Nutrition and Nutritional Supplements

Anthocyanin supplementation improves serum LDL- and HDL-cholesterol concentrations associated with the inhibition of cholesteryl ester transfer protein in dyslipidemic subjects

Qin Y, Xia M, Ma J, et al (Sun Yat-Sen Univ (Northern Campus), Guangzhou, China)

Am J Clin Nutr 90:485-492, 2009

Background.—Anthocyanins have been shown to exert benefits on the lipid profile in many animal models. Whether these molecules have similar beneficial effects in humans is currently unknown.

Objective.—The objective was to investigate the effects of berry-derived anthocyanin supplements on the serum lipid profile in dyslipidemic patients.

Design.—A total of 120 dyslipidemic subjects (age 40–65 y) were given 160 mg anthocyanins twice daily or placebo for 12 wk in a double-blind, randomized, placebo-controlled trial.

Results.—Anthocyanin consumption increased HDL-cholesterol concentrations (13.7% and 2.8% in the anthocyanin and placebo groups, respectively; $P < 0.001$) and decreased LDL-cholesterol concentrations (13.6% and −0.6% in the anthocyanin and placebo groups, respectively; $P < 0.001$). Cellular cholesterol efflux to serum increased more in the anthocyanin group than in the placebo group (20.0% and 0.2%, respectively; $P < 0.001$). Anthocyanin supplementation decreased the mass and activity of plasma cholesteryl ester transfer protein (CETP) (10.4% and 6.3%, respectively, in the anthocyanin group and −3.5% and 1.1%, respectively, in the placebo group; $P < 0.001$). In the anthocyanin group, the change in HDL cholesterol was negatively correlated with the change in CETP activity ($r_s = -0.330$). The change in LDL cholesterol was positively correlated with the change in CETP mass ($r_s = 0.354$). The change in cellular cholesterol efflux to serum was positively correlated with the change in HDL cholesterol ($r_s = 0.485$). In vitro, cyanidin 3-O-β-glucosides dose-dependently lowered CETP activity in human HepG2 cells.

Conclusions.—Anthocyanin supplementation in humans improves LDL- and HDL-cholesterol concentrations and enhances cellular cholesterol efflux to serum. These benefits may be due to the inhibition of CETP (Tables 1 and 2).

▶ A variety of nutrients are purported to beneficially impact serum lipid levels. This is an important issue, given the fact that a significant percentage of patients are opposed to taking medication for dyslipidemia and/or do not tolerate them due to such side effects as myalgia or hepatotoxicity. Among the most important with established evidence for inducing changes in lipid fractions are fish oils, niacin, and phytosterols. Numerous prospective trials studying whether or not vitamins E and C beneficially impact risk for cardiovascular risk have been negative. Clinical trials with folate and vitamins B6 and B12 used to

TABLE 1.—Anthropometric Characteristics of the Dyslipidemic Patients at Baseline and During the 12-wk Intervention by Group[1]

	Placebo ($n = 60$)				Anthocyanin ($n = 60$)				
	Baseline	4 wk	8 wk	12 wk	Baseline	4 wk	8 wk	12 wk	P^2
Weight (kg)	66.1 ± 10.1	66.5 ± 10.1	66.0 ± 10.0	66.4 ± 10.3	63.7 ± 9.7	65.0 ± 9.7	64.1 ± 9.7	63.8 ± 9.5	0.327
BMI (kg/m^2)	26.7 ± 4.0	27.4 ± 4.2	27.5 ± 4.1	26.8 ± 3.9	25.5 ± 3.1	26.2 ± 3.1	25.8 ± 3.0	25.5 ± 2.9	0.063
Waist circumference (cm)	89.7 ± 9.6	89.9 ± 10.2	89.8 ± 10.6	89.5 ± 10.8	87.1 ± 7.1	87.1 ± 7.1	86.8 ± 6.4	86.4 ± 7.2	0.159
Hip circumference (cm)	98.9 ± 6.4	99.4 ± 6.6	98.8 ± 6.8	98.5 ± 6.2	97.5 ± 6.7	97.8 ± 6.0	97.1 ± 6.0	97.5 ± 6.0	0.306
Waist-to-hip ratio	0.91 ± 0.06	0.88 ± 0.06	0.91 ± 0.06	0.91 ± 0.08	0.90 ± 0.06	0.89 ± 0.06	0.89 ± 0.05	0.88 ± 0.06	0.598
Systolic blood pressure (mm Hg)	129.1 ± 19.0	124.2 ± 17.0	123.7 ± 16.5	124.8 ± 17.0	126.5 ± 17.8	124.4 ± 17.3	121.7 ± 17.0	125.3 ± 20.0	0.888
Diastolic blood pressure (mm Hg)	82.4 ± 10.6	80.5 ± 9.4	77.7 ± 10.6	81.6 ± 10.6	82.7 ± 10.0	79.0 ± 9.9	79.8 ± 11.7	82.7 ± 11.1	0.343

[1]All values are means ± SDs. There were no significant differences between the 2 groups at baseline for any variable by the independent-samples *t* test.
[2]The intervention had no significant effect on anthropometric characteristic by repeated-measures ANCOVA with the baseline value as covariate.

TABLE 2.—Mean Daily Intake of Nutrients by the Subjects at Baseline and at 12 wk by Group[1]

	Placebo ($n = 60$)		Anthocyanin ($n = 60$)		
	Baseline	12 wk	Baseline	12 wk	P^2
Energy (kcal/d)	2168 ± 98	2199 ± 133	2145 ± 95	2189 ± 111	0.726
Protein					
(g/d)	88.8 ± 5.1	87.0 ± 4.3	89.8 ± 6.0	86.9 ± 4.5	0.648
(% of energy)	17.5 ± 2.2	17.2 ± 3.2	17.5 ± 2.0	17.3 ± 3.0	0.846
Total carbohydrate					
(g/d)	269 ± 18	270 ± 22	272 ± 19	267 ± 21	0.098
(% of energy)	51.8 ± 1.4	51.4 ± 2.8	51.8 ± 1.4	51.6 ± 2.7	0.809
Total fat					
(g/d)	85.0 ± 2.9	83.0 ± 4.5	85.3 ± 3.2	82.6 ± 3.9	0.363
(% of energy)	31.9 ± 1.5	31.1 ± 1.6	31.7 ± 1.4	31.2 ± 1.6	0.516
Cholesterol (mg/d)	325 ± 17	326 ± 19	327 ± 21	325 ± 21	0.295
Fiber (g/d)	22.0 ± 22.3	22.3 ± 2.4	22.0 ± 2.1	22.1 ± 2.1	0.669

[1]All values are means ± SDs. There were no significant differences between the 2 groups at baseline for any variable by the independent-samples *t* test.

[2]The intervention had no significant effect on mean daily intake of nutrients by one-factor ANCOVA with the baseline value as covariate.

reduce serum homocysteine levels have also been negative. An intriguing area of ongoing investigation is whether or not plant-derived compounds, such as resveratrol, quercetin, and the anthocyanins, provide benefit, given their potent antioxidant capacity. The anthocyanins are plant pigments and provide characteristic colors for fruits such as berries.

In this study, patients were treated with either anthocyanins derived from bilberries and black currants or placebo. The anthocyanins included glycosylated derivatives of cyanidin, peonidin, delphinidin, petunidin, and malvidin. Subjects were well matched between groups both demographically and for baseline serum chemistries, including lipid profiles. Treatment groups were also well matched by dietary composition and caloric intake at baseline and after 12 weeks of treatment (Table 1). Treatment with anthocyanins significantly increased serum levels of apoAI and high-density lipoprotein cholesterol (HDL-C) and decreased apoB and low-density lipoprotein cholesterol (LDL-C) (Table 2). The 13.7% rise in serum HDL-C is striking. This correlates with significant reductions in cholesteryl ester transfer protein (CETP) activity and mass. Consistent with the rise in HDL-C and apoAI, the serum of anthocyanin-treated subjects increased cholesterol mobilization from cultured macrophage J774 cells by 20%. The serum of subjects treated with placebo was not associated with any change in capacity for cholesterol mobilization from macrophages after 3 months.

It remains to be determined whether or not CETP inhibition is therapeutically beneficial. CETP inhibition with torcetrapib was associated with increased mortality, but there is suspicion that this is due to off target toxicity, such as the increased aldosterone production and elevated blood pressure.[1] Studies with dalcetrapib and anacetrapib are ongoing.[2,3] The observation that the serum of anthocyanin-treated subjects had augmented capacity to induce the mobilization of intracellular cholesterol from macrophages suggests that the treatment is associated with the formation of functional HDL. Additional work will need to be performed to ascertain if this also correlates with increased rates of reverse cholesterol transport. A nearly 14% drop in LDL-C could augment diet and other established therapies for achieving significant LDL-C reduction. These findings certainly support the need to evaluate anthocyanins in a larger end point–driven study. Furthermore, delineating whether or not anthocyanins confer benefit independent of lipid modification (ie, their anti-oxidative capacity) and establishing the dose-response relationship between the various anthocyanins and maximal lipid modification warrant further study.

P. P. Toth, MD, PhD

References

1. Toth PP. Torcetrapib and atherosclerosis: what happened and where do we go from here? *Future Lipidol.* 2007;2:277-284.
2. Toth PP. Novel therapies for increasing serum levels of HDL. *Endocrinol Metab Clin North Am.* 2009;38:151-170.
3. Davidson MH, Toth PP. High-density lipoprotein metabolism: potential therapeutic targets. *Am J Cardiol.* 2007;100:n32-n40.

Association between n–3 fatty acid consumption and ventricular ectopy after myocardial infarction

Smith PJ, Blumenthal JA, Babyak MA, et al (Duke Univ, Durham, NC)
Am J Clin Nutr 89:1315-1320, 2009

Background.—n–3 (omega-3) Fatty acids are associated with a reduced risk of cardiovascular disease; however, the relation between dietary intake of n–3 fatty acids and ventricular arrhythmias has not been investigated among acute post-myocardial infarction (AMI) patients—a group at elevated risk of malignant arrhythmias.

Objective.—The objective was to examine the association between n–3 fatty acid consumption and ventricular ectopy among AMI patients.

Design.—In 260 AMI patients, dietary intake of n–3 fatty acids was assessed by using the Harvard food-frequency questionnaire, and ventricular ectopy was estimated from 24-h electrocardiograph recordings.

Results.—A greater intake of n–3 fatty acids (eicosapentaenoic acid + docosahexaenoic acid + docosapentaenoic acid + α-linolenic acid) was associated with lower ventricular ectopy ($\beta = -0.35$, $P = 0.011$), and this effect remained after cardiovascular comorbidities were controlled for ($\beta = -0.47$, $P = 0.003$). Higher concentrations of both marine-based (eicosapentaenoic acid + docosahexaenoic acid) ($\beta = -0.21$, $P = 0.060$) and plant-based (α-linolenic acid) ($\beta = -0.33$, $P = 0.024$) fatty acids remained associated with lower ventricular ectopy after cardiovascular comorbidities were controlled for.

Conclusion.—These findings extend existing evidence linking n–3 fatty acid consumption to a reduced risk of ventricular arrhythmias by showing

that a greater intake of n–3 fatty acids may be associated with low ventricular ectopy among AMI patients.

▶ The ingestion of omega-3 fatty acids derived from fish (ie, fish oils) is associated with reduced risk for cardiovascular events. American Heart Association guidelines recommend that patients with established coronary artery disease (CAD) consume 2 oily fish meals weekly or take 1 g daily of purified fish oil enriched with eicosapentaenoic acid (EPA) and docosahexaenoic acid (DHA).[1] The Physicians' Health Study showed that high serum levels of EPA and DHA are associated with a 90% lower risk for sudden death compared with low levels.[2] In the Gruppo Italiano per lo Studio della Sopravennivenza nell' Infarto Miocardio (GISSI)-Prevenzione trial, subjects with myocardial infraction (MI) were treated with usual care with or without 850 mg of EPA/DHA daily and were followed up for 3.5 years. The addition of fish oil to usual care reduced total mortality and risk for sudden death by 28% and 47%, respectively.[3] It is believed that fish oils reduce risk for sudden death by suppressing ectopy and increasing the ventricular fibrillation threshold. In the Japan EPA Lipid Intervention Study (JELIS), 19 800 Japanese subjects were given statin therapy with or without the addition of 1800 mg daily of EPA.[4] The addition of EPA resulted in an additional 19% reduction in cardiovascular events over 4.6 years of follow-up. EPA and DHA are also known to reduce hepatic triglyceride biosynthesis, decrease hepatic very low-density lipoprotein (VLDL) secretion, and promote lipoprotein lipase-dependent triglyceride hydrolysis in serum. Fish oil supplementation is thus an important therapy for managing hypertriglyceridemia.

In this study, the investigators evaluated the association between ventricular ectopy following an MI and dietary ingestion of omega-3 fatty acids (EPA/DHA and plant-derived alpha-linolenic acid). Ectopy was evaluated with Holter monitoring. Increased omega-3 fatty acid correlated with reduced ventricular ectopy and remained significant even after controlling for cardiovascular comorbidities, such as gender, severity of CAD, and left ventricular ejection fraction (Fig 1 in the original article).

Patients who sustain an MI are at increased risk for arrhythmogenesis, including ventricular tachycardia and ventricular fibrillation. Increased ventricular ectopy is associated with increased mortality from sudden cardiac death. This study confirms that EPA/DHA is protective against ventricular ectopy in the post-MI period. Importantly, this study also suggests that dietary sources of alpha-linolenic acid are as well. This has been less well established. These data also lend support to the current recommendation that high-risk patients with established CAD take 1 g of fish oil supplements or consume fish enriched with EPA/DHA. Much basic scientific work remains to be done to establish the precise cellular and molecular mechanisms by which the omega-3 fatty acids stabilize the electrical properties of myocardial conduction pathways.

P. P. Toth, MD, PhD

References

1. Kris-Etherton PM, Harris WS, Appel LJ, et al. for the Nutrition Committee. AHA scientific statement. Fish consumption, fish oil, omega-3 fatty acids, and cardiovascular disease. *Circulation.* 2002;106:2747-2757.
2. Albert CM, Campos H, Stampfer MJ, et al. Blood levels of long-chain n-3 fatty acids and the risk of sudden death. *N Engl J Med.* 2002;346:1113-1118.
3. GISSI-Prevenzione Investigators. Dietary supplementation with n-3 polyunsaturated fatty acids and vitamin E after myocardial infarction: results of the GISSI-Prevenzione trial. *Lancet.* 1999;354:447-455.
4. Yokoyama M, Origasa H, Matsuzaki M, et al. for the Japan EPA Lipid Intervention Study (JELIS) Investigators. Effects of eicosapentaenoic acid on major coronary events in hypercholesterolemic patients (JELIS): a randomized open-label, blinded endpoint analysis. *Lancet.* 2007;369:1090-1098.

Pleiotropic Effects of Statin Therapy

Impact of Prior Statin Therapy on Arrhythmic Events in Patients With Acute Coronary Syndromes (from the Global Registry of Acute Coronary Events [GRACE])

Vedre A, for the GRACE Investigators (Univ of Michigan, Ann Arbor; et al)
Am J Cardiol 104:1613-1617, 2009

Animal models of myocardial ischemia have demonstrated reduction in arrhythmias using statins. It was hypothesized that previous statin therapy before hospitalization might be associated with reductions of in-hospital arrhythmic events in patients with acute coronary syndromes. In this multinational, prospective, observational study (the Global Registry of Acute Coronary Events [GRACE]), data from 64,679 patients hospitalized for suspected acute coronary syndromes (from 1999 to 2007) were analyzed. The primary outcome of interest was in-hospital arrhythmic events in previous statin users compared with nonusers. The 2 primary end points were atrial fibrillation and the composite end point of ventricular tachycardia, ventricular fibrillation, and/or cardiac arrest. In-hospital death was also examined. Of the 64,679 patients, 17,636 (27%) had received previous statin therapy. Those taking statins had higher crude rates of histories of angina (69% vs 46%), diabetes (34% vs 22%), heart failure (15% vs 8.4%), hypertension (74% vs 58%), atrial fibrillation (9.3% vs 7.0%), and dyslipidemia (85% vs 35%). Patients previously taking statins were less likely to have in-hospital arrhythmias. In propensity-adjusted multivariable models, previous statin use was associated with a lower risk for ventricular tachycardia, ventricular fibrillation, or cardiac arrest (odds ratio 0.81, 95% confidence interval 0.72 to 0.96, $p = 0.002$); atrial fibrillation (odds ratio 0.81, 95% confidence interval 0.73 to 0.89, $p < 0.0001$); and death (odds ratio 0.82, 95% confidence interval 0.70 to 0.95, $p = 0.010$). In conclusion, patients previously taking statins had a lower incidence of in-hospital arrhythmic events after acute coronary syndrome than those not previously taking statins. Our study suggests

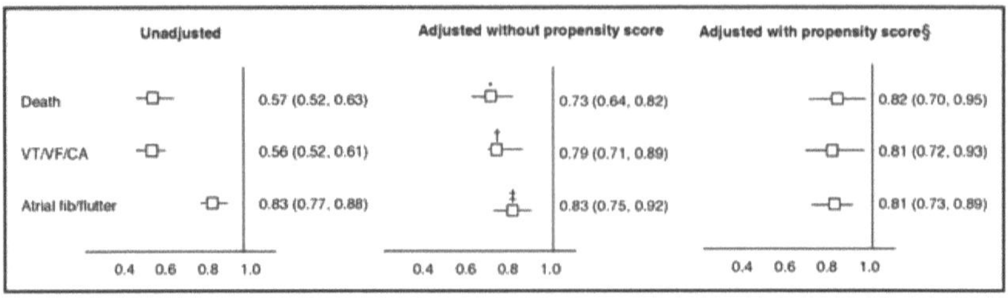

FIGURE 3.—Unadjusted and adjusted odds ratios (95% confidence intervals) for in-hospital outcomes (previous statin users vs nonusers). Unadjusted: n = 64,650 for death; n = 64,043 for VT, VF, and/or CA; and n = 64,277 for AF or atrial flutter. *Adjusted for country, GRACE risk score variables (age, Killip class, CA, systolic blood pressure, pulse, creatinine concentration, ST-segment change, positive initial cardiac biomarkers) (n = 39,844). †Adjusted for age, female gender, country, Killip class, systolic blood pressure, pulse, creatinine concentration, ST-segment change, positive initial cardiac biomarkers, previous therapy (aspirin, amiodarone, or digoxin), and medical history (percutaneous coronary intervention, angina, major bleeding, or stress test) (n = 39,306). ‡Adjusted for age, female gender, country, Killip class, systolic blood pressure, pulse, creatinine concentration, ST-segment change, positive initial cardiac biomarkers, previous therapy (aspirin, warfarin, digoxin, amiodarone, or thienopyridines), and medical history (hypertension, myocardial infarction, dyslipidemia, coronary artery bypass grafting, transient ischemic attack or stroke, smoking, or stress test) (n = 39,462). §Each outcome is adjusted for the same variables as the corresponding outcomes to the left plus propensity score. Corresponding samples sizes are equal. (Reprinted from Vedre A, for the GRACE Investigators. Impact of prior statin therapy on arrhythmic events in patients with acute coronary syndromes (from the Global Registry of Acute Coronary Events [GRACE]). *Am J Cardiol.* 2009;104:1613-1617, with permission from Elsevier.)

TABLE 3.—In-Hospital Outcomes According to Previous Statin Use

Variable	Previous Statin Use (n = 17,636)	No Previous Statin Use (n = 47,043)	p Value
Death	560 (3.2%)	2,563 (5.5%)	<0.0001
Heart failure or pulmonary edema	1,967 (11%)	6,727 (14%)	<0.0001
Cardiogenic shock	453 (2.6%)	2,180 (4.7%)	<0.0001
CA or VF	517 (3.0%)	2,553 (5.5%)	<0.0001
Sustained VT	754 (4.3%)	3,448 (7.4%)	<0.0001
AF or atrial flutter	1,203 (6.9%)	3,830 (8.2%)	<0.0001
Renal failure	685 (3.9%)	1,868 (4.0%)	0.60
Myocardial infarction >24 hours after hospitalization or reinfarction*	263 (2.3%)	616 (2.5%)	0.36

*For myocardial infarction >24 hours after hospitalization or reinfarction, n = 879 for previous statin use and n = 35,680 for no previous statin use.

another possible benefit from appropriate primary and secondary prevention therapy with statins (Fig 3, Table 3).

▶ In recent years, a number of studies have been published suggesting that statin therapy is associated with a lower frequency of new onset or recurrent atrial fibrillation in a variety of settings, including the postoperative period following coronary artery bypass grafting,[1] cardioversion for atrial fibrillation,[2] and in patients with left ventricular systolic dysfunction.[3] The precise mechanism(s) for this protective effect awaits more basic scientific investigation.

Among the hypotheses entertained are: (1) reduction in small vessel disease potentially preserving pacemaking activity in both the sinoatrial and atrioventricular nodes; (2) reduction in adverse remodeling and abnormal intercellular matrix deposition; and (3) maintenance of appropriate ion channel activity and transmembrane ion fluxes, among others.

The Global Registry of Acute Coronary Events (GRACE) is a multinational (14 nations), prospective, observational cohort study of patients hospitalized for suspected acute coronary syndromes (ACSs). In this study, risk for developing cardiac arrhythmias among 64 679 patients admitted for ACS (unstable angina, non ST segment elevating myocardial infarction [NSTEMI], or ST segment elevating MI [STEMI]) was analyzed. The comparison groups were comprised of patients who were or were not taking statin therapy at the time of admission. Statin therapy before admission was associated with statistically significant reductions in mortality, heart failure and pulmonary edema, cardiogenic shock, cardiac arrest, sustained ventricular tachycardia, ventricular fibrillation, as well as atrial fibrillation and atrial flutter (Table 3). In propensity adjusted multivariable models (performed to adjust for bias potentially arising from the nonrandom observational design of the study), previous statin use is associated with a 19% lower risk for atrial fibrillation, ventricular tachycardia, ventricular fibrillation, and cardiac arrest and an 18% lower risk for death (Fig 3).

Statin administration in the setting of an ACS and in secondary prevention, in general, is well established and considered to be the standard of care. The development of cardiac arrhythmias in the setting of an ACS is associated with increased morbidity and mortality. Moreover, new onset arrhythmias may also require chronic treatment with anticoagulation and/or antiarrhythmic agents, which increase expense and risk for adverse side effects. This evaluation from the GRACE study suggests that statins beneficially impact risk for both atrial and ventricular arrhythmogenesis in a population highly vulnerable to these complications, and accentuates the critical importance of early and sustained statin therapy in these patients, irrespective of baseline lipid profile. Data from a committed, adequately powered, prospective randomized study using arrhythmia suppression as a prespecified end point would provide more definitive evidence for this benefit from statin therapy. However, in the current climate of severe funding constraints, such a trial is unlikely to see the light of day.

P. P. Toth, MD, PhD

References

1. Marin F, Pascual DA, Roldan V, et al. Statins and postoperative risk of atrial fibrillation following coronary artery bypass grafting. *Am J Cardiol.* 2006;97:55-60.
2. Ozaydin M, Varol E, Aslan SM, et al. Effect of atorvastatin on the recurrence rates of atrial fibrillation after electrical cardioversion. *Am J Cardiol.* 2006;97:1490-1493.
3. Hanna IR, Heeke B, Bush H, et al. Lipid-lowering drug use is associated with reduced prevalence of atrial fibrillation in patients with left ventricular systolic dysfunction. *Heart Rhythm.* 2006;3:881-886.

Statin use is associated with lower risk of atrial fibrillation in women with coronary disease: the HERS trial

Pellegrini CN, Vittinghoff E, Lin F, et al (Univ of California, San Francisco)
Heart 95:704-708, 2009

Objective.—To determine the efficacy of statin treatment in atrial fibrillation (AF) prevention in women.

Design.—Cohort study using data obtained in the Heart and Estrogen/Progestin Replacement Study (HERS).

Setting.—Secondary analysis of a multicentre, randomised controlled clinical trial.

Patients.—2673 Postmenopausal women with coronary disease.

Main outcome measures.—AF prevalence at baseline and incident AF over a mean follow-up of 4.1 years.

Results.—88 Women with AF were identified: 29 at baseline and 59 during follow-up. Women with AF were significantly less likely to be taking a statin at study enrolment than those without AF (22% vs 37%, $p = 0.003$). Baseline statin use was associated with a 65% lower odds of having AF at baseline after controlling for age, race, history of myocardial infarction or revascularisation and history of heart failure (odds ratio 0.35, 95% confidence interval (CI) 0.13 to 0.93, $p = 0.04$). The risk of developing AF during the study among those free from AF at baseline, adjusted for the same covariates, was 55% less for those receiving statin treatment (hazard ratio 0.45, 95% CI 0.26 to 0.78, $p = 0.004$).

Conclusions.—Statin treatment is associated with a lower prevalence and incidence of AF after adjustment for potential confounders in postmenopausal women with coronary disease (Fig 2).

▶ The Heart and Estrogen/Progestin Replacement Study (HERS) demonstrated that combination estrogen/progesterone supplementation therapy in

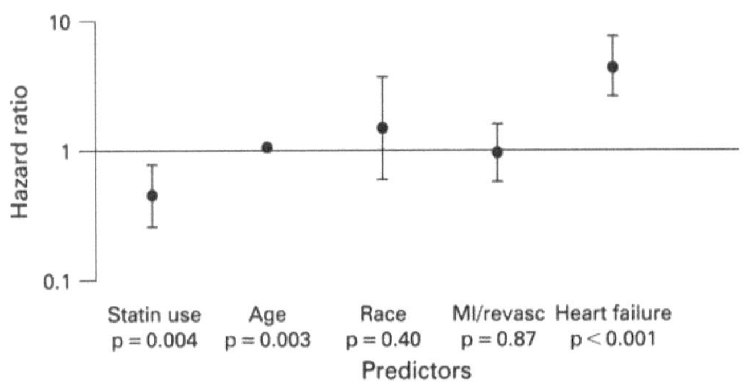

FIGURE 2.—Incidence of atrial fibrillation at follow-up based on presence of predictors. Points display hazard ratios, with adjustment for potential confounders. Bars represent 95% confidence intervals. Age, 10-year increase in age; race, Causcasian compared with all others; MI/revasc, history of myocardial infarction or revascularisation. (Reprinted from Pellegrini CN, Vittinghoff E, Lin F, et al. Statin use is associated with lower risk of atrial fibrillation in women with coronary disease: the HERS trial. *Heart*. 2009;95:704-708, with permission from the BMJ Publishing Group, Ltd.)

postmenopausal women with coronary heart disease (CHD) offered no benefit for reducing primary or secondary cardiovascular end points compared with placebo.[1] In this post hoc analysis from HERS, the impact of statin therapy on risk for atrial fibrillation (AF) in women with CHD was evaluated. After adjusting for confounders, statin usage was associated with lower baseline rates of AF at time of randomization (65%) as well as incident AF (55%) during the course of the trial (Fig 2). The data were adjusted for a variety of confounders, including antiarrhythmic agent usage. This is the only study of its kind done in a population of women, and lends additional confirmation of the relationship between statin usage in patients with CHD and reduction in risk for AF. At minimum, this study reinforces the need to treat women with CHD with statin therapy.

P. P. Toth, MD, PhD

Reference

1. Hulley S, Grady D, Bush T, et al. Randomized trial of estrogen plus progestin for secondary prevention of coronary heart disease in postmenopausal women. Heart and Estrogen/progestin Replacement Study (HERS) Research Group. *JAMA*. 1998;280:605-613.

Effects of Statin Therapy According to Plasma High-Sensitivity C-Reactive Protein Concentration in the Controlled Rosuvastatin Multinational Trial in Heart Failure (CORONA): A Retrospective Analysis

McMurray JJV, for the CORONA Study Group (Univ of Glasgow, UK; et al)

Circulation 120:2188-2196, 2009

Background.—We examined whether the antiinflammatory action of statins may be of benefit in heart failure, a state characterized by inflammation in which low cholesterol is associated with worse outcomes.

Methods and Results.—We compared 10 mg rosuvastatin daily with placebo in patients with ischemic systolic heart failure according to baseline high sensitivity-C reactive protein (hs-CRP) <2.0 mg/L (placebo, $n = 779$; rosuvastatin, $n = 777$) or ≥ 2.0 mg/L (placebo, $n = 1694$; rosuvastatin, $n = 1711$). The primary outcome was cardiovascular death, myocardial infarction, or stroke. Baseline low-density lipoprotein was the same, and rosuvastatin reduced low-density lipoprotein by 47% in both hs-CRP groups. Median hs-CRP was 1.10 mg/L in the lower and 5.60 mg/L in the higher hs-CRP group, with higher hs-CRP associated with worse outcomes. The change in hs-CRP with rosuvastatin from baseline to 3 months was −6% in the low hs-CRP group (27% with placebo) and −33.3% in the high hs-CRP group (−11.1% with placebo). In the high hs-CRP group, 548 placebo-treated (14.0 per 100 patient-years of follow-up) and 498 rosuvastatin-treated (12.2 per 100 patient-years of follow-up) patients had a primary end point (hazard ratio of placebo to rosuvastatin, 0.87; 95% confidence interval, 0.77 to 0.98; $P = 0.024$). In the low hs-CRP group, 175 placebo-treated (8.9 per 100 patient-years

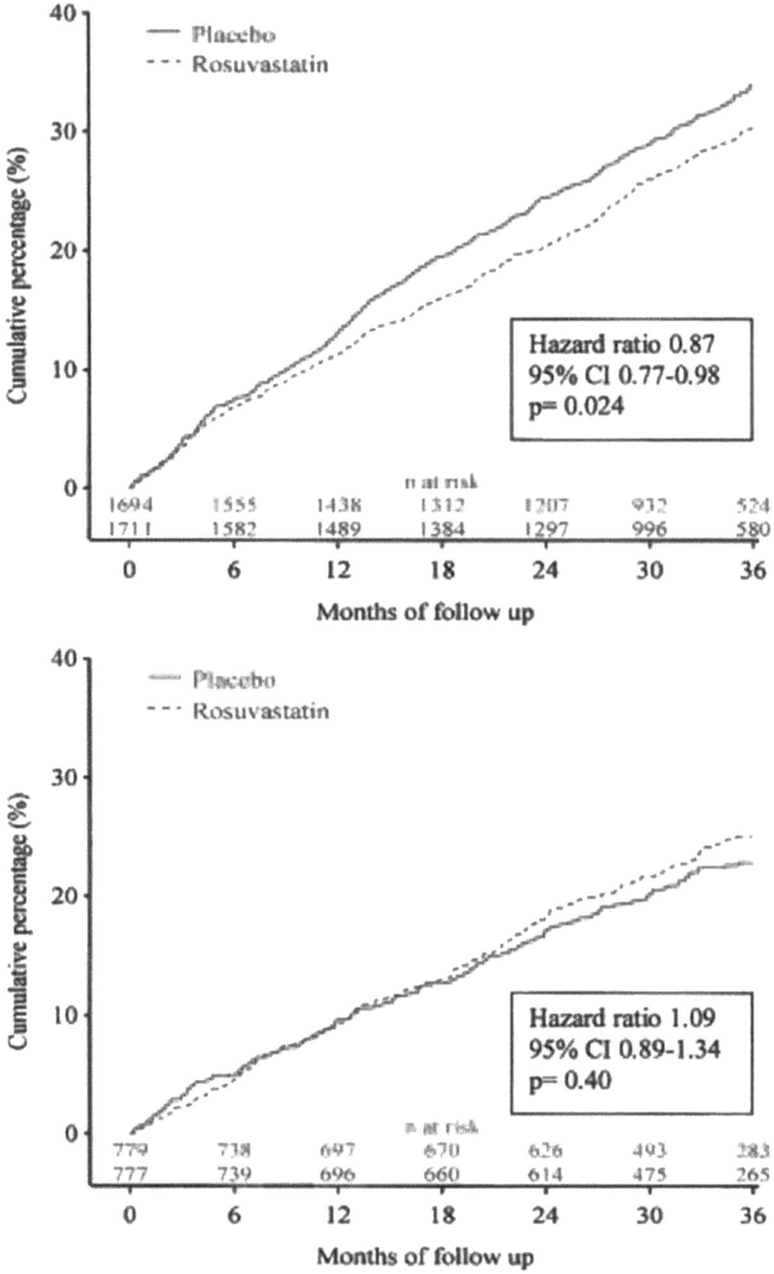

FIGURE 1.—Kaplan-Meier estimates for the primary end point in the 2 hs-CRP subgroups: hs-CRP ≥2.0 mg/L (top) and <2.0 mg/L (bottom). (Reprinted from McMurray JJV, for the CORONA Study Group. Effects of statin therapy according to plasma high-sensitivity C-reactive protein concentration in the Controlled Rosuvastatin Multinational Trial in Heart Failure (CORONA): a retrospective analysis. *Circulation*. 2009;120:2188-2196.)

of follow-up) and 188 rosuvastatin-treated (9.8 per 100 patient-years of follow-up) patients experienced this outcome (hazard ratio, 1.09; 95% confidence interval, 0.89 to 1.34; $P > 0.2$; P for interaction = 0.062). The numbers of deaths were as follows: 581 placebo-treated (14.1 per 100 patient-years of follow-up) and 532 rosuvastatin-treated (12.6 per 100 patient-years) patients in the high hs-CRP group (hazard ratio, 0.89; 95% confidence interval, 0.79 to 1.00; $P = 0.050$) and 170 placebo-treated (8.3 per 100 patient-years) and 192 rosuvastatin-treated (9.7 per 100 patient-years) patients in the low hs-CRP group (hazard ratio, 1.17; 95% confidence interval, 0.95 to 1.43; $P = 0.14$; P for interaction = 0.026).

Conclusion.—In this retrospective hypothesis-generating study, we found a significant interaction between hs-CRP and the effect of rosuvastatin for most end points whereby rosuvastatin treatment was associated with better outcomes in patients with hs-CRP ≥2.0 mg/L.

Clinical Trial Registration Information.—URL: http://www.clinicaltrials.gov. Unique identifier: NCT00206310 (Fig 1).

▶ The Controlled Rosuvastatin Multinational Trial in Heart Failure (CORONA) study evaluated whether or not treatment with rosuvastatin 10 mg daily versus placebo in patients >60 years with chronic New York Heart Association (NYHA) class II to IV heart failure of ischemic origin and an ejection fraction of <40% (<35% if NYHA class II) would reduce risk for cardiovascular events. The primary composite end point for this study (cardiovascular mortality, nonfatal myocardial infarction, or stroke) showed a trend toward benefit but did not achieve statistical significance (hazard ratio [HR] = 0.92, $P = .12$). This was a surprising result given the fact that in a variety of post hoc analyses and observational studies, statin therapy appears to be protective in the setting of heart failure. Moreover, statin therapy is consistently beneficial in patients with ischemic heart disease. In one study by Horwich et al,[1] statin therapy was associated with lower mortality in patients with advanced heart failure. In a post hoc analysis of the Prospective Randomized Amlodipine Survival Evaluation Study (PRAISE) trial, statin therapy was associated with a 62% lower incidence of mortality in patients with advanced heart failure.[2] In contradistinction to these analyses of statin-treated patients, among patients with advanced heart failure not treated with statins, low serum cholesterol is paradoxically associated with increased mortality.[3] This may be due to the advanced state of their disease and onset of cachexia, a poor prognostic indicator. Statin therapy may beneficially impact heart failure because these drugs have been shown to reverse endothelial dysfunction, better balance sympathetic/parasympathetic inputs into myocardium, reduce systemic inflammatory tone, and positively impact cardiac remodeling among other effects.

Inflammation plays a significant role in heart failure. It is well established that there is an increased level of expression of inflammatory cytokines and interleukins. The CORONA investigators dichotomized their analysis according to whether or not patients at study entry had a high-sensitivity C-reactive protein (hsCRP) above or below 2.0 mg/L. In the Justification for the Use of Statins in

Primary Prevention: An Intervention Trial Evaluating Rosuvastatin (JUPITER) trial, an hsCRP ≥2.0 mg/L identified patients with normal lipid profiles but who significantly benefit from rosuvastatin therapy. Among patients with heart failure and a hsCRP >2.0 mg/L, the primary composite end point was reduced significantly (HR = 0.87, P = .024), whereas patients with hsCRP <2.0 mg/L did not (Fig 1). Patients with hsCRP ≥2.0 mg/L experienced significant reductions in any coronary end point, hospitalization for worsening heart failure, and the composite of hospitalization for heart failure and mortality. The reduction for total mortality just missed significance, with a trend for an 11% reduction (P = .056, confidence interval [CI] 0.89-1.00).

Although these findings warrant confirmation in a prospective randomized clinical trial, it is possible that hsCRP screening can be used to identify patients with ischemic heart failure who benefit from statin therapy, irrespective of baseline lipid status. Given the marked elevation in 5-year mortality among these patients, this would be a valuable trial to conduct as it could potentially impact millions of patients with heart failure throughout the world.

P. P. Toth, MD, PhD

References

1. Horwich TB, MacLellan WR, Fonarow GC. Statin therapy is associated with improved survival in ischemic and non-ischemic heart failure. *J Am Coll Cardiol.* 2004;43:642-648.
2. Mozaffarian D, Nye R, Levy WC. Statin therapy is associated with lower mortality among patients with severe heart failure. *Am J Cardiol.* 2004;93:1124-1129.
3. Horwich TB, Hamilton MA, Maclellan WR, et al. Low serum total cholesterol is associated with marked increase in mortality in advanced heart failure. *J Card Fail.* 2002;8:216-224.

Pharmacologic Therapy

1,25(OH)$_2$ Vitamin D Inhibits Foam Cell Formation and Suppresses Macrophage Cholesterol Uptake in Patients With Type 2 Diabetes Mellitus

Oh J, Weng S, Felton SK, et al (Washington Univ, St Louis, MO; et al)
Circulation 120:687-698, 2009

Background.—Cardiovascular disease is the leading cause of death among those with diabetes mellitus. Vitamin D deficiency is associated with an increased risk of cardiovascular disease in this population. To determine the mechanism by which vitamin D deficiency mediates accelerated cardiovascular disease in patients with diabetes mellitus, we investigated the effects of active vitamin D on macrophage cholesterol deposition.

Methods and Results.—We obtained macrophages from 76 obese, diabetic, hypertensive patients with vitamin D deficiency (25-hydroxyvitamin D <80 nmol/L; group A) and 4 control groups: obese, diabetic, hypertensive patients with normal vitamin D (group B; n = 15); obese, nondiabetic, hypertensive patients with vitamin D deficiency (group C; n = 25); and nonobese, nondiabetic, nonhypertensive patients with vitamin D deficiency (group D; n = 10) or sufficiency (group E; n = 10). Macrophages from the same patients in all groups were cultured in vitamin D—deficient or 1,25-dihydroxyvitamin D_3 [1,25$(OH)_2D_3$] –supplemented media and exposed to modified low-density lipoprotein cholesterol. 1,25$(OH)_2D_3$ suppressed foam cell formation by reducing acetylated or oxidized low-density lipoprotein cholesterol uptake in diabetic subjects only. Conversely, deletion of the vitamin D receptor in macrophages from diabetic patients accelerated foam cell formation induced by modified LDL. 1,25$(OH)_2D_3$ downregulation of c-Jun N-terminal kinase activation reduced peroxisome proliferated–activated receptor-γ expression, suppressed CD36 expression, and prevented oxidized low-density lipoprotein–derived cholesterol uptake. In addition, 1,25$(OH)_2$ D_3 suppression of macrophage endoplasmic reticulum stress improved insulin signaling, downregulated SR-A1 expression, and prevented oxidized and acetylated low-density lipoprotein–derived cholesterol uptake.

Conclusion.—These results identify reduced vitamin D receptor signaling as a potential mechanism underlying increased foam cell formation and accelerated cardiovascular disease in diabetic subjects.

▶ The relationship between vitamin D (vit D) deficiency and risk for cardiovascular disease is a fascinating one. Recent studies show associations between vit D deficiency and risk for myocardial infarction,[1] heart failure and mortality,[2] and coronary atherosclerotic plaque calcification.[3] Vitamin D deficiency is highly prevalent, at least partly because of reduced exposure of skin to ultraviolet radiation. Vitamin D receptor-dependent signaling regulates the expression of at least 200 genes.

Macrophages in the subendothelial space arise from blood-borne monocytes. Macrophages are a source of interleukins and cytokines that potentiate atherosclerosis. In addition, they sequester oxidatively modified low-density lipoprotein (LDL) particles by expressing a variety of scavenging receptors, including cluster of differentiation 36 (CD36) and scavenger receptor A (SR-A).[4] As the macrophage takes up more lipid and cholesterol, it forms lipid inclusion droplets ultimately forming a foam cell. Foam cells undergo apoptosis and the resulting histologic debris can coalesce to form fatty streaks and frank atherosclerotic plaques.

This study by Oh and colleagues is fascinating and quite well done. Vitamin D deficiency potentiates risk for cardiovascular disease in diabetics. These investigators isolated macrophages from vit D deficient diabetic patients and a variety of controls. Vitamin D deficiency in the culture medium or deletion of the macrophage vit D receptor, both facilitated increased expression of CD36 and uptake of modified LDL. Vitamin D supplementation reduced modified LDL uptake, decreased CD36 and SR-A expression, and improved insulin signaling. In addition, peroxisomal proliferator activated receptor-gamma (PPAR-γ) expression was also reduced by vit D supplementation. This makes some sense because PPAR-γ regulates cell surface expression of the adenosine triphosphate (ATP) binding membrane cassette transport proteins A1 and G1, which translocate intracellular cholesterol to the extracellular milieu to lipidate high-density lipoprotein (HDL) particles and potentiate reverse cholesterol transport. In the setting of vit D supplementation, less lipid is being internalized and, consequently, there would be less need to stimulate expression of cassette transport proteins to reduce cholesterol loading.

There are many unanswered questions concerning the relationship between vit D deficiency and increased risk for cardiovascular disease. This study explores what may be an important mechanism by which vit D deficiency increases risk for atherosclerotic disease. It is crucial to evaluate in a randomized prospective fashion whether or not normalizing serum levels of 25-hydroxyvitamin D in patients with and without diabetes mellitus reduces risk for atherosclerotic disease as well as cardiovascular morbidity and mortality. The relationship between vit D deficiency and cardiovascular disease is likely to be a complex one involving many genes and intracellular signaling pathways.

P. P. Toth, MD, PhD

References

1. Giovannucci E, Liu Y, Hollis BW, Rimm EB. 25-hydroxyvitamin D and risk of myocardial infarction in men: a prospective study. *Arch Intern Med.* 2008;168: 1174-1180.
2. Pilz S, Marz W, Wellnitz B, et al. Association of vitamin D deficiency with heart failure and sudden cardiac death in a large cross-sectional study of patients referred for coronary angiography. *J Clin Endocrinol Metab.* 2008;93:3927-3935.
3. Watson KE, Abrolat ML, Malone LL, et al. Active serum vitamin D levels are inversely correlated with coronary calcification. *Circulation.* 1997;96:1755-1760.
4. Tabas I. Consequences and therapeutic implications of macrophage apoptosis in atherosclerosis: the importance of lesion stage and phagocytic efficiency. *Arterioscler Thromb Vasc Biol.* 2005;25:2255-2264.

Cardiovascular Benefit of Magnitude of Low-Density Lipoprotein Cholesterol Reduction: A Comparison of Subgroups by Age

Rahilly-Tierney CR, Lawler EV, Scranton RE, et al (Massachusetts Veterans Epidemiology and Res Information Ctr, Boston, MA; et al)
Circulation 120:1491-1497, 2009

Background.—We examined the effect of the magnitude of low-density lipoprotein cholesterol (LDL-C) reduction across subjects of various ages in a retrospective cohort study.

Methods and Results.—We selected 20 132 male veterans at high risk for an acute cardiovascular event and who had 2 or more LDL-C measurements before their first documented acute myocardial infarction, revascularization, death, or censoring date. LDL-C reduction was categorized as no reduction (<10 mg/dL; reference), small reduction (between 10 and 40 mg/dL), moderate reduction (between 40 and 70 mg/dL), or large reduction (≥70 mg/dL). The primary outcome was combined acute myocardial infarction or revascularization. The first and last LDL-C levels in the databases were used to calculate the LDL-C reduction in patients who experienced no outcome or who died. Within each age quartile and

TABLE 4.—Unadjusted and Multivariate-Adjusted* HRs (95% CI) for Each Category of LDL-C Reduction, by Age Quartile

Category of LDL-C Reduction	<61.1 y	61.1 to 69.3 y	69.3 to 75.3 y	≥75.3 y
Small: 10–40 mg/dL				
Unadjusted	0.87 (0.76–1.00)	0.69 (0.59–0.79)	0.77 (0.66–0.90)	0.72 (0.61–0.85)
Multivariate adjusted	0.73 (0.64–0.84)	0.67 (0.58–0.78)	0.70 (0.60–0.82)	0.64 (0.54–0.76)
Moderate: 40–70 mg/dL				
Unadjusted	0.68 (0.59–0.79)	0.57 (0.48–0.67)	0.65 (0.55–0.77)	0.73 (0.60–0.87)
Multivariate adjusted	0.50 (0.43–0.58)	0.45 (0.37–0.52)	0.45 (0.39–0.56)	0.53 (0.44–0.64)
Large: ≥70 mg/dL				
Unadjusted	0.73 (0.61–0.87)	0.57 (0.47–0.68)	0.53 (0.42–0.66)	0.54 (0.42–0.0.70)
Multivariate adjusted	0.37 (0.31–0.45)	0.29 (0.24–0.37)	0.26 (0.20–0.34)	0.38 (0.30–0.49)

*Adjusted for age, gender, current smoking status, body mass index, statin use, nonstatin cholesterol-modifying therapy use, hypertension, cerebrovascular disease, thyroid disease, and renal disease.

in a subgroup of patients ≥80 years of age, a Cox proportional hazards model was used to determine hazard ratios for each category of LDL-C reduction compared with the reference category, with adjustment for age, body mass index, current smoking status, medications, and comorbidities. In all age groups, the magnitude of LDL-C reduction was proportional to the magnitude of cardiovascular risk reduction. Risk reduction for the combined outcome in patients who achieved a large LDL-C reduction was similar in all age quartiles, with multivariate-adjusted hazard ratios of approximately 0.30.

Conclusions.—In a cohort of veterans at high risk for cardiovascular events, patients of all ages, including those 80 years or older, benefitted the most from large reductions in LDL-C (Table 4).

▶ Questions that continue to be asked frequently are whether or not older patients derive as much benefit from lipid lowering as younger patients, and is there an "older limit" above which you should not treat patients for their dyslipidemia. The Pravastatin in Elderly Individuals at Risk of Vascular Disease (PROSPER)[1] trial, post hoc evaluations of data from the Heart Protection Study[2] (HPS), and the Long-Term Intervention with Pravastatin in Ischaemic Disease (LIPID)[3,4] trial all showed that older patients (>70 years) experience significant reductions in risk for acute cardiovascular events when treated with statin therapy. The issue concerning an upper limit on age appears best left to one's judgment. If a patient is 80 or 85 years old, is functional, and wants to reduce risk for myocardial infarction (MI) and stroke, then there should be little reluctance to start appropriate lipid-lowering therapy in the setting of dyslipidemia. If, on the other hand, the patient is demented or poorly functional, then decision making will be significantly influenced by the patient's comorbidities.

This retrospective cohort study by Rahilly-Tierney and coworkers lends important support to the conclusion reached by the PROSPER, LIPID, and HPS investigators, namely that lipid-lowering therapy confers just as much benefit to older high-risk patients as it does for younger ones. These investigators included 20132 high-risk men who had been receiving care within the Veteran's Affairs health system. Within each age quartile, the percentage of patients with acute cardiovascular events (MI or revascularization) decreased with increasing magnitude of low-density lipoprotein-cholesterol (LDL-C) reduction. In all age quartiles, patients who achieved an LDL-C reduction of > 70 mg/dL had the lowest event rates. The unadjusted and multivariate-adjusted hazard ratios for a given intensity of LDL-C reduction compared with the reference within each age quartile are shown in Table 4. After adjustment for age, body mass index (BMI), current smoking status, angiotensin-converting enzyme inhibitor use, aspirin use, beta-blocker use, and comorbidities, any LDL-C reduction was associated with a decreased risk for the combined outcome. The magnitude of benefit increased as the magnitude of LDL-C reduction increased. Interestingly, additional adjustment for either statin or nonstatin cholesterol-modifying therapy did not change the results. Among the patients > 75years, a 70 mg/dL reduction in serum LDL-C was associated with an approximately 70% reduction in risk for MI and need for revascularization, an effect size identical to that seen for younger patients.

Clearly, lipid lowering in high-risk patients is beneficial irrespective of age. Lipid-lowering therapy should not be withheld from patients at risk for cardiovascular events based on age alone. One limitation of these data is that women were not included in this study. However, given the fact that both HPS and Justification for the Use of Statins in Primary Prevention: An Intervention Trial Evaluating Rosuvastatin trials (JUPITER)[5] showed that women derive as much benefit from statin therapy as do men, it would be unreasonable to not treat older high-risk women with lipid-lowering therapy.

P. P. Toth, MD, PhD

References

1. Shepherd J, Blauw GJ, Murphy MB, et al. Pravastatin in elderly individuals at risk of vascular disease (PROSPER): a randomised controlled trial. *Lancet.* 2002;360: 1623-1630.
2. Heart Protection Study Collaborative G. MRC/BHF Heart Protection Study of cholesterol lowering with simvastatin in 20,536 high-risk individuals: a randomised placebo-controlled trial [see comment][summary for patients in Curr Cardiol Rep. 2002 Nov;4(6):486-7; PMID: 12379169]. *Lancet.* 2002;360:7-22.
3. Prevention of cardiovascular events and death with pravastatin in patients with coronary heart disease and a broad range of initial cholesterol levels. The Long-Term Intervention with Pravastatin in Ischaemic Disease (LIPID) Study Group. *N Engl J Med.* 1998;339:1349-1357.
4. Hunt D, Young P, Simes J, et al. Benefits of pravastatin on cardiovascular events and mortality in older patients with coronary heart disease are equal to or exceed those seen in younger patients: results from the LIPID trial. *Ann Intern Med.* 2001; 134:931-940.
5. Ridker PM, Danielson E, Fonseca FA, et al. Reduction in C-reactive protein and LDL cholesterol and cardiovascular event rates after initiation of rosuvastatin: a prospective study of the JUPITER trial. *Lancet.* 2009;373:1175-1182.

Prevention of Atherosclerosis

Arterial Structure and Function After Recovery From the Metabolic Syndrome: The Cardiovascular Risk in Young Finns Study

Koskinen J, Magnussen CG, Taittonen L, et al (Univ of Turku, Finland; Vaasa Central Hosp and Univ of Oulu, Finland; et al)

Circulation 121:392-400, 2010

Background.—The reversibility of ultrasonographic vascular changes associated with the metabolic syndrome (MetS) recovery is unknown. We examined whether spontaneous recovery from MetS (according to the International Diabetes Federation definition) has a favorable effect on vascular properties and evaluated the associations between lifestyle factors and MetS recovery.

Methods and Results.—We measured carotid artery intima-media thickness, distensibility, and brachial low-mediated dilatation by ultrasound in 1673 subjects of the Young Finns Study cohort (age, 31.5 ± 5.0 years in 2001) who participated in follow-up studies in 2001 and 2007. At baseline, no differences in intima-media thickness, carotid artery distensibility, or flow-mediated dilatation were observed between the recovery group (baseline-only MetS) and those with incident (only at follow-up) or persistent (both at baseline and follow-up) MetS. After 6 years, the recovery group had smaller intima-media thickness (mean ± SEM, 0.62 ± 0.01 versus 0.68 ± 0.01 mm; $P = 0.0009$) and higher carotid artery distensibility (1.98 ± 0.07%/mm Hg versus 1.56 ± 0.04%/mm Hg; $P = 0.001$) compared with the persistent group and higher flow-mediated dilatation compared with the control group (9.91 ± 0.51% versus 8.57 ± 0.12%; $P = 0.03$). The recovery group had reduced intima-media thickness progression compared with the persistent group (0.036 ± 0.005 versus 0.079 ± 0.010 mm; $P = 0.001$) and reduced carotid artery distensibility change compared with the incident group (−0.12 ± 0.05%/mm Hg versus −0.38 ± 0.10%/mm Hg; $P = 0.03$) over the 6-year follow-up. Differences in carotid artery distensibility levels were attenuated ($P = 0.11$) after the inclusion of weight change in the models. MetS recovery was paralleled with significant reductions in waist circumference that independently correlated with increased physical activity and increased attention paid to health habits during the follow-up.

Conclusion.—Recovery from the MetS was associated with positive effects on vascular properties during a 6-year follow-up period of young adults.

▶ Metabolic syndrome (MS) is highly prevalent throughout the world. Hypertriglyceridemia, hyperinsulinemia, hyperglycemia, hypertension, obesity, and low levels of high-density lipoprotein-cholesterol (HDL-C) are defining features of MS. The MS is associated with premature, accelerated atherogenesis, loss of vascular compliance, and endothelial dysfunction with compromised vasoreactivity. The insulin resistance that is etiologic for MS is a consequence of obesity, dysregulated/dysfunctional adipose tissue, and the formation of ectopic steatosis in skeletal, the liver, and epicardium. MS is an important precursor to diabetes mellitus and acute cardiovascular events. The various metabolic features of insulin resistance can be normalized through lifestyle modification, weight loss, smoking cessation, and dietary revision.

In this analysis of follow-up data from the Young Finns Study cohort (1673 patients, mean age 31.5 years at time of baseline measurements) the investigators demonstrate that patients who recover from MS through exercise, dietary modification, and weight loss also experience important changes in metabolic features as well as carotid arterial histology and physiology. In the recovery group, weight, serum insulin, glucose, and triglycerides, all decreased significantly. There was also a trend toward slight reduction in systolic blood pressure. HDL-C increased significantly. In the group persistent for MS, metabolic parameters continued to deteriorate over the 6 years of follow-up. In parallel with these changes, the recovery group experienced a significant decrease in carotid intima media thickness (CIMT) and an increase in carotid distensibility compared with baseline. In contrast, the patients with persistent MS had a higher rate of progression of CIMT and a greater rate of loss of carotid distensibility.

This study confirms that accelerated and adverse forms of carotid arterial remodeling occur in young patients with MS. It also demonstrates that CIMT can be reversed and carotid distensibility improved by relieving insulin resistance through lifestyle modification alone. These results extend findings from previous investigations supporting the front line role of lifestyle modification when managing insulin resistance and cardiometabolic risk.[1] It remains particularly important to intercept this process in younger patients.

P. P. Toth, MD, PhD

Reference

1. Tuomilehto J, Lindstrom J, Eriksson JG, et al. Prevention of type 2 diabetes mellitus by changes in lifestyle among subjects with impaired glucose tolerance. *N Engl J Med.* 2001;344:1343-1350.

Dysfunctional Proinflammatory High-Density Lipoproteins Confer Increased Risk of Atherosclerosis in Women With Systemic Lupus Erythematosus

McMahon M, Grossman J, Skaggs B, et al (Univ of California, Los Angeles; et al)

Arthritis Rheum 60:2428-2437, 2009

Objective.—Women with systemic lupus erythematosus (SLE) have an increased risk of atherosclerosis. Identification of at-risk patients and the etiology underlying atherosclerosis in SLE remain elusive. The antioxidant capacity of normal high-density lipoproteins (HDLs) is lost during inflammation, and these dysfunctional HDLs might predispose individuals to atherosclerosis. The aim of this study was to determine whether dysfunctional proinflammatory HDL (piHDL) is associated with subclinical atherosclerosis in SLE.

Methods.—Carotid artery ultrasound was performed in 276 women with SLE to identify carotid plaques and measure intima-media thickness (IMT). The antioxidant function of HDL was measured as the change in oxidation of low-density lipoprotein after the addition of HDL cholesterol. Two antiinflammatory HDL components, paraoxonase 1 and apolipoprotein A-I, were also measured.

Results.—Among the SLE patients, 48.2% were determined to have piHDL on carotid ultrasound, while 86.7% of patients with plaque had piHDL compared with 40.7% of those without plaque ($P < 0.001$). Patients with piHDL also had a higher IMT ($P < 0.001$). After multivariate analysis, the only factors found to be significantly associated with plaque were the presence of piHDL (odds ratio [OR] 16.1, $P < 0.001$), older age (OR 1.2, $P < 0.001$), hypertension (OR 3.0, $P = 0.04$), dyslipidemia (OR 3.4, $P = 0.04$), and mixed racial background (OR 8.3, $P = 0.04$). Factors associated with IMT measurements in the highest quartile were the presence of piHDL (OR 2.5, $P = 0.02$), older age (OR 1.1, $P < 0.001$), a higher body mass index (OR 1.07, $P = 0.04$), a cumulative lifetime prednisone dose ≥20 gm (OR 2.9, $P < 0.04$), and African American race (OR 8.3, $P = 0.001$).

Conclusion.—Dysfunctional piHDL greatly increases the risk of developing subclinical atherosclerosis in SLE. The presence of piHDL was associated with an increased prevalence of carotid plaque and with a higher IMT. Therefore, determination of piHDL may help identify patients at risk for atherosclerosis.

▶ The functionality of high-density lipoprotein (HDL) particles is an area of intensive investigation. The negative relationship between serum levels of HDL cholesterol (HDL-C) and risk for atherosclerotic disease is substantiated by epidemiologic studies conducted throughout the world. HDL particles harbor a large proteosome of 75 or more different proteins and enzymes.[1] The protein cargo of HDL can vary significantly in response to in vivo conditions. For example, if there is increased systemic inflammation or if there is increased expression of acute phase proteins, atheroprotective molecules, such as paraoxonase, apoprotein A-I (apoA-I), and cholesterol ester transfer protein can be displaced from the particle by other proteins, including serum amyloid A or ceruloplasmin. This adversely impacts the functionality of the HDL particle and can be associated with pro-oxidative activity and accelerated atherogenesis. Both paraoxonase and apoA-I protect low-density lipoprotein (LDL) particles from oxidation. Oxidized LDL particles are the preferred substrate for foam cell formation by macrophages in the subendothelial space. A pro-inflammatory and pro-oxidative state can also be associated with increased expression of myeloperoxidase, an enzyme that can alter the 3-dimensional conformation of apoA-I and compromise the ability of HDL to bind to both macrophages and hepatocytes. This results in reduced reverse cholesterol transport.[2]

Rheumatologic disease is associated with heightened systemic inflammation and increased risk for premature coronary artery disease (CAD). Atherosclerosis is an inflammatory disorder.[3] Measurements of carotid intima media thickness (CIMT) are a well-documented surrogate of CAD. In this study, the investigators evaluated the presence of dysfunctional proinflammatory HDL (piHDL) in women with systemic lupus erythematosis (SLE). The presence of piHDL was highly correlated with thicker CIMT and established carotid plaque. On logistic regression analysis, the odds ratio associated with piHDL was dramatically higher (16.1) compared with other established risk factors, such as older age (1.2), hypertension (3.0), or dyslipidemia (3.4). HDL-C levels between groups did not correlate with risk for carotid disease.

This study provides important new information about the mechanistic basis for how rheumatologic disease, and specifically SLE, may accelerate the development of atherosclerosis. In this study, piHDL was shown to be a highly prevalent and valuable predictive biomarker of risk for carotid disease. This study highlights the importance of evaluating the functionality of HDL particles and how this functionality is compromised by specific inflammatory states. Much work remains to be done on how and when HDL particles make the phenotypic transition to becoming proatherogenic. It is likely that, in the future, as more practical and readily applicable assays become available, we will measure both HDL-C and HDL functionality in patients at risk for CAD. Treatment with statins and niacin has been shown to convert dysfunctional HDL to functionally more protective HDL.[4]

P. P. Toth, MD, PhD

References

1. Heinecke JW. The HDL proteome: a marker–and perhaps mediator–of coronary artery disease. *J Lipid Res.* 2009;50:S167-171.
2. Shao B, Oda MN, Oram JF, Heinecke JW. Myeloperoxidase: an inflammatory enzyme for generating dysfunctional high density lipoprotein. *Curr Opin Cardiol.* 2006;21:322-328.
3. Libby P, Ridker PM, Hansson GK. Inflammation in atherosclerosis: from pathophysiology to practice. *J Am Coll Cardiol.* 2009;54:2129-2138.
4. Green PS, Vaisar T, Pennathur S, et al. Combined statin and niacin therapy remodels the high-density lipoprotein proteome. *Circulation.* 2008;118:1259-1267.

3 Obesity

Introduction

Excessive body adipose tissue is deleterious to health and is conveniently measured by the body mass index (BMI). BMI over 30 is considered obesity, and the prevalence of obesity in the United States has increased steadily over the past several decades. In fact, after a period of relative stability between the years 1960 to 1980, the prevalence of obesity suddenly increased dramatically in the 1980s and 1990s. The latest NHANES data analysis now shows that prevalence of obesity may be entering another phase of stability after a period of steady movement upward. This latest tendency may help us further define the causes of the increase in prevalence of obesity; these have been purported to be an increase in energy intake and a decrease in energy expenditure attributed to the advent of fast food and technological advances that result in less physical movement in general.

We can surmise that what happened after 1980 was a societal solution for our fast-paced lifestyle in fast food and fast eating, including drive-through restaurants serving large portions of food and drink for bargain prices. Another purported cause of the epidemic has been the introduction of sugar-sweetened beverages as an accompaniment to any meal, and not just as a treat, which also occurred after 1980.

Our society most likely will have great difficulty retracing steps toward lower BMIs because of the food industry as well as our fast-paced lifestyle. However, the food industry may be swayed by consumer opinion and action, as evidenced by the successful efforts at education regarding tobacco. Because of strong campaigns to educate the consumer on the deleterious effects of tobacco, smoking rates have declined and this has had positive effects on longevity. Now obesity threatens that longevity, according to a study reported in this chapter. Can we learn from the successful anti-tobacco campaign in the United States and project this onto the obesity epidemic?

Perhaps we can target one item to be taxed as tobacco has been taxed? Should it be sugar-sweetened soda? Should it be fast food? Candy? The problem is that not all food is bad for health as opposed to the way all tobacco is bad for health. However, removing candy and sugar-sweetened beverages from the school vending machines was a step in the right direction. A new way of classifying foods based on nutrient value to calorie density is a good way to create "bad" versus "good" categories of foods.

It makes more sense to educate the public toward healthy eating and living than to spend enormous amounts of money finding cures for obesity in surgical and medical approaches. However, better treatments are needed in the short run for those who suffer from obesity now. Preventive efforts can certainly address childhood obesity, but these will take time and money as well. The next few years will see more anti-obesity drugs come to the market, as well as new procedures to simulate bariatric surgery. But the cornerstones of obesity treatment—good nutrition and physical activity—remain the biggest predictors of longevity and health.

Caroline M. Apovian, MD

Epidemiology and Complications of Obesity

Prevalence and Trends in Obesity Among US Adults, 1999-2008

Flegal KM, Carroll MD, Ogden CL, et al (Ctrs for Disease Control and Prevention, Hyattsville, MD)

JAMA 303:235-241, 2010

Context.—The prevalence of obesity increased in the United States between 1976-1980 and 1988-1994 and again between 1988-1994 and 1999-2000.

Objective.—To examine trends in obesity from 1999 through 2008 and the current prevalence of obesity and overweight for 2007-2008.

Design, Setting, and Participants.—Analysis of height and weight measurements from 5555 adult men and women aged 20 years or older obtained in 2007-2008 as part of the National Health and Nutrition Examination Survey (NHANES), a nationally representative sample of the US population. Data from the NHANES obtained in 2007-2008 were compared with results obtained from 1999 through 2006.

Main Outcome Measure.—Estimates of the prevalence of overweight and obesity in adults. Overweight was defined as a body mass index (BMI) of 25.0 to 29.9. Obesity was defined as a BMI of 30.0 or higher.

Results.—In 2007-2008, the age-adjusted prevalence of obesity was 33.8% (95% confidence interval [CI], 31.6%-36.0%) overall, 32.2% (95% CI, 29.5%-35.0%) among men, and 35.5% (95% CI, 33.2%-37.7%) among women. The corresponding prevalence estimates for overweight and obesity combined (BMI ≥25) were 68.0% (95% CI, 66.3%-69.8%), 72.3% (95% CI, 70.4%-74.1%), and 64.1% (95% CI, 61.3%-66.9%). Obesity prevalence varied by age group and by racial and ethnic group for both men and women. Over the 10-year period, obesity showed no significant trend among women (adjusted odds ratio [AOR] for 2007-2008 vs 1999-2000, 1.12 [95% CI, 0.89-1.32]). For men, there was a significant linear trend (AOR for 2007-2008 vs 1999-2000, 1.32 [95% CI, 1.12-1.58]); however, the 3 most recent data points did not differ significantly from each other.

Conclusions.—In 2007-2008, the prevalence of obesity was 32.2% among adult men and 35.5% among adult women. The increases in the prevalence of obesity previously observed do not appear to be continuing at the same rate over the past 10 years, particularly for women and possibly for men.

▶ Obesity is a worldwide public health issue with extensive medical, social, and economic consequences, and has been associated with increased risk for developing many chronic medical conditions, including cardiovascular disease, certain cancers, and diabetes mellitus.[1,2] In the past few years, the rising trend in obesity has been subject to much attention, and rightfully so, considering the epidemic rise in prevalence previously reported poses an enormous threat to public welfare and an already overburdened United States health care system. Gaining insight into the changing prevalence in overweight and obesity across the population, in addition to understanding the demographic characteristics of the affected population, is of paramount importance if we are to potentially identify subgroups of Americans who should be targeted for intervention and counterbalance this rise through changes in public health policy and cultural attitudes.

Prevalence rates of overweight (body mass index [BMI] 25-29.9 kg/m^2) have remained largely stable over the past 50 years, with approximately one-third of the United States population being consistently overweight since the original NHES I survey (1960-1962) was conducted.[3] This study reports that 34.4% of Americans are overweight, after adjusting for age, race, and sex. Therefore, the significant rise in total overweight (BMI > 25 kg/m^2) reported since the 1960s can be attributed to staggering increases in the prevalence of obesity (BMI > 30 kg/m^2). The data published in the 2005-2006 update from the National Health And Nutrition Examination Survey (NHANES) suggested that obesity rates had stabilized since the 2002-2003 report, although this finding was lacking appropriate statistical power.[4] This current analysis overcomes this issue, and in comparing data from the 2007-2008 NHANES cohort with past trends among the United States population during each 2-year survey period over the last decade (1999-2008), has similarly concluded that rising rates of obesity have leveled off among women and are increasing at a drastically lower rate among men.

In the 2007-2008 NHANES survey, minority groups, including non-Hispanic blacks and Hispanics were oversampled to provide adequate sample size for analyses, as they have previously been under-represented despite showing the highest rates of obesity. In subgroup analyses within racial and ethnic groups (adjusted for age), the authors found the highest rates of grades 1 to 3 obesity in both men and women of non-Hispanic black origin. Relative to non-Hispanic whites, the likelihood of being obese was significantly greater among non-Hispanic blacks (odds ratio [OR] for men, 1.13; 95% confidence interval [CI], 1.01-1.27; OR for women, 2.26; 95% CI, 2.02-2.51) and for Mexican American women (OR, 1.53; 95% CI, 1.31-1.78), but not for Mexican American men (OR, 1.01; 95% CI, 0.85-1.19). The likelihood of being obese was also significantly higher across all ethnic and race groups in anyone over the age of 40, but particularly in the age group of 40 to 59 years (OR for men, 1.46; 95% CI, 1.29-1.66; OR for women, 1.50 95%CI, 1.31-1.72).

One of the major limitations in this study is inherent to its nature as a population survey, whereby it is subject to sampling (and non-sampling) error. It is hard to imagine that the 5555 men and women who met inclusion criteria from the 2007-2008 NHANES survey are a perfect representation of the over 300 million Americans who could have potentially responded to the survey, especially when considering racial and ethnic minority groups were targeted for oversampling and less than half of people included in this analysis were non-Hispanic whites. The relatively small sample size relative to the population also limits the power of the study to detect small changes in prevalence, particularly, among subgroups defined by age, sex, and racial and ethnic groups. Additionally, this study identifies non-Hispanic blacks as having the highest rates of obesity, regardless of age or sex, of all the ethnic and racial subgroups, but this finding should be interpreted with some caution. Several previous studies have shown that black men and women tend to have higher lean and lower fat mass at the same BMI relative to non-Hispanic whites, and it is unclear at present whether the relative health risks at a given BMI may be lower in blacks.[5,6]

The United States population has already failed to meet goals set forth by the National Institute of Health in its Healthy People 2010 campaign, and rates of obesity are unacceptably high, even if they have stabilized, considering obesity is a potentially preventable or reversible disease. This study provides important information regarding changes in patterns of obesity, and identifies certain age and racial subgroups with the highest prevalence of obesity that could potentially be targeted for intervention. However, the origin of these fluctuations is unclear and probably reflects multifactorial influence of public policy, environmental, and individual factors, which this study is unable to capture. Therefore, it is impossible to predict future trends with any degree of certainty. Regardless of whether trends are increasing or decreasing, there needs to be a shift in our current paradigm toward preventive measures to address the present excess in obesity prevalence.

A. Port, MD

References

1. Must A, Spadano J, Coakley EH, Field AE, Colditz G, Dietz W. The disease burden associated with overweight and obesity. *JAMA*. 1999;282:1523-1529.
2. Field AE, Coakley EH, Must A, et al. Impact of overweight on the risk of developing common chronic diseases during a 10-year period. *Arch Intern Med*. 2001;161:1581-1586.
3. Flegal KM, Carol MD, Kuczmarski RJ, Johnson CL. Overweight and obesity in the United States: prevalence and trends, 1960-1994. *Int J Obes Relat Metab Disord*. 1998;22:39-47.
4. Ogden CL, Carroll MD, Curtin LR, McDowell MA, Tabak CJ, Flegal KM. Prevalence of overweight and obesity in the United States, 1999–2004. *JAMA*. 2006;295:1549-1555.
5. Fernandez JR, Heo M, Heymsfield SB, et al. Is percentage body fat differentially related to body mass index in Hispanic Americans, African Americans, and European Americans? *Am J Clin Nutr*. 2003;77:71-75.
6. Rahman M, Temple JR, Breitkopf CR, Berenson AB. Racial differences in body fat distribution among reproductive-aged women. *Metabolism*. 2009;58:1329-1337.

Excessive Gestational Weight Gain and Postpartum Weight Retention Among Obese Women

Vesco KK, Dietz PM, Rizzo J, et al (Ctr for Health Res, Portland, OR; Ctrs for Disease Control and Prevention, Atlanta, GA)

Obstet Gynecol 114:1069-1075, 2009

Objective.—To evaluate the incremental effect of weight gain above that recommended for term pregnancy (15 pounds) on postpartum weight retention at 1 year among obese women.

Methods.—In a retrospective cohort study, we identified 1,656 singleton gestations resulting in live births among obese women (body mass index at or above 30 kg/m^2) between January 2000 and December 2005 in Kaiser Permanente Northwest. Pregnancy weight change (last available pre-delivery weight minus weight at pregnancy onset) was categorized as less than 0, 0–15, greater than 15 to 25, greater than 25 to 35, and greater than 35 pounds. Postpartum weight change (weight at 1 year postpartum minus weight at pregnancy onset) was defined as less than 0, 0–10, and greater than 10 pounds.

Results.—Total gestational weight gain was −33.2 (weight loss) to +98.0 pounds (weight gain). Nearly three fourths gained greater than 15 pounds, and they were younger and weighed less at baseline than women who gained 15 pounds or less. Pregnancy-related weight change showed a significant relationship with postpartum weight change. For each pound gained during pregnancy, there was a 0.4-pound increase above baseline weight at 1 year postpartum. In adjusted logistic regression models, the risk of a postpartum weight greater than 10 pounds over baseline was twofold higher for women gaining greater than 15 to 25 pounds compared with women gaining 0–15 pounds (odds ratio [OR] 2.18, 95% confidence interval [CI] 1.54–3.10), fourfold higher for women gaining greater than 25 to 35 pounds (OR 3.91, 95% CI 2.75–5.56), and almost eightfold higher for women gaining greater than 35 pounds (OR 7.66, 95% CI 5.36–10.97).

Conclusion.—Incremental increases in gestational weight gain beyond the current recommendation for obese women substantially increase the risk of weight retention at 1 year postpartum.

Level of Evidence.—II.

▶ The prevalence of overweight and obesity in women of childbearing age has increased markedly during the last 30 years. Approximately 25% of women in the United States who become pregnant are obese. Obese pregnant women are at higher risk of maternal and fetal complications. Adverse maternal outcomes include an increased risk of gestational diabetes, hypertension, preeclampsia and eclampsia, and retention of more postpartum weight. The incidence of fetal macrosomia and congenital malformations is higher in obese pregnant women compared with normal-weight pregnant women. Both maternal and fetal complications lead to a higher rate of cesarean section among obese women.

Vesco et al conducted a retrospective study to evaluate whether weight gain measured at term in obese women who exceeded the 1990 Institutes of Medicine (IOM) recommendation (15 pounds) was related to greater weight retention 1-year postpartum. Data from 1656 obese pregnant women insured by Kaiser Permanente Northwest, a group practice Health Maintenance Organization (HMO), including only singleton gestations with a live birth between January 2000 and December 2005 were included. Seventy-one percent of obese pregnant women gained more than 15 lb, with 21% gaining more than 35 lb (Table 1 in the original article). Postpartum women who gained more than 15 lb during pregnancy were at increased risk of weighing more than 10 lb above their pre-pregnancy weight. Weight retention was greater in obese women who gained more weight during pregnancy (Fig 2 in the original article).

Recently, the IOM updated the recommendations for weight gain during pregnancy. The recommended weight gain during pregnancy depends on the pre-pregnancy weight; the pre-pregnancy BMI is measured and women are stratified as underweight (BMI < 18.5 kg/m^2), normal weight (18.5-24.9 kg/m^2), overweight (25-29.9 kg/m^2) or obese (BMI$\geq$30 kg/m^2).[1] The recommended weight gain at term for obese women with singleton pregnancies should be 11 to 20 lb. It is possible that even a smaller weight gain may be appropriate, as shown by a Swedish study of 298 648 singleton pregnancies in which women with a BMI of 30 kg/m^2 or greater, who gained less than 13 lb during pregnancy had the lowest risk of adverse obstetric and neonatal outcomes.[2] In view of the increasing prevalence of obesity in women of childbearing age, prospective studies should evaluate the safety of minimal weight gain during pregnancy. Furthermore, counseling obese women to lose weight before pregnancy and emphasizing the importance of weight loss postpartum may decrease adverse outcomes in subsequent pregnancies.

R. Ness-Abramof, MD

References

1. Institute of Medicine. Weight gain during pregnancy: reexamining the guidelines. *Natl Acad of Sci.* 2009; 2009.
2. Cedergreen MI. Optimal gestational weight gain for body mass index categories. *Obstet Gynecol.* 2007;110:1153-1161.

The Effect of Excess Weight Gain in Teenage Pregnancies

Haeri S, Masouem S, Baker AM, et al (Univ of North Carolina School of Medicine, Chapel Hill; Washington Hosp Ctr)
Am J Perinatol 27:15-18, 2010

Excess weight gain in pregnancy, as defined by the Institute of Medicine (IOM), has been linked to adverse obstetrical outcomes. However, this relationship has not been examined in the younger maternal population. Our aim was to study excess weight gain in our inner-city teenage population. In this retrospective cohort study, we reviewed all nulliparous teenage deliveries between 2000 and 2004. The groups were divided by IOM criteria into "underweight" (body mass index [BMI] <20 kg/m^2; n = 58), "normal" (BMI, 20 to 26.0 kg/m^2; n = 255), "overweight" (BMI, 26.1 to 29.0 kg/m^2; n = 54), and "obese" (BMI > 29.0 kg/m^2; n = 89). The groups were then compared according to normal (control, n = 257) and excess weight gain (n = 199). Frequencies and odds ratios (ORs) for adverse outcomes were calculated. Excess weight gain was associated with an increased risk for cesarean delivery (OR 1.96, 95% confidence interval [CI], 1.28 to 3.01) and postpartum fever (OR, 2.46; 95% CI, 1.13 to 5.35). Significant neonatal findings included higher birthweight (3199 g versus 2864 g; $p < 0.0001$) and increased risk of macrosomia (OR, 8.18; 95% CI, 2.02 to 32.99) in the excess weight gain group. We concluded that excess weight gain places teen mothers at increased risk for cesarean delivery, postpartum febrile morbidity, and macrosomia. Interventions aimed at optimal weight gain in teen pregnancies are warranted.

▶ Although the incidence of birth rates for teenagers 15 to 19 years has declined in the United States from 1991-2005, since 2006 there is an unexpected rise in its incidence.[1,2] Teenage pregnant girls pose specific nutritional challenges. Pregnancy sometimes occurs at the time of active growth; furthermore, many teenagers suffer from nutritional deficiencies (iron, calcium, and vitamins, particularly folic acid) and poor nutritional habits. The prevalence of overweight or obesity is growing in children and posing additional health-related issues to pregnancy. Obese teenagers have a higher risk of glucose intolerance, type 2 diabetes, and hypertension with its known effects on maternal and fetal outcomes. Recently, the Institute of Medicine (IOM) has published recommendations concerning weight gain in which there is a recommended weight gain during pregnancy according to the prepregnancy body mass index (BMI). Specific recommendations for teenage pregnant women were not available in 1990, and unfortunately, the recent guidelines were not able to issue specific recommendations for pregnant teenagers either. Clinicians are instructed to use BMI cutoffs for teenage girls, similar to the adult population, because the pediatric growth chart is not used in obstetric practices, and there is no specific nutritional care to this group.

Haeri et al designed a retrospective study of nulliparous pregnant women younger than 18 years to evaluate the impact of weight gain during pregnancy on adverse obstetric outcomes, including preterm birth, gestational hypertension and preeclampsia, gestational diabetes, and the need for postdate induction of labor. Intrapartum and postpartum outcomes were also evaluated, including the rate of cesarean section, postpartum hemorrhage, clinical chorioamnionits or endometritis, and postpartum fever. Neonatal outcomes included mean birthweight, low birthweight defined as < 2500 g, and macrosomia. The prepregnancy weight was self-reported, and the maximal desired amount of weight gain was based on the 1990 guidelines. According to this study, excessive weight gain in teenage pregnancies was associated with a higher risk for cesarean section, febrile morbidity, and macrosomia.

This study represents mainly an inner city population of African American teenage girls with the inclusion of few Hispanics and just 1 white girl; therefore, it is questionable whether its conclusions can be extended to other races or populations. Nevertheless, 44% of the teenagers gained more weight than recommended, and in this group there were more maternal and fetal adverse outcomes. There is an urgent need for studies to evaluate the appropriate management of teenage pregnancies to improve outcome and reduce its related morbidity.

R. Ness-Abramof, MD

References

1. Paranjothy S, Broughton H, Adappa R, Fone D. Teenage pregnancy: who suffers? *Arch Dis Child.* 2009;94:239-245.
2. Martin JA, Hamilton BE, Sutoon PD, et al. Division of Vital Statistics. Centers for Disease Control and Prevention Web site. www.cdc.gov/nchs/births.htm. Accessed March 1, 2010.

The Obesity Paradox: Body Mass Index and Outcomes in Patients Undergoing Nonbariatric General Surgery

Mullen JT, Moorman DW, Davenport DL (Beth Israel Deaconess Med Ctr and Harvard Med School, Boston, MA; Univ of Kentucky, Lexington)
Ann Surg 250:166-172, 2009

Objective.—We sought to examine the effect of body mass index (BMI) on 30-day morbidity and mortality in a large cohort of patients undergoing nonbariatric general surgery.

Summary Background Data.—Obesity has long been considered a risk factor for poor outcomes from a variety of surgical procedures, yet recent studies of critically and chronically ill patients suggest that overweight and obese patients may paradoxically have better outcomes than "normal" weight patients.

Methods.—A prospective, multi-institutional, risk-adjusted cohort study of 118,707 patients undergoing nonbariatric general surgery who were included in the National Surgical Quality Improvement Program Participant Use database in 2005 and 2006 was performed. Outcomes and risk variables were compared across NIH-defined BMI class using analysis of variance, Bonferroni multiple comparisons of means tests, and multivariable logistic regression.

Results.—After adjusting for all significant perioperative risk factors, the risk of death according to BMI exhibited a reverse J-shaped relationship, with the highest rates in the underweight and morbidly obese extremes and the lowest rates in the overweight and moderately obese. Overweight (odds ratio, 0.85; 95% CI, 0.75–0.99) and moderately obese (odds ratio, 0.73; 95% CI, 0.57–0.94) patients had a significantly lower risk of death than normal weight patients. There was a progressive increase in the likelihood of a complication with increasing BMI class, almost entirely due to increasing rates of wound infection.

Conclusions.—Overweight and moderately obese patients undergoing nonbariatric general surgery have paradoxically "lower" crude and adjusted risks of mortality compared with patients at a "normal" weight. This finding is in contrast to observations from the general population, confirming the existence of an "obesity paradox" in this patient population.

▶ Although obesity is frequently considered a preoperative risk factor, there are surprisingly few studies that have examined how obesity directly affects surgical outcomes, and those that have offer conflicting results.[1,2] The American College of Surgeons National Surgical Quality Improvement Program (ACS NSQIP) is a meticulously collected, prospective, large, and multicenter database of variables, including preoperative risk factors, intraoperative variables, and 30-day morbidity and mortality outcomes for patients undergoing a variety of surgical procedures and is, therefore, capable of providing highly reliable and statistically relevant information. It is not surprising that the authors found extremes of weight, both underweight and class III obesity (body mass index [BMI] >40), to be associated with greater morbidity and mortality when compared with normal weight individuals, as these conditions are both independently associated with known surgical risk factors and underlying medical disease. The interesting finding here is that, relative to normal weight individuals, patients who were overweight or moderately obese (BMI 30-39.9) had a paradoxically lower crude and adjusted rate of death despite a slight increase in overall adjusted risk of morbidity (Fig 1 in the original article). This may reflect their finding that poorer morbidity outcomes in the overweight and the obese were largely because of increased rates of wound occurrences but were not strongly associated with any other negative outcome. In fact, they reported that relative to normal weight individuals, overweight patients had a significantly lower percentage of pulmonary events, class I obese patients had significantly less sepsis or septic shock, and both groups had decreased frequency of returning to the operating room, shorter length of hospital stay, lower rates of perioperative blood transfusion, and similar levels of other major reported outcomes, including renal failure, cardiac arrest, pneumonia, and urinary tract infection (UTI). Perhaps then, despite an increase in overall morbidity, overweight and obese persons have lower rates of potentially life-threatening postoperative complications relative to normal weight persons, which could explain this discrepancy.

The authors identified several variables that were associated with different BMI groups and could potentially be confounding factors in their analysis. For example, obese patients were the least likely to have suffered a recent weight loss of greater than 10% of body weight, to have disseminated cancer, to have a platelet count of less than 150 000, to smoke, to be on steroids for a chronic condition, to undergo a complicated operation, or to have ascites. They also found that mean albumin level was significantly lower among underweight and class III obese patients, and was significantly higher in the overweight and class I obese patients when compared with the normal weight patients. After adjustment to account for major confounding factors that were related to BMI class, the strength of the association between BMI and mortality was attenuated, but the reverse J-shaped relationship (as seen in Fig 1 in the original article) persisted. Similar findings have been reported in meta-analyses of critically ill patients, whereby modest obesity appears to positively impact 30-day mortality. Akkinusi et al[3] found that in a pooled sample of over 60 000 critically ill patients, obesity (BMI > 30) and morbid obesity (BMI > 40) were not associated with increased intensive care unit (ICU) mortality, but the mild to moderately obese subgroup (BMI 30.0-39.9) actually had improved survival outcomes (relative risk [RR], 0.86; 95% confidence interval [CI], 0.81-0.91; $P < .001$) relative to normal weight individuals.

Unfortunately, this study is unable to capture the complex interplay of the various independent risk factors, which cannot be generalized to each BMI class, and, therefore, these factors cannot be completely accounted for in the analysis. The other major limitation of this study is that outcome measures were only followed for 30 days postoperatively, and so delayed complications, such as incisional hernias, which occur more frequently among the obese, are likely to be missed.[4] It is unclear whether mild degrees of excess adiposity might be protective, or if there is some other contributing factor that is yet to be identified. Often, surgical and critically ill patients receive inadequate or no nutrition support, especially within the first 48 hours of hospitalization, for a multitude of reasons, including anticipation of further surgery, lack of appropriate access for feeding, patient intolerance of tube feeding volumes, or prioritization of other aspects of care, such as hemodynamic management of shock. None of these studies report daily caloric intake or percentage of estimated caloric needs met. This raises the possibility that perhaps an inherent advantage could be conferred by the adipose tissue itself, whereby it acts as a reservoir during the fasted state for endogenous fuel and provides substrate needed for synthesis of inflammatory mediators, neurotransmitters, and hormones which are essential during times of physiologic stress, including surgery.

Fully understanding why these individuals have a significantly lower risk of mortality and seemingly equivalent risk of morbidity (with the exception of wound complications) has enormous implications with regard to preoperative and postoperative management and risk stratification for all surgical patients, and warrants further investigation in the future.

A. Port, MD

References

1. Mullen JT, Davenport DL, Hutter MM, et al. Impact of body mass index on perioperative outcomes in patients undergoing major intra-abdominal cancer surgery. *Ann Surg Oncol.* 2008;15:2164-2172.
2. Dossett LA, Dageforde LA, Swenson BR, et al. Obesity and site-specific nosocomial infection risk in the intensive care unit. *Surg Infections.* 2009;10:137-143.
3. Akkinusi ME, Pineda LA, El Sohl AA. Effect of obesity on intensive care morbidity and mortality: a meta-analysis. *Crit Care Med.* 2008;36:151-158.
4. Alexander JW. Wounds in the morbidly obese. *Obesity Surgery.* 2005;15: 1276-1277.

Are Metabolically Normal but Obese Individuals at Lower Risk for All-Cause Mortality?

Kuk JL, Ardern CI (York Univ, Toronto, Canada)

Diabetes Care 32:2297-2299, 2009

Objective.—The clinical relevance of the metabolically normal but obese phenotype for mortality risk is unclear. This study examines the risk for all-cause mortality in metabolically normal and abnormal obese (MNOB and MAOB, respectively) individuals.

Research Design and Methods.—The sample included 6,011 men and women from the Third National Health and Nutrition Examination Survey (NHANES III) with public-access mortality data linkage (follow-up = 8.7 ± 0.2 years; 292 deaths). Metabolically abnormal was defined as insulin resistance (IR) or two or more metabolic syndrome (MetSyn) criteria (excluding waist).

Results.—A total of 30% of obese subjects had IR, and 38.4% had two or more MetSyn factors, whereas only 6.0% (or 1.6% of the whole population) were free from both IR and all MetSyn factors. By MetSyn factors or IR alone, MNOB subjects (hazard ratio $[HR]_{MetSyn}$ 2.80 [1.18–6.65]; HR_{IR} 2.58 [1.00–6.65]) and MAOB subjects (HR_{MetSyn} 2.74 [1.46–5.15]; HR_{IR} 3.09 [1.55–6.15]) had similar elevations in mortality risk compared with metabolically normal, normal weight subjects.

Conclusions.—Although a rare phenotype, obesity, even in the absence of overt metabolic aberrations, is associated with increased all-cause mortality risk.

▶ Obesity is a known risk factor for diabetes, cardiovascular disease, and hypertension. It is recommended that obese subjects lose weight, independent of cardiovascular risk factors. There are specific subgroups that have unexpected metabolic profiles. The first group described is the metabolically obese, normal-weight (MONW) individuals.[1] The MONW individuals are normal weight or overweight individuals with a BMI of 20 to 27 kg/m^2 who have insulin resistance (IR) and a metabolic profile resembling obese individuals, with an increased risk of diabetes and premature cardiovascular disease. On the other side of the spectrum, we can find the metabolically normal obese (MNOB) individuals. These patients are obese, but don't exhibit the classical "obese" metabolic profiles, such as elevated glucose, triglycerides, and blood pressure or low HDL. The proportion of each particular phenotype within a specific population depends on the criteria used. According to Wildman et al,[2] in the United States, 23.5% of normal-weight adults were metabolically abnormal, while 31.7% of obese adults were metabolically healthy. Specific factors determining a healthier overweight or obese individual were younger age, ethnicity (black non-Hispanic), higher level of physical activity, and a smaller waist circumference.

The study by Kuk and Ardern evaluated the mortality rate of the MNOB in 6011 subjects included in the Third National Health and Nutrition Examination Survey (NHANES III). Abnormal metabolic profile was defined as having IR

(HOMA > 2.5), or 2 or more metabolic syndrome criteria (excluding waist). According to this criteria, just 6% of the obese population (1.3% or the total population) were metabolically normal. Obese patients who were metabolically normal had the same mortality risk as the obese metabolically abnormal subjects (Fig 1 in the original article).

The lower prevalence of MNOB in this study is due to the fact that IR was measured and included as a criterion. If patients were categorized by metabolic syndrome criteria only, 38.4% of obese subjects had less than 1 metabolic syndrome risk factor, and would be classified as MNOB.

MNOG subjects were younger and had a lower BMI. It is possible that this group was relatively healthier due to their younger age and lesser degree of obesity, and will develop the abnormal metabolic profile when they get older and heavier. Furthermore, it is possible that the mortality rate is not due to higher metabolic risk but is biased by other important health-related issues, such as health care use or availability. This study reinforces the present recommendations for weight loss in all obese subjects, regardless of additional risk factors.

R. Ness-Abramof, MD

References

1. Ruderman N, Chisholm D, Pi-Sunyer X, Schneider S. The metabolically obese, normal-weight individual revisited. *Diabetes*. 1998;47:699-713.
2. Wildman RP, Muntner P, Reynolds K, et al. The obese without cardiometabolic risk factor clustering and the normal weight with cardiometabolic risk factor clustering: prevalence and correlates of 2 phenotypes among the US population (NHANES 1999-2004). *Arch Intern Med*. 2008;168:1617-1624.

Diet and Obesity

Effect of Moderate Diet-Induced Weight Loss and Weight Regain on Cardiovascular Structure and Function

de las Fuentes L, Waggoner AD, Mohammed BS, et al (Washington Univ School of Medicine, St Louis, MO; et al)
J Am Coll Cardiol 54:2376-2381, 2009

Objectives.—The objective of this prospective, single-site, 2-year dietary intervention study was to evaluate the effects of moderate weight reduction and subsequent partial weight regain on cardiovascular structure and function.

Background.—Obesity is associated with adverse cardiac and vascular structural and functional alterations.

Methods.—Sixty obese subjects (age 46 ± 10 years, body mass index 37 ± 3 kg/m^2) were evaluated during their participation in a weight loss study. Cardiac and vascular ultrasound studies were performed at baseline and at 3, 6, 12, and 24 months after start of intervention.

Results.—Forty-seven subjects (78%) completed the entire 2-year follow-up. Average weight loss was 7.3 ± 4.0%, 9.2 ± 5.6%, 7.8 ± 6.6%, and 3.8 ± 7.9% at 3, 6, 12, and 24 months, respectively.

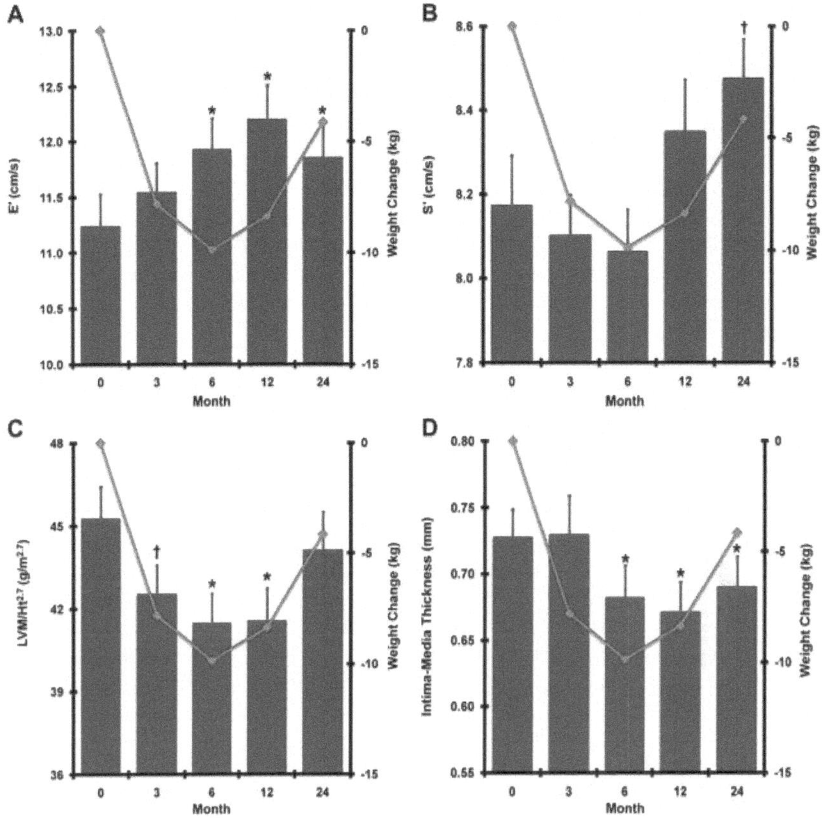

FIGURE 1.—Cardiovascular structure-function response to weight loss. Mean (± SEM) change in (**A**) early diastolic myocardial velocity (E'), (**B**) systolic myocardial velocity (S'), (**C**) left ventricular mass indexed to height$^{2.7}$ (LVM/Ht$^{2.7}$), and (**D**) carotid intima-media thickness in the combined cohort (**blue bars**) with weight change (**red line**) shown for reference. The combined group had 60 subjects at baseline and 3 months, 56 subjects at 6 months, and 47 subjects at 12 and 24 months. There was no significant difference between diet groups for any of these phenotypes. *Adjusted $p \leq 0.005$; †adjusted $p \leq 0.05$ versus baseline. For interpretation of the references to color in this figure legend, the reader is referred to web version of this article. (Reprinted form de las Fuentes L, Waggoner AD, Mohammed BS, et al. Effect of moderate diet-induced weight loss and weight regain on cardiovascular structure and function. *J Am Coll Cardiol.* 2009;54:2376-2381, with permission from the American College of Cardiology Foundation.)

Age- and sex-adjusted mixed linear models revealed that the follow-up time was significantly associated with decreases in weight ($p < 0.0001$), left ventricular (LV) mass ($p = 0.001$), and carotid intima-media thickness ($p < 0.0001$); there was also significant improvement in LV diastolic ($p \leq 0.0001$) and systolic ($p = 0.001$) function. Partial weight regain diminished the maximal observed beneficial effects of weight loss, however cardiovascular parameters measured at 2 years still showed a net benefit compared with baseline.

Conclusions.—Diet-induced moderate weight loss in obese subjects is associated with beneficial changes in cardiovascular structure and function. Subsequent weight regain is associated with partial loss of these beneficial effects. (The Safety and Effectiveness of Low and High Carbohydrate Diets; NCT00079547) (Fig 1).

▶ This study examines the effect of weight loss on cardiovascular structure and function, and whether this effect is sustained in patients who regain weight. Several abnormalities in cardiovascular structure and function have been associated with obesity, including left ventricular (LV) hypertrophy and LV systolic and diastolic dysfunction, all of which are known to be independent risk factors for development of heart failure.[1-3] Previous work has demonstrated that weight loss promotes cardiac remodeling and improves related measures of cardiac function.[4,5] However, most of the available data come from studies in class III obese patients undergoing bariatric surgery who experience considerable weight loss following surgery (often >20% body weight) and often show resolution of underlying medical diseases known to increase cardiovascular risk, such as diabetes mellitus or hypertension. Therefore, improvements in cardiac function in patients following bariatric surgery may not be applicable to patients with more modest degrees of weight loss.

This prospective study follows a cohort of 60 patients randomly assigned to follow 1 of 2 calorie-restricted diets (low-carbohydrate or low-fat diet) over a 2-year period. Subjects also participated in weekly group counseling sessions and were encouraged to begin walking regularly. There were no significant differences between diet treatment groups in terms of baseline characteristics, weight loss, or primary outcome measures, and therefore data analyses were performed on the entire pooled sample. Patients lost an average of about 5% to 10% of their initial body weight during the study, with maximal weight loss occurring at 6 months and weight regain noted at 12 and 24 months, although mean weight at completion remained below baseline levels. In Fig 1, authors show that weight loss was significantly correlated with improvements in LV diastolic relaxation (E′ [early diastolic myocardial velocity]) at 6, 12, and 24 months, improvement in LV systolic function (S′ [systolic myocardial velocity]) at 24 months, decreased LV mass ($LVM/Ht^{2.7}$ [LVM indexed to $height^{2.7}$]) at 3, 6, and 12 months, and decreased carotid intima-media wall thickness at 6, 12, and 24 months. These favorable changes in cardiac structure and function appear to lag behind achievement of maximal weight loss by about 3 to 6 months. Subsequent weight regain was associated with worsening of LVM, diastolic function, and vascular hypertrophy, although improvements in LV systolic function persisted at 24 months.

It is impossible to know whether these effects would last if an additional 3 to 6 months of time passed or if patients were followed after returning to their baseline weight. Another limitation of this study is that patients were encouraged, but not required, to participate in cardiovascular exercise, such as regular walking, and because patient exercise was neither supervised nor recorded in this study, its role as a confounding factor on outcomes cannot be accounted for. It would be premature to conclude that the improvements in cardiovascular function and structure can be attributed to weight loss alone. Additionally, it is unclear whether transient improvements in cardiac function associated with modest weight loss will show any sustained benefit and/or translate into meaningful improvements in clinical outcomes (eg, decreased hospitalizations for heart failure) over time. What is encouraging about this study is that the authors have shown that with modest weight loss (5%-10% of baseline weight), many of the changes seen in cardiomyopathy of obesity can be reversed. Weight regain attenuates the maximal observed benefit of these effects, although improvements in cardiac outcomes persist well beyond this period. Further studies to investigate the long-term effects of weight loss and gain on improvements in cardiovascular structure and function and the specific mechanisms underlying these changes are warranted.

A. Port, MD

References

1. Wong CY, O'Moore-Sullivan T, Leano R, Byrne N, Beller E, Marwick TH. Alterations of left ventricular myocardial characteristics associated with obesity. *Circulation.* 2004;110:3081-3087.
2. Alpert MA. Obesity cardiomyopathy: pathophysiology and evolution of the clinical syndrome. *Am J Med Sci.* 2001;321:225-236.
3. Kenchaiah S, Evans JC, Levy D, et al. Obesity and the risk of heart failure. *N Engl J Med.* 2002;347:305-313.
4. Alpert MA, Terry B, Lambert CR, et al. Factors influencing left ventricular systolic function in nonhypertensive morbidly obese patients, and effect of weight loss induced by gastroplasty. *Am J Cardiol.* 1993;71:733-737.
5. Ippisch HM, Inge TH, Daniels SR, Wang B, Khoury PR, Witt SA. Reversibility of cardiac abnormalities in morbidly obese adolescents. *J Am Coll Cardiol.* 2008;51: 1342-1348.

Eating Slowly Increases the Postprandial Response of the Anorexigenic Gut Hormones, Peptide YY And Glucagon-Like Peptide-1

Kokkinos A, Le Roux CW, Alexiadou K, et al (Athens Univ Med School, Athens, Greece; Hammersmith Hosp, London, UK)
J Clin Endocrinol Metab 95:333-337, 2010

Context.—The rate at which people eat has been suggested to be positively associated with obesity, although appetite and related gut hormones have not been measured.

Objective.—The objective of the study was to determine whether eating the same meal at varying speeds elicits different postprandial gut peptide responses.

Design and Setting.—This was a crossover study at a clinical research facility.

Study Participants.—Seventeen healthy adult male volunteers participated in the study.

Intervention.—A test meal consisting of 300 ml ice cream (675 kcal) was consumed in random order on two different sessions by each subject: meal duration took either 5 or 30 min.

Main Outcome Measures.—The postprandial response of the orexigenic hormone ghrelin and the anorexigenic peptides peptide YY and glucagon-like peptide-1 over 210 min was assessed. Visual analog scales for the subjective feelings of hunger and fullness were completed throughout each session.

Results.—Peptide YY area under the curve (AUC) was higher after the 30-min meal than after the 5-min meal (mean ± SEM AUC 5 min meal: 4133 ± 324, AUC 30 min meal: 5250 ± 330 pmol/liter · min, $P = 0.004$), as was glucagon-like peptide-1 AUC (mean ± SEM AUC 5 min meal: 6219 ± 256, AUC 30 min meal: 8794 ± 656 pmol/liter · min, $P = 0.001$). There was a trend for higher visual analog scale fullness ratings immediately after the end of the 30-min meal compared with immediately after the 5-min meal. There were no differences in ghrelin response.

Conclusions.—Eating at a physiologically moderate pace leads to a more pronounced anorexigenic gut peptide response than eating very fast.

▶ The increased prevalence of obesity is best explained by a positive caloric balance. Dieters are advised to eat slowly, using strategies such as prolonged chewing and putting down the fork between bites. Whether these recommendations indeed increase satiety and whether there is a scientific explanation behind these popular strategies was investigated in the above study.

Kokkinos et al conducted a prospective study to evaluate whether eating a test meal consisting of 300 ml of ice cream (675 kcal, 59% of kcal fat, 33% carbohydrates, 8% protein) consumed quickly (within 5 minutes) or slowly (within 30 minutes) would impact satiety (subjective feel of hunger and fullness) and the secretion of orexigenic (ghrelin) and anorexigenic (peptide YY and glucagon-like-peptide-1) gut hormones. Seventeen healthy males were recruited. Blood samples were withdrawn before the meal and every 30 minutes for 210 minutes. Visual assessment of the subjective feelings of hunger and fullness were completed at the meal and thereafter for every 30 minutes. There was a trend toward higher fullness after the 30-minute meal compared with the 5-minute meal but no difference in hunger at the same point (Fig 1 in the original article). The areas under the curve (AUC) for PYY and GLP-1 over 210 minutes were significantly greater after the 30-minute meal (Fig 2 in the original article). Ghrelin levels were not significantly different among groups. Insulin and glucose levels were also similar in both groups.

This interesting study is the first to evaluate the physiological mechanism behind eating slowly. A rise in the anorexigenic peptides PYY and GLP-1 may explain part of the mechanism associated with increased satiety when eating slowly. It is important to evaluate whether the same effect will be reproduced in female subjects and in obese individuals. Nevertheless, now we have some physiological base for the beneficial effect of eating slowly.

R. Ness-Abramof, MD

Physical Activity and Obesity

The Impact of Exercise Training Compared to Caloric Restriction on Hepatic and Peripheral Insulin Resistance in Obesity

Coker RH, Williams RH, Yeo SE, et al (Univ of Arkansas for Med Sciences, Little Rock)

J Clin Endocrinol Metab 94:4258-4266, 2009

Context.—It has been difficult to distinguish the independent effects of caloric restriction versus exercise training on insulin resistance.

Objective.—Utilizing metabolic feeding and supervised exercise training, we examined the influence of caloric restriction *vs.* exercise training with and without weight loss on hepatic and peripheral insulin resistance.

Design, Participants, and Intervention.—Thirty-four obese, older subjects were randomized to: caloric restriction with weight loss (CR), exercise training with weight loss (EWL), exercise training without weight loss (EX), or controls. Based on an equivalent caloric deficit in EWL and CR, we induced matched weight loss. Subjects in the EX group received caloric compensation. Combined with [6,6$^2H_2$]glucose, an octreotide, glucagon, multistage insulin infusion was performed to determine suppression of glucose production (SGP) and insulin-stimulated glucose disposal (ISGD). Computed tomography scans were performed to assess changes in fat distribution.

Results.—Body weight decreased similarly in EWL and CR, and did not change in EX and controls. The reduction in visceral fat was significantly greater in EWL (-71 ± 15 cm^2) compared to CR and EX. The increase in SGP was also almost 3-fold greater (27 ± 2%) in EWL. EWL and CR promoted similar improvements in ISGD [+2.5 ± 0.4 and 2.4 ± 0.9 mg · kg fat-free mass (FFM)$^{-1}$ · min^{-1}], respectively.

Conclusions.—EWL promoted the most significant reduction in visceral fat and the greatest improvement in SGP. Equivalent increases in ISGD were noted in EWL and CR, whereas EX provided a modest improvement. Based on our results, EWL promoted the optimal intervention-based changes in body fat distribution and systemic insulin resistance.

▶ The increased caloric intake and reduced physical activity are the main culprits for the obesity epidemic. Obesity is the most common cause of insulin resistance carrying a higher risk to develop type 2 diabetes mellitus and cardiovascular disease. Diabetes was shown to be delayed or prevented by lifestyle changes, including weight loss and exercise. The Diabetes Prevention Program (DPP) enrolled 3232 patients with impaired glucose tolerance to metformin, lifestyle changes, or control group.[1] Patients on lifestyle modification program had a goal to lose at least 7% of basal weight and to exercise at least 150 minutes per week. The incidence of diabetes was reduced by 58% in the lifestyle change group and by 31% on the metformin group compared with the placebo group. A 10-year follow-up of patients from the DPP trial still showed protective effect of lifestyle changes and metformin in the incidence of type 2 diabetes.[2]

Most weight loss programs combine dietary restriction and increased physical activity. Although an increase in physical activity would not promote a significant weight loss, it improves insulin sensitivity.[3] Coker et al designed a study to evaluate the effectiveness of weight loss through caloric restriction (CR), exercise training with weight loss (EWL), and exercise training without weight loss (EX) on hepatic and peripheral insulin resistance. They measured insulin-stimulated glucose disposal (ISGD) and determined the suppression of glucose production (SGP) in 34 obese patients. Weight decreased in both the CR and EWL group and remained unchanged in the EX and control group. The EWL group had the greatest reduction in visceral fat as assessed by computed tomography. The SGP was higher in the EWL group and ISGD was similar in the EWL and CR group. According to this study, EWL promoted the highest reduction in visceral fat and improvement in hepatic insulin resistance. EWL and CR both increased peripheral insulin sensitivity, whereas EX alone provided just a modest improvement.

The improvement in hepatic insulin sensitivity in this study was higher than that found with CR only, a finding that needs to be revalidated.

R. Ness-Abramof, MD

References

1. Diabetes Prevention Program Research, G. Reduction in the incidence of type 2 diabetes with lifestyle intervention or metformin. *N Engl J Med.* 2002;346:393-403.
2. Diabetes Prevention Program Research, G. 10-year follow-up of diabetes incidence and weight loss in the Diabetes Prevention Program Outcomes Study. *Lancet.* 2009;374:1677-1686.
3. O'Gorman DJ, Krook A. Exercise and the treatment of diabetes and obesity. *Endocrinol Metab Clin North Am.* 2008;37:887-903.

Dual-process action of exercise on appetite control: Increase in orexigenic drive but improvement in meal-induced satiety

King NA, Caudwell PP, Hopkins M, et al (Univ of Technology, Brisbane, Australia; Univ of Leeds, UK; Trinity and All Saints Colleges, Leeds, UK)

Am J Clin Nutr 90:921-927, 2009

Background.—Exercise could contribute to weight loss by altering the sensitivity of the appetite regulatory system.

Objective.—The aim of this study was to assess the effects of 12 wk of mandatory exercise on appetite control.

Design.—Fifty-eight overweight and obese men and women [mean ($\pm$SD) body mass index (in kg/m^2) = 31.8 ± 4.5, age = 39.6 ± 9.8 y, and maximal oxygen intake = $29.1 \pm 5.7\ mL \cdot kg^{-1} \cdot min^{-1}$] completed 12 wk of supervised exercise in the laboratory. The exercise sessions were designed to expend 2500 kcal/wk. Subjective appetite sensations and the satiating efficiency of a fixed breakfast were compared at baseline (week 0) and at week 12. An Electronic Appetite Rating System was used to measure subjective appetite sensations immediately before and after the fixed breakfast in the immediate postprandial period and across the whole day. The satiety quotient of the breakfast was determined by calculating the change in appetite scores relative to the breakfast's energy content.

Results.—Despite large variability, there was a significant reduction in mean body weight (3.2 ± 3.6 kg), fat mass (3.2 ± 2.2 kg), and waist circumference (5.0 ± 3.2 cm) after 12 wk. The analysis showed that a reduction in body weight and body composition was accompanied by an increase in fasting hunger and in average hunger across the day ($P < 0.0001$). Paradoxically, the immediate and delayed satiety quotient of the breakfast also increased significantly ($P < 0.05$).

Conclusions.—These data show that the effect of exercise on appetite regulation involves at least 2 processes: an increase in the overall (orexigenic) drive to eat and a concomitant increase in the satiating efficiency of a fixed meal.

▶ Appetite is regulated by a complex network in which the central nervous, adipose, and gastrointestinal systems interact to maintain body weight. Exercise induces a negative energy balance, increases free fat mass, and decreases fat mass. It is incorporated into all weight loss programs to improve and maintain weight loss, but exercise without energy restriction would not lead to a substantial weight loss in spite of the negative energy balance. The effect of exercise on appetite is not well understood. It is possible that it differs according to gender, body mass index, and amount and intensity of exercise performed. An in-depth review of exercise on appetite was recently published by Martins et al.[1]

King et al conducted a prospective study to evaluate the effect of exercise on satiety. Fifty-eight overweight and obese men and women were recruited and enrolled on a 12-week supervised exercise program designed to spend 2500 kcal/wk (500 kcal per session). Appetite and satiety sensations of a fixed breakfast were compared at baseline and at 12 weeks. The subjective appetite sensation was measured before and immediately after the breakfast and across the whole day. Although a great variability was found within subjects, overall there was a decrease in weight, fat mass, and waist circumference at 12 weeks. The weight loss and change in body composition was accompanied by an increase in hunger (fasting and average hunger across the day), but there was also an increase in satiety. According to this study, exercise has a dual effect on overweight and obese subjects, increasing hunger but also increasing satiety. Eventually, the net effect, although not similar in all individuals, seems to produce a negative energy balance and explains the crucial effect of exercise on weight loss promotion and weight loss maintenance.

R. Ness-Abramof, MD

Reference

1. Martins C, Morgan L, Truby H. A review of the effects of exercise on appetite regulation: an obesity perspective. *Int J Obes.* 2008;32:1337-1347.

Pharmacological Treatment of Obesity

Effects of liraglutide in the treatment of obesity: a randomised, double-blind, placebo-controlled study

Astrup A, on behalf of the NN8022-1807 Study Group (Univ of Copenhagen, Denmark; et al)

Lancet 374:1606-1616, 2009

Background.—The frequency of obesity has risen dramatically in recent years but only few safe and effective drugs are currently available. We assessed the effect of liraglutide on bodyweight and tolerability in obese individuals without type 2 diabetes.

Methods.—We did a double-blind, placebo-controlled 20-week trial, with open-label orlistat comparator in 19 sites in Europe. 564 individuals (18–65 years of age, body-mass index 30–40 kg/m^2) were randomly assigned, with a telephone or web-based system, to one of four liraglutide doses (1·2 mg, 1·8 mg, 2·4 mg, or 3·0 mg, n=90–95) or to placebo (n=98) administered once a day subcutaneously, or orlistat (120 mg, n=95) three times a day orally. All individuals had a 500 kcal per day energy-deficit diet and increased their physical activity throughout the trial, including the 2-week run-in. Weight change analysed by intention to treat was the primary endpoint. An 84-week open-label extension followed. This study is registered with ClinicalTrials.gov, number NCT00422058.

Findings.—Participants on liraglutide lost significantly more weight than did those on placebo (p=0·003 for liraglutide 1·2 mg and p<0·0001 for liraglutide 1·8–3·0 mg) and orlistat (p=0·003 for

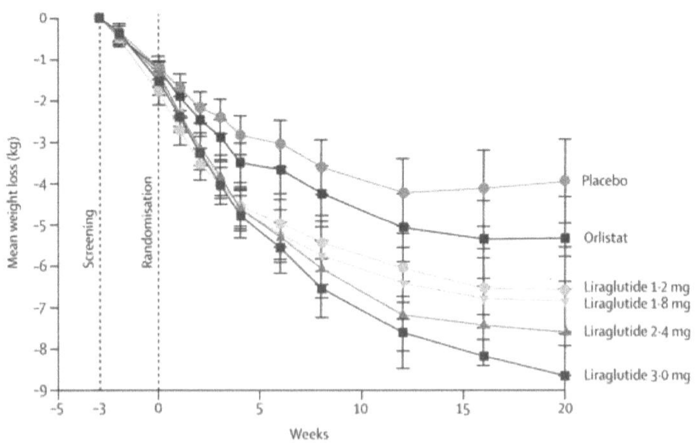

FIGURE 2.—Change in bodyweight. Data are mean (95% CI) (ANCOVA estimate) for the intention-to-treat population with the last observation carried forward. (Reprinted from Astrup A, on behalf of the NN8022-1807 Study Group. Effects of liraglutide in the treatment of obesity: a randomised, double-blind, placebo-controlled study. *Lancet.* 2009;374:1606-1616, with permission from Elsevier.)

liraglutide 2·4 mg and $p<0·0001$ for liraglutide 3·0 mg). Mean weight loss with liraglutide 1·2–3·0 mg was 4·8 kg, 5·5 kg, 6·3 kg, and 7·2 kg compared with 2·8 kg with placebo and 4·1 kg with orlistat, and was 2·1 kg (95% CI 0·6–3·6) to 4·4 kg (2·9–6·0) greater than that with placebo. More individuals (76%, n=70) lost more than 5% weight with liraglutide 3·0 mg that with placebo (30%, n=29) or orlistat (44%, n=42). Liraglutide reduced blood pressure at all doses, and reduced the prevalence of prediabetes (84–96% reduction) with 1·8–3·0 mg per day. Nausea and vomiting occurred more often in individuals on liraglutide than in those on placebo, but adverse events were mainly transient and rarely led to discontinuation of treatment.

Interpretation.—Liraglutide treatment over 20 weeks is well tolerated, induces weight loss, improves certain obesity-related risk factors, and reduces prediabetes (Fig 2).

▶ The prevalence of obesity has increased markedly during the last 30 years. More than 50% of the adult population in the United States and in some European countries is either overweight or obese. Obesity increases the risk of diabetes, hypertension, cardiovascular disease, some cancers, obstructive sleep apnea, and many other diseases. Lifestyle changes are the cornerstone in the treatment and prevention of obesity. Unfortunately, weight loss promoted by hypocaloric diets is mild and the rate of recidivism approaches 95%.

Pharmacotherapy is an important tool in the management of the obese patient. Although many drugs are being investigated as weight loss medications, presently, only orlistat and sibutramine are approved for long-term use. Orlistat and sibutramine promote an additional 3 to 4-kg weight loss compared with placebo in overweight/obese patients on a hypocaloric diet. Recently, sibutramine was withdrawn from the European Union because of new data from the Sibutramine Cardiovascular Outcome trial (SCOUT).[1] The SCOUT study was designed to investigate whether patients with a high cardiovascular risk would benefit from weight loss with sibutramine therapy. Patients were assigned to sibutramine or placebo in addition to lifestyle changes. The sibutramine group had an increased risk of heart attacks and stroke compared with the placebo group. The Food and Drug Administration (FDA) decided not to withdraw sibutramine from the market but demanded that the manufacturer emphasize the known risks for some patients, such as cardiovascular disease, arrhythmias, and uncontrolled hypertension, in which the drug is contraindicated.

Glucagon-like peptide-1 (GLP-1) is a hormone secreted from the gastrointestinal tract in response to nutrient ingestion. GLP-1 increases insulin secretion in a glucose-dependent manner. In pharmacological doses, GLP-1 suppresses glucagon secretion, which slows gastric emptying and gut motility, delaying nutrient absorption, decreasing postprandial glucose levels, and increasing satiety. GLP-1 is rapidly metabolized by dipeptidyl peptidase (DPP) 4 with a half-life of 1 to 2 min.[2] Liraglutide is a GLP-1 analogue, with a 97% homology to human GLP-1. It has a half-life of 13 hours, allowing for a daily subcutaneous injection. It is approved for the treatment of diabetes mellitus in doses up to 1.8 mg/d. Liraglutide was shown to improve glycemic control and promote weight loss in patients with type 2 diabetes. Its weight loss effect is mediated through the gastrointestinal system and possibly through a central effect. In clinical trials, liraglutide improved glucose control and β-cell function, promoted weight loss, and decreased blood pressure. The main side effects were gastrointestinal, mainly nausea and vomiting, that generally subsided after 4 weeks of therapy. Safety concerns are related to data derived from rodent studies in which liraglutide was associated with an increased risk of thyroid C-cell focal hyperplasia and C-cell tumors. Calcitonin, a biomarker for the detection of medullary thyroid cancer, was followed in clinical trials, without evidence of a significant increase in its level. Another concern is the increased risk of pancreatitis arising from postmarketing reports attributed to the use of exenatide, a GLP-1 analog, and sitagliptin, a DPP-4 inhibitor, submitted to the FDA. Whether the cases of pancreatitis are related to the GLP-1 pathway or casualty is difficult to assess due to the relatively small number of cases.[3]

Another potential use for liraglutide is as a weight-loss medication. The study by Astrup et al is the first in which GLP-1 analogues were evaluated for use in weight loss. Five hundred sixty-four obese individuals were randomized to different doses of liraglutide, placebo, or orlistat and followed for 20 weeks. The different doses of liraglutide and placebo were double blinded, whereas the orlistat comparator was open-label. Patients treated with liraglutide at any dose lost more weight than placebo-treated patients. Compared with orlistat, weight loss was greater for the higher doses of liraglutide, 2.4 and 3 mg daily (Fig 2). The liraglutide group had more nausea and vomiting, but it was mostly transient and generally did not lead to discontinuation of therapy.

Liraglutide reduced blood pressure in all doses, an effect observed in previous clinical trials of GLP-1 agonists. At the highest liraglutide doses (1.8, 2.4, and 3 mg), there was a marked decrease in the prevalence of prediabetes.

According to the above data, liraglutide appears to be an effective drug for the treatment of obesity, in conjunction with lifestyle changes. Long-term safety is the primary concern. Data will be obtained from the 84-week extension of this study and future studies should be designed to evaluate the efficacy and safety of this new class of drugs for the treatment of obesity.

R. Ness-Abramof, MD

References

1. Van Gaal LF, Caterson ID, Coutinho W, et al. Weight and blood pressure response to weight management and sibutramine in diabetic and non-diabetic high-risk patients: an analysis from the 6-week lead-in period of the sibutramine cardiovascular outcomes (SCOUT) trial. *Diabetes Obes Metab.* 2009;12:26-34.
2. Chia CW, Egan JM. Incretin-based therapies in type 2 diabetes mellitus. *J Clin Endocrinol Metab.* 2008;93:3703-3716.
3. Parks M, Rosebraugh C. Weighing risks and benefits of liraglutide – the FDA's review of a new antidiabetic therapy. *N Engl J Med.* 2010;362:774-777.

New Developments in Obesity

Normalization of obesity-associated insulin resistance through immunotherapy

Winer S, Chan Y, Paltser G, et al (Univ of Toronto Depts of Pediatrics & Immunology, Ontario, Canada; et al)
Nat Med 15:921-929, 2009

Obesity and its associated metabolic syndromes represent a growing global challenge, yet mechanistic understanding of this pathology and current therapeutics are unsatisfactory. We discovered that $CD4^+$ T lymphocytes, resident in visceral adipose tissue (VAT), control insulin resistance in mice with diet-induced obesity (DIO). Analyses of human tissue suggest that a similar process may also occur in humans. DIO VAT-associated T cells show severely biased T cell receptor V_α repertoires, suggesting antigenspecific expansion. $CD4^+$ T lymphocyte control of glucose homeostasis is compromised in DIO progression, when VAT accumulates pathogenic interferon-γ (IFN-γ)-secreting T helper type 1 (T_H1) cells, overwhelming static numbers of T_H2 ($CD4^+$GATA-binding protein-3 $(GATA\text{-}3)^+$) and regulatory forkhead box P3 $(Foxp3)^+$ T cells. $CD4^+$ (but not $CD8^+$) T cell transfer into lymphocyte-free Rag1-null DIO mice reversed weight gain and insulin resistance, predominantly through T_H2 cells. In obese WT and *ob/ob* (leptin-deficient) mice, brief treatment with CD3-specific antibody or its F(ab′)$_2$ fragment, reduces the predominance of T_H1 cells over $Foxp3^+$ cells, reversing insulin resistance for months, despite continuation of a high-fat diet. Our data suggest that the progression of obesity-associated metabolic abnormalities is under the pathophysiological control of $CD4^+$ T cells. The eventual failure of this control, with expanding adiposity and pathogenic VAT T cells, can successfully be reversed by immunotherapy.

► In recent years, accumulating evidence indicates that adipose tissue inflammation contributes to the metabolic pathogenesis of obesity.[1] Inflammation directly affects metabolic abnormalities of obesity, including disruption of insulin signalling[1] and endothelial dysfunction.[2] There is strong evidence to support an active role for macrophages in these processes; however, there is limited data to support participation of lymphocytes or the adaptive immune response. T cells recognize and remember distinct antigens and coordinate with the adaptive immune system to mount and then resolve an appropriate immune response. Derangements in T cell function are responsible for the pathogenesis of inflammatory autoimmune disease, such as rheumatoid arthritis and ulcerative colitis. However, their role in adipose tissue inflammation is poorly understood. Winer et al present one of the first studies to demonstrate that specific subsets of T cells contribute to obesity-associated adipose tissue inflammation. The authors reported that in both human and mouse visceral adipose tissue, there was an increased accumulation of T helper type 1 (T_H1) cells (proinflammatory T cells) and fewer regulatory T cells (inflammatory suppressing cells). Thus, T cells are important regulators of inflammation in visceral adipose tissue. Winer et al also provide evidence indicating that regulatory T cells present in adipose tissue may protect against the adverse metabolic consequences of obesity-associated insulin resistance. In addition, this study indicates that there may be specific adipose tissue antigens that drive selection of T cell receptors (TCRs). Overall, this study presents a novel perspective on the pathogenic process of adipose tissue inflammation and provides the first evidence that regulatory T cells contribute to whole body insulin sensitivity and glucose tolerance. Further research is necessary to identify specific antigenic components of visceral adipose tissue, which may lead to the development of immunotherapies aimed at minimizing the metabolic consequences of adipose tissue inflammation.

M. Ruth, PhD

References

1. Hotamisligil GS. Inflammation and metabolic disorders. *Nature*. 2006;444: 860-867.
2. Rizvi AA. Cytokine biomarkers, endothelial inflammation, and atherosclerosis in the metabolic syndrome: emerging concepts. *Am J Med Sci*.. 2009;338:310-318.

Hypothalamic Leptin Signaling Regulates Hepatic Insulin Sensitivity via a Neurocircuit Involving the Vagus Nerve

German J, Kim F, Schwartz GJ, et al (Univ of Washington, Seattle; Albert Einstein College of Medicine, Bronx, NY; et al)

Endocrinology 150:4502-4511, 2009

Recent evidence suggests that hormones such as insulin and leptin act in the hypothalamus to regulate energy balance and glucose metabolism. Here we show that in leptin receptor-deficient Koletsky (fa^k/fa^k) rats, adenovirally induced expression of leptin receptors in the area of the hypothalamic arcuate nucleus improved peripheral insulin sensitivity via enhanced suppression of hepatic glucose production, with no change of insulin-stimulated glucose uptake or disposal. This effect was associated with increased insulin signal transduction via phosphatidylinositol-3-OH kinase (as measured by pY-insulin receptor substrate-1 and pS-PKB/Akt) in liver, but not skeletal muscle, and with reduced hepatic expression of the gluconeogenic genes, glucose-6-phosphatase and phosphoenolpyruvate kinase. Moreover, the beneficial effects of hypothalamic leptin signaling on hepatic insulin sensitivity were blocked by selective hepatic vagotomy. We conclude that hypothalamic leptin action increases peripheral insulin sensitivity primarily via effects on the liver and that the mechanism underlying this effect is dependent on the hepatic branch of the vagus nerve.

▶ Because of our hunter-gatherer ancestry, the central nervous system (CNS) has evolved with an extremely complex redundant mechanism for keeping track of its available energy supply, including both stored fat and circulating forms, so that energy balance can be closely regulated as a means of promoting survival. We are just beginning to understand the intricate pathways by which nutrition-related and gut- and fat-derived hormone signals, notably insulin and leptin, stimulate key areas of the brain, such as the hypothalamus, to activate pathways that regulate: (1) appetite and satiety, and ultimately control food intake, (2) metabolism and thermogenesis, (3) insulin sensitivity and therefore glucose homeostasis, and (4) autonomic nervous function.

Through selective restoration of leptin receptor (LR) expression in LR knockout rats, the authors were able to investigate the role of leptin signaling exclusively in the arcuate nucleus of the hypothalamus (ARC), which acts on the liver by way of signaling along the hepatic branch of the vagus nerve. It appears that intact parasympathetic tone along the vagus nerve has no role on hepatic insulin sensitivity independent of leptin, which is supported by the fact that control rats in which leptin signaling was not restored showed no difference in liver gluconeogenesis levels, regardless of whether they had undergone hepatic vagotomy. This pathway is probably redundant, as hepatic vagotomy in genetically normal rats has not been shown to affect liver glucose metabolism, probably because of some alternate compensatory mechanism.[1,2] Additionally, insulin resistance was only partially reversed by recovery of leptin function in the ARC, which argues that leptin targets in other areas of the brain (unstimulated here due to lack of functioning LR) may also play an important role in regulation of glucose homeostasis. Further studies are warranted to better understand the significance of this hypothalamus-liver neurocircuit and the role of the ARC and vagus nerve in controlling hepatic glucose metabolism.

This study offers further insight into the mechanism of leptin-regulated hypothalamic signaling and its effects on insulin sensitivity and glucose homeostasis throughout the body. Better understanding of this pathway, which ultimately regulates energy intake, appetite, satiety, and glucose homeostasis, in addition to better understanding the mechanism for leptin resistance in the obese, may provide a number of potential targets for future development of antiobesity or antidiabetes drugs. Unlike the incretin analogs, recombinant leptin has had limited success as a therapeutic agent thus far because of its short half-life in circulation and issues with drug delivery into the CNS as a result of impaired transport across the blood-brain barrier (BBB) in the obese.[3] Leptin continues to be explored as a potential drug target, with some groups chemically altering its structure to make it increasingly stable in plasma and more permeable to the BBB, whereas others are examining the use of leptin in combination with other injectable hormones.[4]

A. Port, MD

References

1. Pocai A, Lam TK, Gutierrez-Juarez R, et al. Hypothalamic K(ATP) channels control hepatic glucose production. *Nature*. 2005;434:1026-1031.
2. Pocai A, Obici S, Schwartz GJ, Rossetti L. A brain-liver circuit regulates glucose homeostasis. *Cell Metab*. 2005;1:53-61.
3. Myers MG, Cowley MA, Münzberg H. Mechanisms of leptin action and leptin resistance. *Annu Rev Physiol*. 2008;70:537-556.
4. Price TO, Farr SA, Yi X, et al. Transport across the blood-brain barrier of pluronic leptin. *J Pharmacol Exp Ther*. 2010; 2010.

Effects of androgens on adipocyte differentiation and adipose tissue explant metabolism in men and women

Blouin K, Nadeau M, Perreault M, et al (Laval Univ Med Res Ctr, Québec, Canada; et al)

Clin Endocrinol 72:176-188, 2010

Objective.—To examine the effects of aromatizable or nonaromatizable androgens on abdominal subcutaneous (SC) and omental (OM) adipose tissue lipid metabolism and adipogenesis in men and women.

Design and subjects.—Primary organ and preadipocyte cultures were established from surgical samples obtained in men ($n = 22$) and women undergoing biliopancreatic diversions ($n = 12$) or gynaecological surgeries ($n = 8$). Cultures were treated with testosterone, dihydrotestosterone (DHT) and methyltrienolone (R1881).

Measurements.—Heparin-releasable lipoprotein lipase (HR-LPL) activity, glycerol release, adiponectin secretion, glycerol-3-phosphate dehydrogenase activity and lipid accumulation were measured.

Results.—In organ cultures from men, DHT had a statistically significant inhibitory effect on HR-LPL activity in the OM compartment. Testosterone significantly inhibited HR-LPL activity in SC and OM cultures. In women, high DHT concentrations tended to inhibit HR-LPL activity in OM cultures. Minor androgenic effects were observed for basal and isoproterenol-stimulated lipolysis as well as adiponectin release in men. On the other hand, adipocyte differentiation was significantly and dose-dependently inhibited by DHT, testosterone and R1881 in SC and OM cultures from both sexes. These effects did not differ according to adipose tissue depot but appeared to be more pronounced in women than in men.

Conclusions.—Androgens slightly decreased HR-LPL activity in adipose tissue organ cultures, but markedly inhibited adipogenesis in SC and OM primary preadipocyte cultures in both sexes. Androgenic effects on adipose tissue in men *vs.* women may not differ in terms of direction but in the magnitude of their negative impact on adipogenesis and lipid synthesis.

▶ Fat distribution is sexually dimorphic. Men accumulate more upper body visceral adipose tissue, while women have greater lower-body (gluteal-femoral) subcutaneous adipose tissue.[1] The lower body fat distribution in females confers protection against metabolic disease, while male-pattern fat distribution favors disease development, including type 2 diabetes and cardiovascular disease.[1] There is an age-associated decline in sex hormones, which is associated with shift toward central adiposity and adverse metabolic consequences.[2] There is evidence to suggest that testosterone replacement may reduce visceral adiposity and improve lean body mass in aging men.[2] However, the mechanisms used by sex steroids to alter adipocyte and adipose tissue metabolisms have not been elucidated.

Blouin et al presented a well-designed study and reported novel findings regarding the role of androgens, testosterone, and dihydrotestosterone (DHT) on subcutaneous and visceral adipose tissue metabolisms. The use of both visceral and subcutaneous human adipose tissues from men and women allowed the authors to determine whether there were depot and/or sex differences in response to androgen exposure. Overall, the authors report that androgens may act to decrease adipose tissue storage by inhibiting lipoprotein lipase (LPL) activity in subcutaneous and visceral adipose tissues in men. However, in women DHT lowered LPL activity in visceral adipose only (not subcutaneous). This suggests that there may be depot differences in DHT activity in women compared with men. Blouin et al also provide evidence that physiological doses of androgens act at the cellular level to inhibit adipogenesis and, thus, expansion of adipose tissue.

Understanding the mechanisms by which androgens modify adipose tissue metabolism will provide a foundation to generate therapeutic strategies aimed at reducing visceral adiposity and confer protection against metabolic disease in overweight and aging populations.

M. Ruth, PhD

References

1. Mayes JS, Watson GH. Direct effects of sex steroid hormones on adipose tissues and obesity. *Obes Rev.* 2004;5:197-216.
2. Allan CA, Strauss BJG, Burger HG, Forbes EA, McLachlan RI. Testosterone therapy prevents gain in visceral adipose tissue and loss of skeletal muscle in non-obese aging men. *J Clin Endocrinol Metab.* 2008;93:139-146.

Cold-Activated Brown Adipose Tissue in Healthy Men

van Marken Lichtenbelt WD, Vanhommerig JW, Smulders NM, et al (Maastricht Univ Med Ctr, the Netherlands)
N Engl J Med 360:1500-1508, 2009

Background.—Studies in animals indicate that brown adipose tissue is important in the regulation of body weight, and it is possible that individual variation in adaptive thermogenesis can be attributed to variations in the amount or activity of brown adipose tissue. Until recently, the presence of brown adipose tissue was thought to be relevant only in small mammals and infants, with negligible physiologic relevance in adult humans. We performed a systematic examination of the presence, distribution, and activity of brown adipose tissue in lean and obese men during exposure to cold temperature. Brown-adipose-tissue activity was studied in relation to body composition and energy metabolism.

Methods.—We studied 24 healthy men — 10 who were lean (body-mass index [BMI] [the weight in kilograms divided by the square of the height in meters], <25) and 14 who were overweight or obese (BMI, ≥25) — under thermoneutral conditions (22°C) and during mild cold exposure (16°C). Putative brown-adipose-tissue activity was determined with the use of integrated ^{18}F-fluorodeoxyglucose positron-emission tomography and computed tomography. Body composition and energy expenditure were measured with the use of dual-energy x-ray absorptiometry and indirect calorimetry.

Results.—Brown-adipose-tissue activity was observed in 23 of the 24 subjects (96%) during cold exposure but not under thermoneutral conditions. The activity was significantly lower in the overweight or obese subjects than in the lean subjects ($P = 0.007$). BMI and percentage of body fat both had significant negative correlations with brown adipose tissue, whereas resting metabolic rate had a significant positive correlation.

Conclusions.—The percentage of young men with brown adipose tissue is high, but its activity is reduced in men who are overweight or obese. Brown adipose tissue may be metabolically important in men, and the fact that it is reduced yet present in most overweight or obese subjects may make it a target for the treatment of obesity.

▶ Brown adipose tissue (BAT) is a metabolically active fat depot characterized by a high concentration of mitochondria. Uncoupling protein-1 (UCP-1) is an established marker of BAT and resides in the inner mitochondrial membrane.[1] In response to sympathetic nervous stimulation, typically due to cold temperatures, UCP-1 induces a leak in the inner mitochondrial membrane that causes energy to be released as heat.[2] The role of BAT in this nonshivering thermogenesis process has been well established in small mammals and infant humans.[1] For several years, researchers postulated that BAT is present in adult humans and that by manipulating this organ, we may be able to positively affect energy regulation in overweight and obese humans. van Marken Lichtenbelt et al present one of the first studies to demonstrate that BAT is present and metabolically active in adult humans and that BAT activity is associated with body-mass index (BMI) (Fig 1 in the original article). With the use of fluorodeoxyglucose (FDG)-positron emission tomography (PET)/X-ray computed tomography (CT) scan, van Marken Lichtenbelt et al identified BAT throughout the body, but the major depot was concentrated in the supraclavicular region in healthy adult males (Fig 1 in the original article). There was a marked increase in FDG uptake with cold exposure, suggesting that a standardized cold temperature exposure may be necessary to adequately quantify BAT activity in humans. The authors also demonstrated that there was significantly higher BAT tissue volume and activity in cold-exposed lean (BMI 21.3-24.5 kg/m^2) relative to overweight or obese (BMI 25.4-38.7 kg/m^2) individuals (Fig 1 in the original article). BMI and percent body fat determined by dual energy X-ray absorptiometry (DXA) were negatively correlated with BAT activity. Moreover, the authors provide some of the first evidence that BAT may contribute to whole body energy expenditure. Although this study provides strong support for the presence of a BAT in adults and that the activity of this BAT is influenced by cold temperatures and BMI, the study was limited by its smaller size ($N = 24$) and select population, young (18-30 years) healthy adult males. There is evidence to suggest that BAT activity may decrease with age 3, indicating that further investigation is warranted in the aging population. This study, as well as 3 others[3-5] printed simultaneously, provide formidable evidence that there are marked quantities of active BAT in adult humans and that it likely contributes to body weight regulation. These studies present BAT as a novel target for development of therapeutic strategies to regulate adiposity and body weight. Future research should be directed at delineating the mechanisms and physiology of BAT as it relates to whole body energy expenditure.

M. Ruth, PhD

References

1. Porter RK. A new look at UCP-1. *Biochimica et Biophysica Acta.* 2006;1757: 446-448.
2. Celi FS. Brown adipose tissue? When it pays to be inefficient. *N Engl J Med.* 2009; 360:1553.
3. Saito M, Okamatsu-Ogura Y, Matsushita M, et al. High incidence of metabolically active brown adipose tissue in healthy adult humans. *Diabetes.* 2009;58: 1526-1531.
4. Cypess AM, Lehman S, Williams G, et al. Identification and importance of brown adipose tissue in adult humans. *N Engl J Med.* 2009;360:1509-1517.
5. Virtanen KA, Lidell ME, Orava J, et al. Functional brown adipose tissue in healthy adults. *N Engl J Med.* 2009;360:1518-1525.

4 Thyroid

Introduction

A number of studies published last year and selected for the 2010 YEAR BOOK have a great impact on endocrine basic research as well as on the clinical practice in endocrinology.

A study by Horie et al[1] investigated the role of Th17 cells in autoimmune thyroiditis (AIT). Interleukin-17 producing T (Th17) cells have recently been identified as a novel T effector subset. The authors observed increased numbers of Th1 and Th17 cells in spleen and accumulation of both types of effector T cells in the thyroid glands of iodine-fed wild-type mice, indicating that Th17 cells as well as Th1 cells constitute thyroid lesions. Together with other phenomena shown in this article, the results indicate that both Th1 and Th17 cells are critical effector T cell subsets for the pathogenesis of spontaneous autoimmune thyroiditis.

Another paper by Brix et al[2] focused on the role of microchimerism in postpartum thyroiditis. Here, the authors compared the frequency of thyroid autoantibodies (TA) in twin individuals from opposite-sex (OS) and monozygotic (MZ) twin pairs. The authors show a higher prevalence of TA in both females and males from opposite-sex twin pairs compared with a control group of twins from MZ pairs matched for sex.

Assuming that the degree of maternal microchimerism (maternal cells in her progeny) is equal for OS and MZ twin pairs, the observed difference in the frequency of TA could be the result of microchimerism due to in utero bidirectional cell trafficking between twin subjects in OS pairs. These data suggest that microchimerism may play a role in the development of thyroid autoimmunity.

Among the thyroid cancer studies, the published article by Schlumberger et al[3] is one of the best. Here, the authors investigated the use of motesanib diphosphate, an oral multikinase inhibitor in progressive metastasized medullary thyroid cancers (MTC). The authors reported a high rate (>80%) of stable disease in patients who had initially progressive MTC. From the point of view of a clinical endocrinologist, these findings are of major importance because they show that multikinase inhibitors are clinically effective in this patient cohort.

In basic science, a number of brilliant articles have also been published. One of those is the article by Neumann et al[4] published in *Proceedings of the National Academy of Science*. The aim of the study was to identify a new small-molecule TSH receptor (TSHR) agonist. The molecule identified is an agonist for a 7-transmembrane- spanning receptor like the TSHR. The authors could demonstrate that binding of this compound to the TSHR results in an increase of thyroglobulin, thyroperoxidase, and sodium-iodide-symporter mRNA levels, as well as an increase of T4 in mice after administration. Even though chemical optimization is needed, such molecules might be used in the future for stimulating (malignant) thyroid cells in vivo instead of using (expensive) recombinant TSH.

These are just a few examples of very good papers published in 2009. I hope you enjoy reading these selections and find them as informative as I did.

Matthias Schott, MD, PhD

References

1. Horie I, Abiru N, Nagayama Y, et al. T helper type 17 immune response plays an indispensable role for development of iodine-induced autoimmune thyroiditis in nonobese diabetic-H2h4 mice. *Endocrinology.* 2009;150:5135-5142.
2. Brix TH, Hansen PS, Kyvik KO, Hegedüs L. Aggregation of thyroid autoantibodies in twins from opposite-sex pairs suggests that microchimerism may play a role in the early stages of thyroid autoimmunity. *J Clin Endocrinol Metab.* 2009;94:4439-4443.
3. Schlumberger MJ, Elisei R, Bastholt L, et al. Phase II study of safety and efficacy of motesanib in patients with progressive or symptomatic, advanced or metastatic medullary thyroid cancer. *J Clin Oncol.* 2009;27:3794-3801.
4. Neumann S, Huang W, Titus S, et al. Small-molecule agonists for the thyrotropin receptor stimulate thyroid function in human thyrocytes and mice. *Proc Natl Acad Sci U S A.* 2009;106:12471-12476.

Hypothyroidism and Thyroid Autoimmune Disease

Epitope recognition patterns of thyroid peroxidase autoantibodies in healthy individuals and patients with Hashimoto's thyroiditis

Nielsen CH, Brix TH, Gardas A, et al (Rigshospitalet Univ Hosp, Copenhagen, Denmark; Odense Univ Hosp, Denmark; Med Centre of Postgraduate Education, Warsaw, Poland)

Clin Endocrinol 69:664-668, 2008

Objective.—Thyroid peroxidase antibodies (TPOAb) are markers of autoimmune thyroid disease (AITD), including Hashimoto's thyroiditis (HT), but naturally occurring TPOAb are also detectable in healthy, euthyroid individuals. In AITD, circulating TPOAb react mainly with two immunodominant regions (IDR), IDR-A and IDR-B. The present study was undertaken in order to compare the epitope recognition pattern of TPOAb in HT patients and healthy subjects.

Design.—Sera from 21 out of 98 healthy controls were selected on the basis of high TPOAb values, required for determination of TPOAb recognition pattern; as were sera from 92 HT patients.

Measurements.—Measurement of IDR-reactivity was possible in 90 patients and 12 controls. IDR-A-, IDR-B- and non-IDR-A/non-IDR-B-Ab constituted 24 ± 11%, 50 ± 15% and 26 ± 12%, respectively, in the patients. The distribution in the controls was distinctly different, only 12 ± 13% being directed against IDR-A ($P < 0\cdot002$) and 66 ± 22% against IDR-B ($P < 0\cdot002$). Half of the healthy individuals, vs. none of the HT patients, lacked IDR-A reactivity completely ($P < 0\cdot0001$). In HT patients, IDR-B-Ab proportions increased slightly with increasing TPOAb levels ($P < 0\cdot05$), while IDR-B-Ab of the controls showed a strong opposite trend ($P < 0\cdot0001$). Accordingly, the proportion of non-A/non-B-Ab correlated with TPOAb levels in the healthy controls ($P < 0\cdot008$), and an inverse correlation was seen in HT patients ($P < 0\cdot02$).

Conclusion.—The data suggest that TPOAb do not differ only in quantity between HT patients and healthy individuals, but may also follow distinct qualitative patterns. Larger studies are required to confirm this, and to determine whether the propensity to produce antibodies to certain TPO epitopes, for example, IDR-A, is of pathogenic relevance.

▶ It is known that circulating anti-TPO-antibodies in patients with autoimmune thyroid disease (AITD) react mainly with 2 immunodominant regions (IDR), IDR-A and IDR-B. The aim of this study by Nielson et al was to investigate epitope recognition pattern of thyroid peroxidase antibodies (TPOAb) in Hashimto's thyroiditis (HT) patients. In the HT patients examined in this study, the distribution of IDR-A-, IDR-B-, and non-IDR-A/non-IDR-B antibodies (24%, 50% and 26%, respectively) accords with the distribution in previous studies.[1] By contrast, TPOAb of the controls exhibited a different overall distribution with a smaller fraction (12%) being directed against IDR-A. In fact, half of the controls with measurable IDR-reactivity had no anti-IDR-A activity at all. Moreover, the epitope recognition pattern of TPOAb from controls with high TPOAb levels differed from that of HT patients by containing a relatively high proportion of TPOAb directed against non-A/non-B epitopes. The HT patients and the healthy controls differed considerably in age, but this difference could not account for the differences in TPOAb reactivity as the epitope recognition patterns of young and elderly patients were essentially identical. Although the authors cannot entirely rule out that the assay used for measurement of IDR-reactivity was biased toward measurement of low fractions of IDR-A-Ab at low TPOAb levels, they regarded it unlikely that such a bias could explain the high prevalence of anti-IDR-A-negative healthy individuals, as 21 ± 18% of the antibody activity was directed against IDR-A in 6 HT patients with TPOAb levels below 160 IU/ml. In summary, the authors conclude that a substantial fraction of healthy euthyroid individuals with high serum TPOAb levels lack antibodies directed against the IDR-A epitope on TPO, and, in contrast with sera from HT patients, exhibit increasing fractions of non-A/non-B antibodies with increasing TPOAb levels. On this basis, the authors put forward the hypothesis that TPOAb from healthy individuals and HT patients differ in recognition patterns. These informations are important for the understanding of the pathogenesis of HT. Nonetheless, much more important, in my eyes, are details of reactions on the cellular level. Almost no data are available on the recognition pattern of cytotoxic T cell infiltrating the thyroid gland. Therefore, tetramer analysis of peripheral CTLs as well as of thyroid infiltrating CD8 +T cells should be performed. This will help to exactly characterize the cellular immune response in HT.

M. Schott, MD, PhD

Reference

1. Jastrzebska-Bohaterewicz E, Gardas A. Proportion of antibodies to the A and B immunodominant regions of thyroid peroxidase in Graves and Hashimoto disease. *Autoimmunity.* 2004;37:211-216.

Aggregation of Thyroid Autoantibodies in Twins from Opposite-Sex Pairs Suggests that Microchimerism May Play a Role in the Early Stages of Thyroid Autoimmunity

Brix TH, Hansen PS, Kyvik KO, et al (Odense Univ Hosp, Denmark; Univ of Southern Denmark, Odense)

J Clin Endocrinol Metab 94:4439-4443, 2009

Context.—Microchimerism is the presence of small populations of cells from one individual in another genetically distinct individual. This phenomenon can arise from pregnancy, blood transfusion, or bidirectional cell trafficking between twins in utero. Microchimerism has recently been proposed to play a role in the pathogenesis of thyroid autoimmunity. In that case, twins from opposite-sex pairs (OS) should have an increased risk of thyroid autoantibodies (TA).

Aim.—The aim of the study was to compare the frequency of TA in twin individuals from OS and monozygotic (MZ) twin pairs.

Design.—This was a case-control study of 240 individuals (120 females and 120 males) from OS twin pairs (cases) and 568 control individuals from MZ pairs (284 females and 284 males).

Methods.—Antibodies toward thyroid peroxidase (TPOAb), thyroglobulin (TgAb), and the TSH receptor (TSHRAb) were measured and considered positive if greater than 60 U/ml, greater than 60 U/ml, and greater than 1.0 U/liter, respectively.

Results.—The frequency of TPOAb, TgAb, and TSHRAb among female cases was 15.0, 5.0, and 4.2%, respectively, which was higher than the corresponding prevalences in the female control population: 7.4% ($P = 0.018$), 1.1% ($P = 0.023$), and 0.7% ($P = 0.026$), respectively. However, when corrected for the number of phenotypes studied (TPOAb, TgAb, TSHRAb, and any thyroid antibody), the association remained significant only in the combined group, $P_{corrected} = 0.012$. Essentially similar results were obtained in males.

TABLE 2.—Unadjusted and Adjusted Odds Ratios with 95% Confidence Intervals for the Association Between TPOAb, TgAb, and TSHRAb and Being a Twin from OS Pairs

Sex	Phenotype	Odds Ratio	*P* Value	Odds Ratio[a]	*P* Value	Odds Ratio[b]	*P* Value
Female	TPOAb	2.2 (1.1 – 4.3)	0.020	2.1 (1.1 – 4.1)	0.034	1.9 (0.9 – 3.9)	0.065
	TgAb	4.9 (1.2 – 20.1)	0.026	4.7 (1.2 – 19.3)	0.031	4.4 (1.1 – 18.1)	0.043
	TSHRAb	6.1 (1.2 – 32.1)	0.032	5.9 (1.1 – 31.2)	0.035	6.0 (1.1 – 31.5)	0.034
	Any thyroid antibody[c]	2.6 (1.4 – 4.8)	0.004	2.4 (1.3 – 4.6)	0.006	2.3 (1.2 – 4.4)	0.011
Male	TPOAb	3.7 (1.0 – 13.3)	0.046	3.3 (0.9 – 12.2)	0.080	3.3 (0.9 – 12.7)	0.077
	TgAb	2.4 (0.7 – 8.5)	0.167	2.9 (0.8 – 10.8)	0.105	3.0 (0.8 – 11.1)	0.104
	TSHRAb	3.2 (0.7 – 14.7)	0.129	4.5 (0.9 – 21.5)	0.063	4.5 (0.9 – 21.5)	0.063
	Any thyroid antibody[c]	4.0 (1.7 – 9.6)	0.002	4.5 (1.8 – 11.1)	0.001	4.6 (1.9 – 11.2)	0.001

[a]Adjusted for age and smoking habits.
[b]Adjusted for age, smoking habits, and serum TSH.
[c]Subjects were considered as antibody positive if TPOAb, TgAb, or TSHRAb was positive.

Conclusion.—Both female and male twins from OS pairs, as opposed to MZ pairs, have an increased frequency of TA, indicating a potential role of microchimerism in developing TA (Table 2).

▶ The aim of this study was to compare the frequency of thyroid autoantibodies (TA) in twin individuals from opposite-sex (OS) and monozygotic (MZ) twin pairs. The authors show a higher prevalence of TA in both females and males from OS twin pairs compared with a control group of twins from MZ pairs matched for sex (Table 2).

Assuming that the degree of maternal microchimerism (maternal cells in her progeny) is equal for OS and MZ twin pairs, the observed difference in the frequency of TA could be the result of microchimerism due to in utero bidirectional cell trafficking between twin subjects in OS pairs. It is, however, important to point out that the authors have not de facto measured or identified the presence of microchimerism in the thyroid. Nonetheless, these data suggest that microchimerism may play a role in the development of thyroid autoimmunity.

M. Schott, MD, PhD

Immune Response of Mice Transgenic for Human Histocompatibility Leukocyte Antigen-DR to Human Thyrotropin Receptor-Extracellular Domain

Inaba H, Pan D, Shin Y-H, et al (Brown Univ, Providence, RI; Univ of Rhode Island; et al)
Thyroid 19:1271-1280, 2009

Background.—Hyperthyroidism of Graves' disease is caused by autoantibodies to human thyrotropin receptor (hTSH-R). To elucidate important T-cell epitopes in TSH-R, we studied three models of immunity to TSH-R in mice.

Methods.—Mice transgenic for histocompatibility leukocyte antigen DR3 or DR2 were immunized with cDNA for hTSH-R-extracellular domain (hTSH-R-ECD), or hTSH-R-ECD protein, or hTSH-R peptide epitopes. Proliferative responses of immunized splenocytes to epitopes derived from the hTSH-ECD sequence, anti-TSH-R antibody responses, serum thyroxine and TSH, and thyroid histology were recorded.

Results.—DR3 mice responded to genomic immunization with proliferative responses to several epitopes, which increased in intensity and spread to include more epitopes, during a 6-week immunization program. DR2 transgenic mice developed weak proliferative responses. Both types of mice developed anti-TSH-R antibodies measured by enzyme-linked immunosorbent assay or TSH-binding inhibition assay in 16–60% of animals. There was evidence of weak thyroid stimulation in one group of animals. Immunization of DR3 transgenic mice to hTSH-R-ECD protein induced a striking response to an epitope with sequence ISRIYVSIDVTLQQLES (aa78–94). Immunization to peptides derived from the TSH-R-ECD sequence (including aa78–94) caused strong responses to the epitopes, and development of immune responses to several other nonoverlapping epitopes within the hTSH sequence (epitope spreading) and antibodies reacting with hTSH-R. This implies that immunization with hTSH-R epitopes produced immunity to mouse TSH-R.

Conclusion.—T-cell and B-cell responses to genetic immunization differ in DR3 and DR2 transgenic mice, and there is less genetic control of antibody than of T-cell responses. During both genomic and peptide epitope immunization there was evidence of epitope spreading during the immunization. Several functionally important epitopes are evident, especially aa78–94. However, if similar progressive epitope recruitment occurs in human disease, epitope-based therapy will be difficult to achieve.

▶ Development of the autoimmune reaction in Graves' disease (GD) involves the uptake and presentation of immunogenic epitopes of human thyrotropin receptor (hTSH-R) by histocompatibility leukocyte antigen (HLA) class II molecules on the surface of antigen-presenting cells. This allows interaction of the DR-epitope complex with the T-cell receptor on $CD4^{+}T$ cells and leads to activation of the T cell, which in turn produces signals that help B cells produce pathogenic antibodies. The aim of the study by Inaba et al was to evaluate the epitope progression in response to cDNA vaccination depending on the HLA type of the mice used. In this study, DR3 transgenic mice responded to immunization using TSH-R-ECD DNA with a much more intense T-cell response to TSH-R epitopes than did DR2+ transgenics, but DR2+ mice produced a similar antibody response (Fig 5 in the original article). The implication of this difference is not certain, but DR3 is associated with GD, and this may imply that the T-cell response is as important in determining GD as is the ability to produce antibodies. The antibodies produced in this study clearly reacted with TSH-R protein and mildly stimulated the thyroid production of T4, but did not cause clear hyperthyroidism, indicating that they are primarily TSH-R-ECD binding, but not stimulating antibodies. DR3+ transgenic mice were studied on the assumption that they would be more prone to develop anti-TSH-R immunity than other mice, in parallel with the known importance of DR3 in propensity to develop GD in humans. DR2+ transgenics were presumed to represent a relatively neutral DR genotype. The difference in the T-cell response between DR3+ and DR2+ mice is quite striking and supports the relative importance of DR3 in the development of anti-TSH-R immunity.

M. Schott, MD, PhD

T Helper Type 17 Immune Response Plays an Indispensable Role for Development of Iodine-Induced Autoimmune Thyroiditis in Nonobese Diabetic-H2^{h4} Mice

Horie I, Abiru N, Nagayama Y, et al (Nagasaki Univ Graduate School of Biomedical Sciences, Japan; et al)
Endocrinology 150:5135-5142, 2009

T helper type 1(Th1)/Th2 paradigm has been expanded by discovery of a novel effector T cell (T_{eff}) subset, Th17 cells, which produce a proinflammatory cytokine IL-17. Th17 cells have recently been shown to play a major role in numerous autoimmune diseases that had previously been thought to be Th1-dominant diseases. We here studied the significance of Th17 cells in iodine-induced autoimmune thyroiditis in nonobese diabetic-H2^{h4} mice, a mouse model of Hashimoto's thyroiditis in humans, which spontaneously develop antithyroglobulin autoantibodies and intrathyroidal lymphocyte infiltration when supplied with iodine in the drinking water. We observed increased numbers of Th1 and Th17 cells in spleen and accumulation of both types of T_{eff} in the thyroid glands of iodine-fed wild-type mice, indicating that Th17 cells as well as Th1 cells constitute thyroid lesions. Furthermore, the incidence and severity of intrathyroidal lymphocyte infiltration, and the titers of antithyroglobulin autoantibodies were markedly reduced in iodine-treated IL-17$^{-/-}$ mice as compared with wild-type mice. Of interest, IL-17$^{+/-}$ mice showed an intermediate phenotype. Therefore, the present study, together with a previous report demonstrating the importance of Th1, not Th2, immune response for developing thyroiditis using mice deficient for interferon-γ or IL-4, clearly indicates that both Th1 and Th17 cells are critical T_{eff} subsets for the pathogenesis of spontaneous autoimmune thyroiditis in nonobese diabetic-H2^{h4} mice.

▶ Regarding CD4^{+} T cells, this T cell subpopulation can largely be divided into 2 different subsets with distinct differentiation profiles and functional characteristics; CD25 negative effector T cells (T_{eff}) and CD25 positive regulatory T cells, which positively and negatively, respectively, regulate immune responses.[1] The former subset has long been thought to be represented by T helper type 1 (Th1) and Th2 cells,[2] but interleukin (IL)-17 producing T (Th17) cells have recently been identified as a novel T_{eff} subset.[3] Although the pathogenesis of most of autoimmune diseases has long been argued on relative balance between Th1 versus Th2, recent studies revealed that Th17 immune responses play a major role in numerous autoimmune diseases, such as multiple sclerosis/experimental autoimmune encephalitis (EAE) and many others. The aim of this study was to investigate the role of Th17 cells in autoimmune thyroiditis (AIT). The authors observed increased numbers of Th1 and Th17 cells in spleen and accumulation of both types of T_{eff} in the thyroid glands of iodine-fed wild-type mice, indicating that Th17 cells and Th1 cells constitute thyroid lesions (Fig 2 in the original article). The thyroiditis score is shown in Fig 1 in the original article. Furthermore, the incidence and severity of intrathyroidal lymphocyte infiltration and the titers of antithyroglobulin autoantibodies were markedly reduced in iodine-treated IL-17 double negative mice as compared with wild-type mice (Fig 3 in the original article). Of interest, IL-17 double negative mice showed an intermediate phenotype. Therefore, this study clearly indicates that both Th1 and Th17 cells are critical T_{eff} subsets for the pathogenesis of spontaneous AIT at least in this type of mouse used for this study.

M. Schott, MD, PhD

References

1. Bettelli E, Oukka M, Kuchroo VK. T(H)-17 cells in the circle of immunity and autoimmunity. *Nat Immunol.* 2007;8:345-350.
2. Mosmann TR, Coffman RL. TH1 and TH2 cells: different patterns of lymphokine secretion lead to different functional properties. *Annu Rev Immunol.* 1989;7: 145-173.
3. Harrington LE, Hatton RD, Mangan PR, et al. Interleukin 17-producing CD4+ effector T cells develop via a lineage distinct from the T helper type 1 and 2 lineages. *Nat Immunol.* 2005;6:1123-1132.

Programmed Death Ligand 1 (*PD-L1*) Gene Variants Contribute To Autoimmune Addison's Disease and Graves' Disease Susceptibility

Mitchell AL, Cordell HJ, Soemedi R, et al (Newcastle Univ, UK; et al)
J Clin Endocrinol Metab 94:5139-5145, 2009

Context.—Despite much investigation, a substantial amount of the genetic susceptibility to autoimmune diseases remains unaccounted for. Recently, a single-nucleotide polymorphism (SNP) in the programmed death ligand 1 (*PD-L1*) gene has been associated with Graves' disease (GD) in a Japanese patient cohort. Our aim was to determine whether variants in *PD-L1* are also associated with autoimmune Addison's disease (AAD) and to replicate the previous association in patients with GD from the United Kingdom.

Design and Patients.—We analyzed eight SNPs within *PD-L1* in a United Kingdom cohort of 315 AAD subjects and 316 healthy controls. We then replicated our experiment in a cohort of 342 Norwegian AAD cases and 379 controls and in 496 United Kingdom GD subjects.

Results.—Three of the eight SNPs studied, part of a haplotype block in the *PD-L1* gene, showed modest association with both AAD and GD in

TABLE 2.—Structure and Frequency of the Two most Common Haplotypes in the Different Populations at the Three most Associated Markers (1, *RS822339*; 3, *RS2282055*; 7, *RS1411262*)

	United Kingdom Cohort			Norwegian Cohort	
Haplotype	AAD (%)	GD (%)	Control (%)	AAD (%)	Control (%)
Markers 1-3-7					
G-T-C	457 (74.6)	703 (76.1)	386 (69.7)	524 (79.2)	526 (74.7)
A-G-T	155 (25.3)	221 (23.9)	168 (30.3)	138 (20.9)	178 (25.2)
P value	0.057	**0.007**		0.052	

P values are shown, with statistically significant results in *bold.*

the United Kingdom cohort, with maximum evidence at the marker *RS1411262* [United Kingdom AAD odds ratio 1.33 (5–95% confidence interval 1.02–1.73), $P_{(genotype)} = 0.028$; GD odds ratio 1.36 (5–95% confidence interval 1.07–1.72), $P_{(genotype)} = 0.033$]. Association with genotypes at the same three markers was confirmed in the Norwegian AAD cohort [$P_{(genotype)} = 0.011–0.020$]. A recessive effect at the most associated alleles was observed in both the AAD and GD cohorts.

Conclusions.—We confirm the role of *PD-L1* variants in GD susceptibility and extend these findings to demonstrate association in two Northern European patient cohorts with AAD. *PD-L1* joins the growing number of known susceptibility loci exerting modest effects in these autoimmune disorders (Table 2).

▶ Graves' disease (GD) is a common autoimmune disease. There are several susceptibility loci known for GD. These susceptibility loci have been discovered, mostly through candidate gene studies. Association with alleles of the major histocompatibility complex region, including human leukocyte antigen (HLA) and variants at other genes located on chromosome 6p21, has been widely reported. In addition, alleles of the cytotoxic T lymphocyte antigen-4 gene (*CTLA4*) and the Fc receptor-like-3 gene (*FCRL3*) have been associated with GD. Additional disease-specific loci have been found, such as the thyroid-stimulating hormone (TSH) receptor and thyroglobulin. Another potential gene locus may represent the programmed death ligand 1 (PD-L1, also called CD274 or B7-H1). It is a ligand for the programmed death 1 (PDCD-1, PD-1) molecule, which is a member of the CD28/CTLA4 costimulatory family of cell surface receptors. The PDCD-1/PD-L1 interaction is thought to have a central role in down regulating cytokine production and T-cell responses and therefore in maintaining immune tolerance. The gene encoding PD-L1 is located on the short arm of chromosome 9 (9p24) spanning 17.9 kb and includes 7 exons, 6 of which are coding. The PD-L1 gene is highly conserved, particularly in higher mammals, with many species having an orthologous gene, suggesting functional importance in multiple species. In humans, the association of PDCD-1 gene polymorphisms with autoimmune disease has been widely reported, for example, in systemic lupus erythematosus, type 1 diabetes mellitus, and rheumatoid arthritis. The aim of this study was to determine whether variants in PD-L1 are also associated with GD and with autoimmune Addison disease. As shown in Table 2, there is a clear association between the 2 common haplotypes. These data confirm that variants within the PD-L1 gene are associated with GD in a large cohort (in the United Kingdom). This report also adds to the growing number of known susceptibility loci exerting modest effects in GD.

M. Schott, MD, PhD

Prevalence and Functional Significance of Thyrotropin Receptor Blocking Antibodies in Children and Adolescents with Chronic Lymphocytic Thyroiditis

Feingold SB, Smith J, Houtz J, et al (Harvard Univ School of Medicine, Boston, MA; Diagnostic Hybrids, Inc., Athens, OH)

J Clin Endocrinol Metab 94:4742-4748, 2009

Context.—TSH receptor (TSHR) blocking antibodies (Abs) inhibit TSH-induced thyroid growth and function insomeadults with chronic lymphocytic thyroiditis (CLT), but their role in the pediatric age range is unknown.

Objectives.—Our objectives were: 1) to determine the prevalence of TSHR blocking Abs in children and adolescents with CLT and 2) assess their functional significance both *in vivo* and *in vitro*.

Design and Setting.—This was a retrospective study in a referral outpatient setting.

Patients.—Sera from a total of 87 CLT patients and 33 controls were studied.

Main Outcome Measures.—TSHR Abs were measured by both ELISA and bioassay.

Results.—Eight of 87 children and adolescents with CLT (9.2%), including one as young as 4 yr of age, had TSHR Abs in serum as measured by ELISA. The prevalence was significantly higher in individuals whose serum TSH concentration was 20 mU/liter or greater within 3 months of study than in less hypothyroid patients (eight of 45 *vs.* none of 42, $P < 0.005$). Conversely, TSHR Ab-positive patients were significantly more hypothyroid at diagnosis but onlywhenthe analysis was restricted to those with severe hypothyroidismwasa decreased prevalence of goiter observed. IgG purified from TSHR Ab sera retained the TSH binding-inhibitory activity and TSHR Ab-positive sera inhibited TSH-induced stimulation of cAMP significantly more than normal.

Conclusions.—TSHR-blocking Abs contribute significantly to the severity of the hypothyroidism in some children with CLT, but as compared with adults, they appear to play less of a role in determining the presence or absence of a goiter.

▶ Although numerous studies have evaluated the prevalence of TSH receptor (TSHR)-blocking antibodies in adults with chronic lymphocytic thyroiditis

(CLT), there are very few data published on children and adolescents. This study by Feingold et al establishes unequivocally that these antibodies occur in the pediatric population as well, including children as young as 4 years of age, and that, as in the adults, they play an important role in the observed hypothyroidism in these individuals. Overall, significant TSH-binding inhibitory activity was observed in 8 of 87 children and adolescents with CLT (9.2%) and only in patients whose serum TSH was 20 mU/L or greater within 3 months of study (Fig 1 in the original article). Furthermore, TSHR antibody-positive patients were significantly more hypothyroid at diagnosis than TSHR antibody-negative individuals strongly supporting an etiological role. These findings are consistent with similar studies in adults in which these antibodies were found almost exclusively in hypothyroid patients[1] and probably explain failure in this study to find TSHR antibodies previously in euthyroid children with CLT.[2] In view of their relatively low prevalence, TSHR-blocking antibodies are but one of a number of immunopathogenic mechanisms contributing to thyroid gland failure in this patient population. A limitation of this retrospective study was that many of the patients included were being treated. Nonetheless, these data suggest that TSHR-blocking antibodies may remain elevated indefinitely in individuals with extremely elevated concentrations in serum. In addition, there appears to be an increased prevalence of TSHR-blocking antibodies in patients with Down syndrome (as shown in this article).

M. Schott, MD, PhD

References

1. Chiovato L, Vitti P, Santini F, et al. Incidence of antibodies blocking thyrotropin effect in vitro in patients with euthyroid or hypothyroid autoimmune thyroiditis. *J Clin Endocrinol Metab.* 1990;71:40-45.
2. Smith J, Brown RS. Persistence of thyrotropin (TSH) receptor antibodies in children and adolescents with Graves' disease treated using antithyroid medication. *Thyroid.* 2007;17:1103-1107.

A Stimulatory Thyrotropin Receptor Antibody (M22) and Thyrotropin Increase Interleukin-6 Expression and Secretion in Graves' Orbital Preadipocyte Fibroblasts

Kumar S, Schiefer R, Coenen MJ, et al (Mayo Clinic, Rochester, MN)
Thyroid 20:59-65, 2010

Background.—Patients with Graves' ophthalmopathy (GO) have circulating autoantibodies directed against the thyrotropin receptor (TSHR) and elevated levels of the proinflammatory cytokine interleukin-6 (IL-6) in both serum and orbital tissues. We hypothesized that these autoantibodies might increase IL-6 expression and secretion in preadipocyte fibroblasts and adipocytes from patients with GO, and thus directly impact the clinical activity of the disease.

Methods.—*IL-6* mRNA levels were measured in cultures of GO orbital preadipocytes ($n = 3$) treated during adipocyte differentiation with a monoclonal stimulatory TSHR antibody (M22; 10 ng/mL), IL-6 (1 ng/mL), or TSH (10 U/L). Additionally, levels of IL-6 protein secretion were assessed after adipocyte differentiation in orbital cultures exposed to TSH or M22 for 24 or 48 hours ($n = 8$). *IL-6* mRNA levels were also measured in orbital adipose tissue specimens from well-characterized GO patients ($n = 9$) and normal individuals ($n = 9$).

Results.—Treatment of GO orbital preadipocyte cultures with IL-6, TSH, or M22 during adipocyte differentiation resulted in increased *IL-6* mRNA levels (3.1-fold, 2.9-fold, and 2.7-fold, respectively; $p < 0.05$). Treatment of orbital cultures with M22 or TSH after adipocyte differentiation enhanced the release of IL-6 protein into the medium at both 24 and 48 hours for TSH (mean 1.9- and 2.3-fold; $p = 0.002$ and 0.015, respectively) and at 48 hours for M22 (mean 2.0-fold; $p = 0.005$). In addition, we found mean IL-6 mRNA levels to be significantly increased in GO orbital adipose tissue specimens (10-fold; $p < 0.01$), primarily attributable to high levels in three of the four patients with clinical activity scores ≥5.

Conclusions.—Both TSH and M22 increase *IL-6* expression in orbital preadipocyte fibroblasts and *IL-6* secretion by mature adipocytes. These results suggest that circulating TSHR autoantibodies in GO might play a direct role in the clinical activity of the disease.

▶ The aim of this study by Kumar et al was to investigate interleukin-6 (IL-6) expression and secretion in preadipocyte fibroblasts and adipocytes from patients with Graves' ophthalmopathy (GO), which may have a direct impact on the clinical activity of the disease. Orbital adipocytes have already been shown to express the TSH receptor (TSHR), and levels of circulating autoantibodies targeting the TSHR have been shown to correlate with the clinical activity score in patients with GO. The authors could demonstrate that treatment with the monoclonal (stimulating) TSHR antibody M22 enhanced both IL-6 mRNA levels during adipocyte differentiation (Fig 1 in the original article) and IL-6 protein secretion by mature adipocytes (Fig 2 in the original article). These findings are consistent with a previous report showing that TSH stimulates IL-6 in cultured 3T3-L1 and human abdominal adipose cells.[1,2] It might be discussed that the possible increase in the clinical activity score observed in some patients with GO in this study is due to the hypothyroidism with elevated TSH levels after radioiodine ablation for hyperthyroidism. Another potential limitation of this study is that the normal control orbital tissue was obtained at very early autopsy from patients (without GO) whose corneas had been harvested for transplantation. Nonetheless, the data show that TSH and the stimulatory TSHR antibody M22 increase IL-6 expression in cultured orbital preadipocytes, and that both TSH and M22 stimulate IL-6 protein secretion by mature orbital adipocytes. These findings suggest that circulating autoantibodies directed against the TSHR in Graves' disease may act to increase IL-6 levels and secretion within the orbit, and that IL-6 in turn may act locally to stimulate its own production. In addition, the B-cell differentiating effects of

IL-6 may lead to further production of TSHR autoantibodies within the orbit in GO.

M. Schott, MD, PhD

References

1. Antunes TT, Gagnon A, Chen B, Pacini F, Smith TJ, Sorisky A. Interleukin-6 release from human abdominal adipose cells is regulated by thyroid-stimulating hormone: effect of adipocyte differentiation and anatomic depot. *Am J Physiol Endocrinol Metab*. 2006;290:E1140-E1144.
2. Bell A, Gagnon A, Sorisky A. TSH stimulates IL-6 secretion from adipocytes in culture. *Arterioscler Thromb Vasc Biol*. 2003;23:e65-e66.

Technical Evaluation of the first fully automated assay for the detection of TSH receptor autoantibodies

Hermsen D, Broecker-Preuss M, Casati M, et al (Univ Hosp Duesseldorf, Germany; Univ Hosp Essen, Germany; San Gerardo Hosp, Monza, Italy; et al)
Clin Chim Acta 401:84-89, 2009

Background.—Graves' disease (GD) is mediated by autoantibodies which bind to the TSH receptor (TRAb). The aim of the present study was to evaluate the technical performance of the first fully automated immunoassay for TRAb detection.

Methods.—The Elecsys® Anti-TSHR immunoassay utilizes a porcine TSH receptor (TSHR) and the human thyroid stimulating monoclonal TSHR autoantibody M22.

Results.—Intraassay and total imprecision CV were determined between 1.4%–14.9%, and 2.4%–28.8%, respectively. Using the 20% CV criteria the functional sensitivity was found at 0.73 IU/L. The median CV at the cut-off (1.75 IU/L) was found to be 11%. Comparison studies with five TRAb immunoassays yielded slopes and intercepts between 1.02–1.48, and −0.74–0.56, respectively. Correlation coefficients were determined between 0.895 and 0.978. ROC plot analysis of patients with GD, patients with other thyroid disorders and healthy controls revealed an AUC of 0.99 resulting in a sensitivity of 97% and a specificity of 99% at a TRAb level of 1.75 IU/L.

Conclusion.—The evaluation of the TRAb immunoassay generated homogeneous performance data and demonstrated a high degree of comparability to established TRAb assays. The automated TRAb assay represents a major improvement of thyroid testing in clinical practice.

▶ Over the last few decades, a great improvement has been achieved with regard to TSH receptor autoantibody (TRAb) detection methodologies.[1-5] At present, the bioassay and competitive TSH-binding inhibition assays are the 2 established principles of TRAb detection (reviewed in Ref 4) with the competitive assays being the only validated routine tests for TRAb analysis.[1,2,6,7] Traditionally, these assays are based on the ability of TRAb to

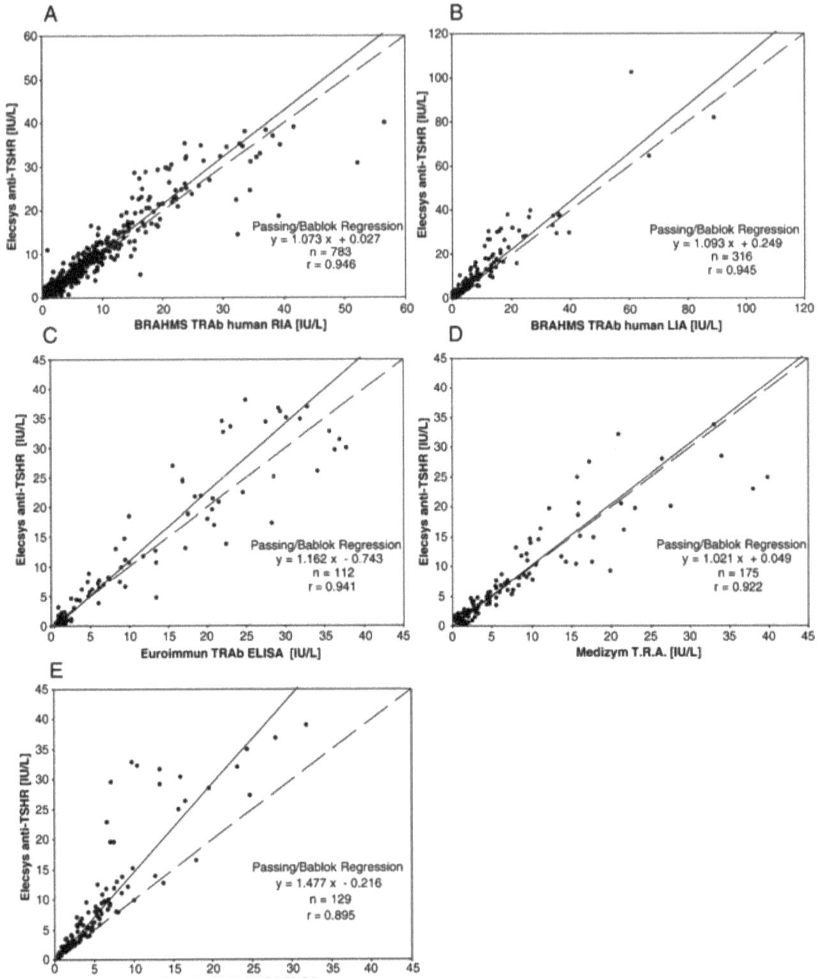

FIGURE 2.—(A–E): Representative plots of the method comparison study. Fig. 2A and B shows pooled comparison data of three sites. (Reprinted from Hermsen D, Broecker-Preuss M, Casati M, et al. Technical evaluation of the first fully automated assay for the detection of TSH receptor autoantibodies. *Clin Chim Acta*. 2009;401:84-89, with permission from Elsevier.)

inhibit TSHR binding by labelled bovine TSH because purified bovine TSH has higher affinity toward the TSH receptor than human TSH and is a more suitable ligand for ^{125}I or biotin labelling.[4] Among those, the recombinant human TSHR-based assay in combination with labelled bovine TSH is still the gold standard with highest sensitivity and specificity,[5,8] even though other TRAb hand assays with solid phase technology have been improved as well.[8] Recently, alternatives to bovine TSH have become available for use in competitive assays.[5,9] In 2002, Sanders et al developed a new assay with labelled mouse thyroid-stimulating monoclonal antibodies, and TSHR binding was

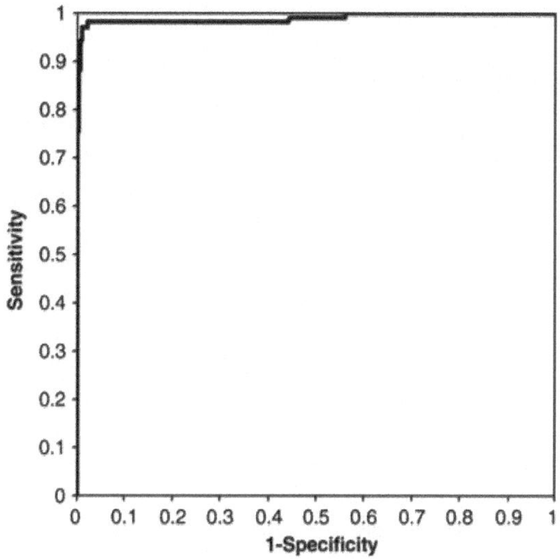

FIGURE 3.—Determination of the cut-off limit for positivity of the Elecsys Anti-TSHR assay. The ROC analysis was performed in 102 patients with untreated Graves' disease (sensitivity cohort), 210 patients with other thyroid diseases and 436 apparently healthy individuals (specificity cohort). The optimal cut off limit was calculated at 1.75 IU/L (sensitivity 97%, specificity 99%). AUC 0.99 (95% CI: 0.98–1.0). (Reprinted from Hermsen D, Broecker-Preuss M, Casati M, et al. Technical evaluation of the first fully automated assay for the detection of TSH receptor autoantibodies. *Clin Chim Acta.* 2009;401:84-89, with permission from Elsevier.)

shown to be inhibited in a similar way to inhibition of labelled bovine TSH binding.[5] More recently, the same group reported a new procedure for measuring TRAb in patient serum.[9] In this new assay system, bound TRAb are detected by their ability to inhibit the binding of labelled human monoclonal thyroid-stimulating antibody (M22) to porcine TSHR-coated ELISA plates. One study of these inventors claimed a 100% specificity and 95% sensitivity for this assay.[9] Moreover, inhibition of M22 binding to the TSHR was closely correlated to inhibition of TSH binding by the sera of tested GD patients. In this study, the inhibition of M22 binding was almost always greater, indicating an improvement of sensitivity and precision.[9] Until now, 3 comparison studies have been published. Two studies were conducted by Kamijo et al who found that the new M22-biotin-based ELISA was superior to TSH-biotin-based second generation porcine ELISA in terms of diagnostic sensitivity and specificity.[10,11] Another evaluation of this assay has, however, revealed a relatively poor precision (CV > 20%) at the recommended cut-off level for positivity.[12]

The drawbacks of all manually performed assays independent of their individual sensitivity, specificity, and intra- and interassay coefficients of variation are, however, the typically long incubation times and the intense manpower needed to perform these assays. Most recently, a new rapid and fully automated TRAb assay has been established.[13] This assay system also uses the M22 human monoclonal antibody for competing against the patient's TSH receptor autoantibodies to be detected. The aim of this study by Hermsen et al was to technically evaluate this new automated system. The authors could demonstrate that this assay has a high sensitivity and specificity as well as homogeneous performance data and a high degree of comparability to the established manual TRAb assays (Fig 2 and Fig 3). In my eyes, this assay may represent the future technology for TRAb detection in clinical practice.

S. Schinner, MD, PhD

References

1. Smith BR, Sanders J, Furmaniak J. TSH receptor antibodies. *Thyroid.* 2007;17: 923-938.
2. Schott M, Scherbaum WA, Morgenthaler NG. Thyrotropin receptor autoantibodies in Graves' disease. *Trends Endocrinol Metab.* 2005;16:243-248.
3. Costagliola S, Morgenthaler NG, Hoermann R, et al. Second generation assay for thyrotropin receptor antibodies has superior diagnostic sensitivity for Graves' disease. *J Clin Endocrinol Metab.* 1999;84:90-97.
4. Morgenthaler NG. New assay systems for thyrotropin receptor antibodies. *Curr Opin Endocrinol Diabetes.* 1999;6:251-260.
5. Sanders J, Jeffreys J, Depraetere H, et al. Thyroid-stimulating monoclonal antibodies. *Thyroid.* 2002;12:1043-1050.
6. Pedersen IB, Knudsen N, Perrild H, Ovesen L, Laurberg P. TSH-receptor antibody measurement for differentiation of hyperthyroidism into Graves' disease and multinodular toxic goitre: a comparison of two competitive binding assays. *Clin Endocrinol (Oxf).* 2001;55:381-390.
7. Cappelli C, Gandossi E, Castellano M, et al. Prognostic value of thyrotropin receptor antibodies (TRAb) in Graves' disease: a 120 months prospective study. *Endocr J.* 2007;54:713-720.
8. Hermsen D, Liu D, Domberg J, et al. Comparison of a solid phase human- versus porcine- thyrotropin receptor-based immunoassay for the measurement of thyrotropin receptor antibodies assays in patients with thyroid diseases. *Exp Clin Endocrinol Diabetes.* 2008;116:S59-63.
9. Smith BR, Bolton J, Young S, et al. A new assay for thyrotropin receptor autoantibodies. *Thyroid.* 2004;14:830-835.
10. Kamijo K. TSH-receptor antibody measurement in patients with various thyrotoxicosis and Hashimoto's thyroiditis: a comparison of two two-step assays, coated plate ELISA using porcine TSH-receptor and coated tube radioassay using human recombinant TSH-receptor. *Endocr J.* 2003;50:113-116.
11. Kamijo K. TSH-receptor antibodies determined by the first, second and third generation assays and thyroid-stimulating antibody in pregnant patients with Graves' disease. *Endocr J.* 2007;54:619-624.
12. Liu C, Hermsen D, Domberg J, et al. Comparison of M22-based ELISA and human-TSH-receptor-based luminescence assay for the measurement of thyrotropin receptor antibodies in patients with thyroid diseases. *Horm Metab Res.* 2008;40:479-483.
13. Gassner D, Golla R, Stock W, Yoshimura Noh J, Sanders J, Smith RB. Development of a new automated assay for thyrotropin receptor autoantibodies on the elecsys system. *Clin Chem.* 2007;53:C-135.

Graves' Orbitopathy Activation after Radioactive Iodine Therapy with and without Steroid Prophylaxis

Vannucchi G, Campi I, Covelli D, et al (Univ of Milan, Italy; et al)

J Clin Endocrinol Metab 94:3381-3386, 2009

Context.—The reactivation of Graves' orbitopathy (GO) after radioiodine (RAI) for Graves' disease (GD) is a known effect, and its clinical relevance is controversial. Prevention of RAI-induced GO activation is possible in at-risk patients with oral glucocorticoids (OGC).

Objectives.—The aim of the study was to analyze the effects of RAI on GO with or without prophylactic steroids based on known risk factors and to compare the effectiveness of prophylaxis with iv glucocorticoids (IVGC) and OGC.

Design.—We conducted a retrospective study in which patients were assessed before and 1–12 months after RAI.

Patients and Setting.—A total of 113 patients were included in the study; 83 underwent RAI without prophylactic steroids for the absence of risk of activation, and 30 were treated with either OGC (n = 21) or IVGC (n = 9).

Main Outcome Measures.—We analyzed the prevalence of GO activation with or without steroid prophylaxis and the difference in the prevalence of GO activation after OGC or IVGC.

Results.—GO activation was observed in 7.2% of patients without and 33.3% of patients with steroid prophylaxis ($P < 0.0001$), for an overall prevalence of 14.6%. GO activation occurred in 47.6% of patients treated with OGC but in none of the nine patients treated with IVGC ($P = 0.0001$). Disease activation was more prevalent in males ($P < 0.02$) and in older patients ($P = 0.04$) with a shorter duration of GD ($P < 0.01$) and time from GO onset ($P < 0.01$).

Conclusions.—GO may occur after RAI in approximately 15% of patients also in the absence of signs of active GO. Prophylactic OGC did not prevent GO activation in a large proportion of patients, compared to IVGC.

▶ The aim of the study by Vannucchi et al was to analyze the effects of radioiodine (RAI) on Graves' orbitopathy (GO) with or without prophylactic steroids based on known risk factors and to compare the effectiveness of prophylaxis with intravenous glucocorticoids (IVGC) and oral glucocorticoids (OGC). This work shows that GO may occur after RAI therapy in approximately 15% of patients with Graves' disease (GD) and also in the absence of signs of GO or of significantly active GO. Although these findings are obtained from a retrospective study, their significance relies on the fact that all patients were studied with the same approach in a standardized method before and after RAI therapy, according to the suggestions of a recent consensus statement (European Group on Graves'Orbitopathy [EUGOGO]).[1] GO activation after RAI therapy has been previously reported in about 15% to 20% of patients by several authors,[2,3] although in most studies patients with or without pre-existing signs of mild and/or minimally active eye disease were not clearly classified. Moreover, a definite assessment of the clinical activity of GO before and after RAI therapy has not been accurately performed.[4] The possibility of predicting, at the time of RAI therapy, which patients are at risk for the occurrence of GO has been a matter of controversy over the last few years. This is mostly due to the lack of controlled studies identifying plausible and consistent risk factors for de novo occurrence or relapse of active GO in GD patients with persistent hyperthyroidism treated with RAI therapy. Another major finding of this work is the observation that prophylactic treatment with OGC prevented GO activation in about 50% of patients compared with successful prevention in all patients with intravenous (IV) steroids (Fig 1 in the original article). Patients with signs of moderately active GO were more prevalent in the IVGC group, as shown by the significantly higher clinical activity score (CAS). Other clinical characteristics of the patients treated with the 2 modalities did not differ, that is, previous therapy for active GO, when present, and interval between such therapy and RAI. Therefore, it might be hypothesized that when given via IV route, steroids have a greater immunosuppressive effect on the thyroid and orbital autoimmune reactions involved in GO activation. In interpreting this finding, which should be confirmed in a randomized controlled study and on a larger series of patients, one also has to consider that patient compliance with OGC may not have been as adequate as with the IV administration route, because of the duration of therapy (up to 8 weeks) and the frequent appearance of side effects.

M. Schott, MD, PhD

References

1. Bartalena L, Baldeschi L, Dickinson A, et al. European Group on Graves' Orbitopathy (EUGOGO). Consensus statement of the European Group on Graves' orbitopathy (EUGOGO) on management of GO. *Eur J Endocrinol.* 2008;158:273-285.
2. Rasmussen AK, Nygaard B, Feldt-Rasmussen U. (131)I and thyroid-associated ophthalmopathy. *Eur J Endocrinol.* 2000;143:155-160.
3. Bonnema SJ, Bartalena L, Toft AD, Hegedus L. Controversies in radioiodine therapy: relation to ophthalmopathy, the possible radioprotective effect of antithyroid drugs, and use in large goitres. *Eur J Endocrinol.* 2002;147:1-11.
4. Sisson JC, Schipper MJ, Nelson CC, Freitas JE, Frueh BR. Radioiodine therapy and Graves' ophthalmopathy. *J Nucl Med.* 2008;49:923-930.

Endothelial Progenitor Cells in Subclinical Hypothyroidism: The Effect of Thyroid Hormone Replacement Therapy

Shakoor SKA, Aldibbiat A, Ingoe LE, et al (Queen Elizabeth Hosp, UK; Newcastle Univ, UK)

J Clin Endocrinol Metab 95:319-322, 2010

Context.—Subclinical hypothyroidism (SCH) is associated with cardiovascular (CV) risk factors, and possibly CV disease. However, its management remains controversial. Endothelial progenitor cells (EPC), expressing both endothelial and stem cell markers, are known to offer a novel CV risk marker.

Objective.—The aim of the study was to ascertain whether EPC count or function is reduced in SCH and whether it improves with T_4 therapy.

Design and Intervention.—EPC were studied in peripheral blood by fluorescence-activated cell sorter and following *in vitro* cultures before and after T_4 together with CV risk factors in 20 SCH and healthy controls (HC).

Main Outcome Measure.—EPC count was measured at baseline and after T_4 replacement in SCH.

Results.—EPC count was significantly reduced in SCH compared to HC: median (range)—CD133+/VEGFR-2+, 0.09 (0.02–0.44) *vs.* 0.47 (0.17–2.12), $P < 0.001$; CD34+/VEGFR-2+, 0.10 (0.04–0.46) *vs.* 0.39 (0.11–2.13), $P < 0.001$; whereas EPC function was similar. There was a significant positive correlation between CD133+/VEGFR-2+ with free T_4 levels ($r = 0.38$; $P = 0.02$); high-density lipoprotein cholesterol levels ($r = 0.51$; $P = 0.001$); and negative correlation with TSH concentrations ($r = -0.64$; $P < 0.001$). After adjustment for conventional CV risk factors, SCH predicted lower EPC count, β coefficient/P value: CD133+/VEGFR-2+ (−0.77/<0.001), and CD34+/VEGFR-2+ (−0.71/<0.001). In SCH participants, EPC count increased and was similar to HC after T_4; CD133+/VEGFR-2+, 0.32 (0.03–0.94) *vs.* 0.09 (0.02–0.44), $P < 0.001$; and CD34+/VEGFR-2+, 0.26 (0.06–0.88) *vs.* 0.10 (0.04–0.46), $P < 0.001$.

Conclusion.—SCH predicted lower EPC count, which improved with T_4 treatment, independent of other CV risk factors, providing additional evidence that T_4 replacement may improve CV risk in SCH.

▶ Subclinical hypothyroidism (SCH) has been associated with atherogenic lipid profile and endothelial dysfunction assessed by flow-mediated dilatation (FMD), which improves with thyroid hormone replacement therapy.[1] The aim of this study was to ascertain whether endothelial progenitor cells (EPC) count or function is reduced in SCH and whether it improves with T4 therapy. The authors report, for the first time, lower circulating EPC count in SCH subjects, which increased significantly with T4 replacement (Fig 1 in the original article). EPC showed significant negative and positive relations between serum TSH and FT4, respectively. The pathogenesis behind lower EPC count in SCH is, however, still unclear. Reduced nitric oxide availability has been suggested to cause endothelial dysfunction in hypothyroidism and SCH, contributing to reversible endothelial dysfunction,[2] which may represent one potential mechanism. The other possible mechanisms for reduced numbers of EPC include direct effects of thyroid hormone on EPC survival. Irrespective of these results, a double-blind controlled study still needs to be performed to investigate the cardiovascular outcomes after T4 replacement therapy.

M. Schott, MD, PhD

References

1. Danese MD, Ladenson PW, Meinert CL, Powe NR. Clinical review 115: effect of thyroxine therapy on serum lipoproteins in patients with mild thyroid failure: a quantitative review of the literature. *J Clin Endocrinol Metab.* 2000;85: 2993-3001.
2. Taddei S, Caraccio N, Virdis A, et al. Impaired endothelium-dependent vasodilatation in subclinical hypothyroidism: beneficial effect of levothyroxine therapy. *J Clin Endocrinol Metab.* 2003;88:3731-3737.

Evidence for a Specific Defect in Hippocampal Memory in Overt and Subclinical Hypothyroidism

Correia N, Mullally S, Cooke G, et al (Adelaide and Meath Hosp, Tallaght, Dublin, Ireland; Trinity College Inst of Neuroscience, Dublin, Ireland)
J Clin Endocrinol Metab 94:3789-3797, 2009

Context.—Declarative memory largely depends upon normal functioning temporal lobes (hippocampal complex) and prefrontal cortex. Animal studies suggest abnormal hippocampal function in hypothyroidism.

Objective.—The aim of the study was to assess declarative memory in overt and subclinical (SCH) hypothyroid patients before and after L-T_4 (LT4) replacement and in matched normal subjects.

Design and Setting.—A prospective, open-labeled interventional study was conducted at a teaching hospital.

Participants and Intervention.—Hypothyroid ($n = 21$) and SCH ($n = 17$) patients underwent neuropsychological tests at baseline and 3 and 6 months after LT4 replacement. Normal subjects were studied at the same time-points.

Main Outcome.—Tests of spatial, verbal, associative, and working memory; attention; and response inhibition and the Hospital Anxiety and Depression Scale were administered.

Results.—Baseline deficits in spatial, associative, and verbal memory, which rely upon the integrity of the hippocampal and frontal areas, were identified in patients with overt hypothyroidism. Spatial and verbal memory were impaired in SCH patients ($P < 0.05$). TSH levels correlated negatively ($P < 0.05$) with these deficits. After LT4 replacement, verbal memory normalized. Spatial memory normalized in the SCH group but remained impaired in the hypothyroid group. Associative memory deficits persisted in the overt hypothyroid group. Hospital Anxiety and Depression Scale scores did not correlate with cognitive function. Measures of attention and response inhibition did not differ from control subjects.

Conclusion.—Cognitive impairment occurs in SCH and more markedly in overt hypothyroidism. These impairments appear predominantly mnemonic in nature, suggesting that the etiology is not indicative of general cognitive slowing. We propose that these deficits may reflect an underlying disruption of normal hippocampal function and/or connectivity.

▶ For a long time, it has been known that the cognitive function in overt hypothyroidism is impaired. Some studies have reported general cognitive slowing,[1] whereas others suggest a more specific mnemonic deficit.[2] Deficits in hippocampal-dependent memory tasks that are reversible with thyroid hormone replacement are apparent in animal models of hypothyroidism, whereas studies in hypothyroid rats have demonstrated impaired hippocampal neurogenesis, providing a potential mechanistic explanation for these mnemonic deficits. To date, it is not known whether similar mnemonic deficits occur in humans.

It is also not known whether the neurocognitive deficits associated with overt hypothyroidism occur in patients with subclinical hypothyroidism (SCH), which is defined as persistently raised serum thyroid-stimulating hormone (TSH) level in the presence of normal free T_4 (FT4) and which occurs in 4% to 10% of the adult population. Although some studies suggest impairment of cognitive function in SCH, there remain inconsistencies in the range and degree of these deficits. The authors of this article hypothesized that specific impairments in hippocampal and, possibly, frontally driven memory processes could be demonstrated in subjects with overt hypothyroidism and to a lesser degree in SCH, and these deficits would improve after L-T_4 (LT4) replacement. Exactly this could now been demonstrated. Summarized data are shown in Fig 3 in the original article. One major drawback of this study is the limited number of patients enrolled. Nonetheless, the data are convincing and should force doctors to prescribe thyroid hormone already at the level of subclinical hypothyroidism with elevated TSH levels.

M. Schott, MD, PhD

References

1. Constant EL, Adam S, Seron X, Bruyer R, Seghers A, Daumerie C. Anxiety and depression, attention, and executive functions in hypothyroidism. *J Int Neuropsychol Soc.* 2005;11:535-544.
2. Miller KJ, Parsons TD, Whybrow PC, et al. Memory improvement with treatment of hypothyroidism. *Int J Neurosci.* 2006;116:895-906.

Impact of Resistance to Thyroid Hormone on the Cardiovascular System in Adults

Pulcrano M, Palmieri EA, Mannavola D, et al (Univ Federico II, Naples, Italy; Centro Traumatologico Ospedaliero, Naples, Italy; Univ of Milan, Italy)
J Clin Endocrinol Metab 94:2812-2816, 2009

Background.—The clinical manifestations of resistance to thyroid hormone (RTH) are highly variable, and the impact of RTH on the cardiovascular system has been poorly investigated.

Aim.—The objective of the study was to evaluate the cardiovascular characteristics of 16 untreated and asymptomatic patients with RTH compared with 16 euthyroid healthy controls to define the cardiovascular involvement in RTH syndrome.

Patients and Methods.—Sixteen untreated and asymptomatic RTH patients (eight males; aged 33 ± 12 yr, range 21–45 yr) and 16 controls (nine males; aged 33 ± 5 yr, range 24–42 yr) were enrolled. Clinical data, thyroid status, and echocardiographic results were recorded.

Results.—Heart rate was comparable with that of controls, whereas arterial pressure was higher than controls. Mean interventricular septum diastolic thickness and mean left ventricular (LV) posterior wall diastolic thickness were significantly lower in RTH patients than controls with a consequent significant decrease of the mean LV mass and LV mass indexed by body surface area. Patients also had abnormalities of myocardial relaxation as indicated by a significant increase of peak A and consequent reduction of the early to late ratio. Finally, systemic vascular resistance was significantly higher in RTH patients than controls.

Conclusions.—Our results suggest the presence of cardiovascular alterations in asymptomatic and untreated RTH patients similar to those reported in hypothyroid patients. Our strict selection likely created a bias in the inclusion of a particular type of RTH patients, who could represent a minority of patients with RTH. However, no correlation was

TABLE 2.—Cardiovascular Characteristics of RTH Patients and Control Subjects

	Control Subjects (n = 16)	RTH Patients (n = 16)	*P* value
HR (bpm)	78 ± 7	80 ± 15	NS
SBP (mm Hg)	117 ± 7	124 ± 9	<0.05
DBP (mm Hg)	73 ± 8	81 ± 9	<0.01
MAP (mm Hg)	87 ± 7	95 ± 8	<0.01
PP (mm Hg)	44 ± 7	43 ± 8	NS
LVEDDi (mm/m^2)	27.7 ± 3.4	28.7 ± 3.0	NS
LVESDi (mm/m^2)	16.9 ± 2.4	18.7 ± 2.3	<0.05
LVEDWTi (mm/m^2)	5.2 ± 0.6	4.6 ± 0.6	<0.01
LVMi (g/m^2)	85 ± 12	69 ± 14	<0.01
RWT	0.38 ± 0.05	0.32 ± 0.04	<0.001
LVEF (%)	69 ± 6	63 ± 7	<0.05
SI (%)	42 ± 8	40 ± 8	NS
E (cm/sec)	77 ± 11	70 ± 18	NS
A (cm/sec)	48 ± 8	58 ± 15	<0.05
E/A (kg)	1.6 ± 0.2	1.3 ± 0.4	<0.01
E-dt (msec)	144 ± 19	123 ± 14	<0.01
CI (liters/m^2)	1.73 ± 0.17	1.65 ± 0.17	NS
SVRi (dyne · sec/cm^{-5} · m^2)	744 ± 160	949 ± 253	<0.05
PP/SI (mm Hg/ml · m^2)	1.09 ± 0.32	1.12 ± 0.26	NS

Data are mean ± SD. The *bold* numbers indicate the parameters that are statistically significant between the two groups studied. HR, Heart rate; SBP, systolic blood pressure; DBP, diastolic blood pressure; MAP, mean arterial pressure; PP, pulse pressure; LVEDDi, left ventricular end-diastolic diameter index; LVESDi, left ventricular end-systolic diameter index; LVEDWTi, left ventricular end-diastolic wall thickness index (as mean value of interventricular septum and posterior wall); LVMi, left ventricular mass index; RWT, relative wall thickness; LVEF, left ventricular ejection fraction; SI, stroke index; E, early transmitral peak inflow velocity from pulsed-wave Doppler imaging; A, late transmitral peak inflow velocity from pulsed-wave Doppler imaging; E-dt, deceleration time of the early transmitral inflow from pulsed-wave Doppler imaging; CI, cardiac index; SVRi, systemic vascular resistance index; PP/SI, pulse pressure/stroke index (total arterial stiffness); NS, not statistically significant.

found between the type of mutation and cardiovascular characteristics of RTH patients (Table 2).

▶ Within this case-control study, the authors assessed cardiac morphology and function in 16 patients with resistance to thyroid hormone (RTH) compared with euthyroid healthy controls. The authors selected a homogeneous RTH group of patients without cardiovascular symptoms and untreated with thyroid or cardiovascular drugs to assess the cardiovascular response to thyroid hormone in RTH syndrome. The results indicate that this dominantly inherited condition of altered tissue responsiveness to thyroid hormone is associated with measurable alterations of left ventricular characteristics and circulatory function (Table 2). These findings reinforce the concept that thyroid hormone plays an important physiologic role in the cardiovascular system.

These results are apparently different from a previous study by Kahaly et al[1] in which a heterogeneous RTH group showed some cardiovascular alterations similar to those found in hyperthyroid subjects, whereas other cardiovascular parameters were comparable with controls. In fact, it is difficult to compare the patients in the present study with the RTH group evaluated by Kahaly et al because the authors used different selection criteria. Indeed, the RTH group by Kahaly et al included patients with and without thyrotoxic cardiovascular symptoms, some patients treated with levothyroxine or antithyroid drugs and patients with a wide age range, including children. Furthermore, Kahaly et al only compared the data of 2 distinct RTH groups (with and without thyrotoxic cardiovascular symptoms) without comparing them to euthyroid subjects; they compared the results of the entire RTH group only with those of euthyroid, hypothyroid, and hyperthyroid subjects. Because of that, the authors selected a homogeneous RTH group of young and middle-aged patients (age range 21-45 yr), without thyrotoxic cardiovascular symptoms and untreated with thyroid or cardiovascular drugs. These strict selection criteria likely created a bias in the inclusion of a particular type of RTH patients, who could represent a minority of patients with RTH. Nonetheless, these results support the concept that thyroid hormone plays an important physiological role in the development of the cardiovascular system.

M. Schott, MD, PhD

Reference

1. Kahaly GJ, Matthews CH, Mohr-Kahaly S, Richards CA, Chatterjee VK. Cardiac involvement in thyroid hormone resistance. *J Clin Endocrinol Metab.* 2002;87: 204-212.

Thyrotoxicosis

Impact of Lithium on Efficacy of Radioactive Iodine for Graves' Disease: A Cohort Study on Cure Rate, Time to Cure, and Frequency of Increased Serum Thyroxine After Antithyroid Drug Withdrawal

Bogazzi F, Giovannetti C, Fessehatsion R, et al (Univ of Pisa, Italy)

J Clin Endocrinol Metab 95:201-208, 2010

Context.—Radioactive iodine (RAI) is a common therapy for hyperthyroidism due to Graves' disease. A small but significant proportion of patients have recurrence of hyperthyroidism after RAI therapy. Lithium might increase RAI effectiveness by increasing RAI retention in the thyroid. However, whether lithium favorably affects the long-term outcome of RAI therapy is still a matter of argument.

Objective.—The objective of the study was to compare the efficacy of RAI given with or without concomitant lithium treatment.

Design.—This was a retrospective cohort study.

Setting.—The study was conducted at a tertiary university center.

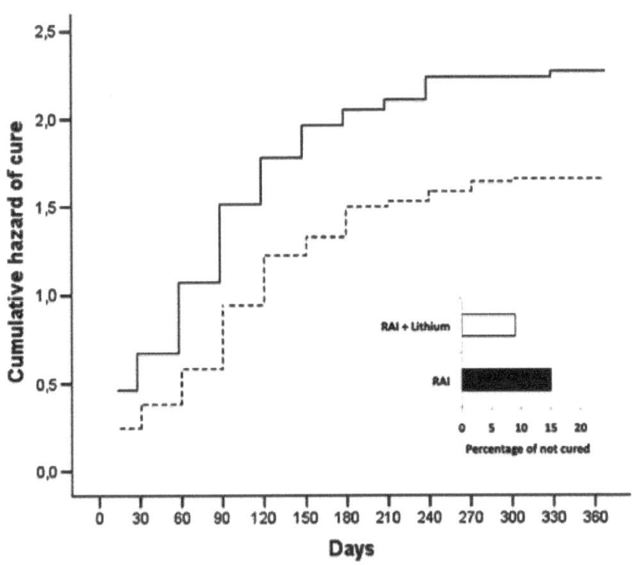

FIGURE 1.—Cumulative hazard of cured patients estimated by the Kaplan-Meier method. The two curves were compared by the log-rank test ($P = 0.000$). Difference in the cure rate at the end of the follow-up period was assessed by Fisher's exact test ($P = 0.030$). The outcome of patients treated with RAI and lithium is indicated by *solid line* and that of patients treated with RAI alone by *dotted line*. The cumulative hazard of cure is related to the cumulative proportion of patients not cured. The *insert figure* shows the percentage of patients not cured in the two groups. (Reprinted from Bogazzi F, Giovannetti C, Fessehatsion R, et al. Impact of lithium on efficacy of radioactive iodine for graves' disease: a cohort study on cure rate, time to cure, and frequency of increased serum thyroxine after antithyroid drug withdrawal. *J Clin Endocrinol Metab*. 2010;95:201-208, with permission from The Endrocrine Society.)

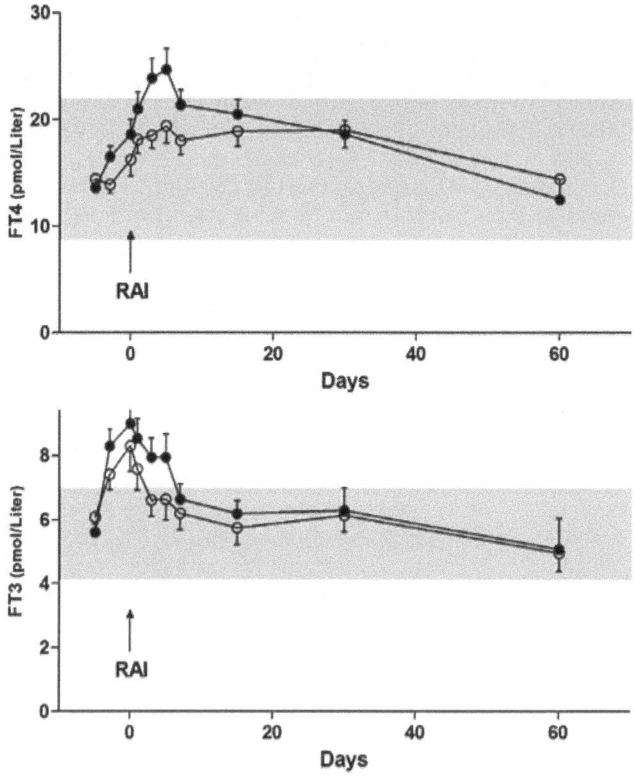

FIGURE 2.—Outcome of serum thyroid hormone concentrations. The *shaded area* shows the normal range for serum FT4 and FT3 levels. Outcome of mean serum FT4 and FT3 concentrations (±SE) in patients treated with RAI and lithium are shown by *white circles* and that in patients treated with RAI alone by *black circles*. Difference in the outcome of serum FT4 concentrations between the RAI plus lithium group and the RAI alone group were different at T + 3 and T + 5 ($P = 0.0139$ and $P = 0.0373$, respectively); on the contrary, mean serum FT3 concentrations, although lower in patients treated with RAI plus lithium, were not significantly different in the two treatment groups. (Reprinted from Bogazzi F, Giovannetti C, Fessehatsion R, et al. Impact of lithium on efficacy of radioactive iodine for graves' disease: a cohort study on cure rate, time to cure, and frequency of increased serum thyroxine after antithyroid drug withdrawal. *J Clin Endocrinol Metab*. 2010;95:201-208, with permission from The Endrocrine Society.)

Patients.—Six hundred fifty-one patients with newly diagnosed Graves' disease participated in the study.

Intervention.—Two hundred ninety-eight patients were treated with RAI plus lithium (900 mg/d for 12 d) and 353 with RAI alone.

Main Outcome Measures.—Proportion of cured patients and time to achieve cure of hyperthyroidism during 1 yr of follow-up was measured.

Results.—Patients treated with RAI plus lithium had a higher cure rate (91.0%) than those treated with RAI alone (85.0%, $P = 0.030$). In addition, patients treated with RAI plus lithium were cured more rapidly (median 60 d) than those treated with RAI alone (median 90 d, $P = 0.000$). Treatment with lithium prevented the serum free T_4 increase after methimazole withdrawal and RAI therapy. Side effects after RAI therapy occurred in a subset of patients and were mild, transient, and without differences in the two groups.

Conclusions.—RAI combined with lithium is safe and more effective than RAI alone in the cure of hyperthyroidism due to Graves' disease.

▶ Radioactive iodine (RAI) is widely used for hyperthyroidism due to Graves' disease either as a first-line treatment or when hyperthyroidism relapses after a course of antithyroid drug treatment.[1] The target of RAI therapy (cure of hyperthyroidism) is a stable restoration of euthyroidism or permanent hypothyroidism. To this purpose, several regimens have been proposed, including, for example, selection of patients and different schedules based on variable RAI doses.[2] Pretreatment with thionamides may reduce RAI efficacy as pointed out in a recent meta-analysis, irrespective of the type of drug and discontinuation protocol.[3] Studies reported variable percentage of failure after RAI therapy, depending on several variables, including 131-I dose, although a recent meta-analysis did not show difference in the outcome of calculated or fixed doses. Lithium accumulates in the thyroid and increases (radio)iodine retention without affecting thyroidal radioiodine uptake (RAIU). The addition of lithium to RAI has been associated with an increase in the radiation dose delivered to the thyroid.[4] Whether this results in a higher cure rate of hyperthyroidism is still a matter of argument. Conflicting results have been reported on this issue. Furthermore, the potential toxicity of lithium raised some concern about its use in combination with RAI for hyperthyroidism.[5] The objective of this study was to compare the efficacy of RAI given with or without concomitant lithium treatment. The protocol, which has been used in the study by Bogazzi et al is shown in Fig 1. It has a good design to avoid interference with antithyroid drugs, and to deliver lithium at the most favorable time. In this study, lithium was given for only 9 days, beginning 5 days before ^{131}I therapy was initiated, and maintained for 7 days thereafter. This is a shorter protocol (12 vs 19 days) than that of a previous pilot study by Bogazzi and associates[4] that found that the effect of lithium on serum thyroid hormone concentrations occurred 3 to 5 days after ^{131}I was administered. Although this is a retrospective study, the scrupulous statistical analysis takes into account the possibility of selection bias by adjusting for confounding variables. Multivariate analysis was performed using both the propensity score and significant covariates to control for possible bias from the nonrandomized assignment of patients to treatment. The main findings of the study were that patients treated with ^{131}I plus lithium had a higher cure rate (91%) than those treated with ^{131}I alone. Treatment with lithium also prevented an increase in serum free T4 and T3 levels after withdrawal of MMI, which had been given for 3 to 6 months before ^{131}I therapy (Fig 2). Side effects of lithium were mild and transient and were not different in the 2 study groups with and without lithium pretreatment for ^{131}I therapy. None of the patients had ophthalmopathy, and the thyroid volume decreased much more rapidly in the patients pretreated with lithium as compared with the group treated with ^{131}I alone.

In summary, this study shows that lithium is of substantial benefit in the treatment of patients with Graves' hyperthyroidism. The authors suggest that a short course of lithium is safe and beneficial for patients treated with ^{131}I, increasing the cure rate for hyperthyroidism and shortening the time for cure, and preventing an abrupt increase in thyroid hormone levels. It is highly likely that this important study will provide a strong impetus for a change in practice paradigms for patients with Graves' hyperthyroidism. It must be kept in mind, however, that all the positive effects of lithium found in this study rely upon careful adherence to a treatment protocol described in this article. Based on that, the present RAI treatment protocols will be changed in the near future.

M. Schott, MD, PhD

References

1. Weetman AP. Radioiodine treatment for benign thyroid diseases. *Clin Endocrinol (Oxf)*. 2007;66:757-764.
2. Allahabadia A, Daykin J, Sheppard MC, Gough SC, Franklyn JA. Radioiodine treatment of hyperthyroidism-prognostic factors for outcome. *J Clin Endocrinol Metab*. 2001;86:3611-3617.
3. Walter MA, Briel M, Christ-Crain M, et al. Effects of antithyroid drugs on radioiodine treatment: systematic review and meta-analysis of randomised controlled trials. *BMJ*. 2007;334:514.
4. Bogazzi F, Bartalena L, Campomori A, et al. Treatment with lithium prevents serum thyroid hormone increase after thionamide withdrawal and radioiodine therapy in patients with Graves' disease. *J Clin Endocrinol Metab*. 2002;87:4490-4495.
5. Dunkelmann S, Kunstner H, Nabavi E, Eberlein U, Groth P, Schumichen C. Lithium as an adjunct to radioiodine therapy in Graves' disease for prolonging the intrathyroidal effective half-life of radioiodine. Useful or not? *Nuklearmedizin*. 2006;45:213-218.

Serum Chromogranin A Concentration in Hyperthyroidism before and after Medical Treatment

Al-Shoumer KAS, Vasanthy BA (Mubarak Al Kabeer Hosp, Kuwait; Kuwait Univ, Jabriya, Safat)

J Clin Endocrinol Metab 94:2321-2324, 2009

Objective.—The aim was to evaluate changes in chromogranin A (CgA) concentration in hyperthyroidism and to assess its metabolic correlations.

Methods.—We studied CgA levels in hyperthyroidism. First, 38 hyperthyroid patients matched with 86 normal controls were studied after an overnight fast. Second, 30 if the 38 patients were followed up for 6 months with medical antithyroid drug therapy (carbimazole). In the first study, after 10–12 h overnight fasting, blood was collected for measurement of CgA, glucose, insulin, intact proinsulin, and thyroid function. These variables were remeasured in the second study for the patients after attainment of euthyroidism with the antithyroid drug carbimazole for 6 months.

Results.—Pretreatment CgA level was significantly higher in patients compared with controls. CgA levels dropped significantly to levels similar to those of controls after antithyroid therapy. Although baseline and follow-up fasting glucose, insulin, and intact proinsulin demonstrated similar pattern of CgA changes before and after medical treatment, CgA did not correlate with any of them. However, CgA levels demonstrated a significant positive correlation with free T_3 and free T_4 only.

Conclusion.—These studies demonstrate that untreated hyperthyroidism is associated with elevated CgA level that changes in parallel to thyroid status. It is therefore possible to use CgA concentration as a potential marker of disease activity in hyperthyroidism.

▶ In this study, the authors investigated the diagnostic value of serum chromogranin A (CgA) in hyperthyroidism. This study demonstrated that untreated hyperthyroid patients exhibited significant elevation in CgA levels that is correlated positively with thyroid hormones (Fig 2 in the original article). The degree of elevation in CgA was correlated with the severity of hyperthyroidism because CgA levels dropped to similar concentrations of controls with achievement of euthyroidism. The mechanism of CgA elevations in hyperthyroidism is unknown. Several symptoms and signs in patients with hyperthyroidism suggest an abnormality of the autonomic nervous system. These are thought to be the result of interaction of thyroid hormones with the sympathetic nervous system. This interaction has resulted from a sympathovagal imbalance, characterized by increased sympathetic activity in the presence of diminished vagal tone, which coincides with increased urinary excretion of catecholamines. Although co-stored in the same vesicles, catecholamines and CgA are not always co-secreted under all conditions. Co-release of catecholamines and CgA does not occur after weak sympathetic activation or after nonexocytotic stimuli, but only after adrenal exocytotic stimuli. Because elevations in plasma adrenomedullin and proadrenomedullin-N terminal 20-peptide have been demonstrated in thyrotoxic Graves' patients,[1] it is possible that thyroid hormone itself increases the production of CgA by increased adrenal exocytotic stimuli or by other unknown mechanisms. Whether synthesis of CgA in thyrotoxicosis is increased in vivo remains to be elucidated. As far as I know, this is the first report to assess CgA levels in hyperthyroid humans showing its elevation. There are no reported studies on the assessment of CgA changes in thyroid dysfunction except for one article demonstrating unchanged CgA in hypothyroidism.[2]

M. Schott, MD, PhD

References

1. Taniyama M, Kitamura K, Ban Y, Sugita E, Ito K, Katagiri T. Elevation of circulating proadrenomedullin-N terminal 20-peptide in thyrotoxicosis. *Clin Endocrinol (Oxf)*. 1997;46:271-274.
2. Nehar D, Lombard-Bohas C, Olivieri S, et al. Interest of Chromogranin A for diagnosis and follow-up of endocrine tumours. *Clin Endocrinol (Oxf)*. 2004;60: 644-652.

Thyroid Nodules

An Ultrasonogram Reporting System for Thyroid Nodules Stratifying Cancer Risk for Clinical Management

Horvath E, Majlis S, Rossi R, et al (Clinica Alemana de Santiago, Chile; et al)

J Clin Endocrinol Metab 94:1748-1751, 2009

Context.—There is a high prevalence of thyroid nodules on ultrasonographic (US) examination. However, most of them are benign. US criteria may help to decide cost-effective management.

Objective.—Our objective was to develop a standardized US characterization and reporting data system of thyroid lesions for clinical management: the Thyroid Imaging Reporting and Data System (TIRADS).

Design.—This was a prospective study using the TIRADS, which is based on the concepts of the Breast Imaging Reporting Data System of the American College of Radiology.

Materials.—A correlation of the US findings and fine needle aspiration biopsy (FNAB) results in 1959 lesions biopsied under US guidance and studied histologically during an 8-yr period was divided into three stages. In the first stage, 10 US patterns were defined. In the second stage, four TIRADS groups were defined according to risk. The percentages of malignancy defined in the Breast Imaging Reporting and Data System were followed: TIRADS 2 (0% malignancy), TIRADS 3 (<5% malignancy), TIRADS 4 (5–80% malignancy), and TIRADS 5 (>80% malignancy).

Results.—The TIRADS classification was evaluated at the third stage of the study in a sample of 1097 nodules (benign: 703; follicular lesions: 238; and carcinoma: 156). Sensitivity, specificity, positive predictive value, negative predictive value, and accuracy were 88, 49, 49, 88, and 94%, respectively. The ratio of benign to malignant or follicular FNAB results currently is 1.8.

Conclusions.—The TIRADS has allowed us to improve patient management and cost-effectiveness, avoiding unnecessary FNAB. In addition, we have established standard codes to be used both for radiologists and endocrinologists (Tables 1 and 2).

▶ The widespread use of imaging ultrasound (US) techniques has generated an overwhelming increase in the recognition of thyroid nodules. Thus, there is a need to establish some basic criteria to select nodules for fine needle aspiration biopsies (FNAB) to minimize costs and maximize benefits. FNAB is the best tool in helping to decide between nodules that require surgery and those that can be followed. The aim of this study was to establish a new concept to US evaluation of thyroid nodules. The authors called it the Thyroid Imaging Reporting and Data System (TIRADS), which is in analogue to the breast imaging reporting and data system (BI-RADS) for breast lesions. Table 1 shows the US characteristics used for the TIRADS system. Some examples are shown in Fig 1 in the original article. Sensitivity, specificity, positive predictive value (PPV), negative predictive value (NPV), and accuracy were 88, 49,

TABLE 1.—US Characteristics of Thyroid Nodules, 10 US Patterns with their Malignancy Risk, and TIRADS Category

Description of US Pattern	US Patterns	Malignancy	TIRADS
Anechoic with hyperechoic spots, nonvascularized lesion.	Colloid type 1		
Nonencapsulated, mixed, nonexpansile, with hyperechoic spots, vascularized lesion, "grid" aspect (spongiform nodule).	Colloid type 2	0%	TIRADS 2: benign findings
Nonencapsulated, mixed with solid portion, isoechogenic, expansile, vascularized nodule with hyperechoic spots.	Colloid type 3		
Hyper, iso, or hypoechoic, partially encapsulated nodule with peripheral vascularization, in Hashimoto's thyroiditis.	Hashimoto pseudonodule	<5%	TIRADS 3: probably benign
Solid or mixed hyper, iso, or hypoechoic nodule, with a thin capsule.	Simple neoplastic pattern	5–10%	TIRADS 4A: undetermined
Hypoechoic lesion with ill-defined borders, without calcifications.	de Quervain pattern		
Hyper, iso, or hypoechoic, hypervascularized, encapsulated nodule with a thick capsule, containing calcifications (coarse or microcalcifications).	Suspicious neoplastic pattern		
Hypoechoic, nonencapsulated nodule, with irregular shape and margins, penetrating. vessels, with or without calcifications	Malignant pattern A	10–80%	TIRADS 4B: suspicious
Iso or hypoechoic, nonencapsulated nodule with multiple peripheral microcalcifications and hypervascularization.	Malignant pattern B	>80%	TIRADS 5: consistent with malignancy
Nonencapsulated, isoechoic mixed hypervascularized nodule with or without calcifications, without hyperechoic spots.	Malignant pattern C Cancer, confirmed by previous biopsy	100%	TIRADS 6: malignant

TABLE 2.—Correlation of TIRADS Categories and Risk of Malignancy in FNAB Histology

FNAB (n = 1097)	TIRADS 2 (n = 62)		TIRADS 3 (n = 326)		TIRADS 4 (n = 642)		TIRADS 5 (n = 67)	
Benign	62 (100%)	62 (100%)	280 (85.9%)	280 (85.9%)	353 (55%)	353 (55%)	7 (10.4%)	7 (10.4%)
Follicular lesion	0%	0%	35 (10.7%)	46 (14.1%)	199 (31%)	289 (45%)	2 (3.1%)	60 (89.6%)
Cancer	0%	0%	11 (3.4%)	46 (14.1%)	90 (14%)	289 (45%)	58 (86.5%)	60 (89.6%)

49, 88, and 94%, respectively. Correlation of TIRADS categories and risk for malignancy in FNAB histology are shown in Table 2. Sensitivity, specificity, PPV, NPV, and accuracy calculated for the TIRADS in this study are, however, biased because follicular lesions are included as "non-benign," knowing that 80% of them are follicular adenomas. Nonetheless, the TIRADS classification allows for a better selection of nodules submitted to FNAB, avoiding unnecessary procedures. These data need to be, however, also reevaluated from other groups.

M. Schott, MD, PhD

Molecular Testing for Mutations in Improving the Fine-Needle Aspiration Diagnosis of Thyroid Nodules

Nikiforov YE, Steward DL, Robinson-Smith TM, et al (Univ of Cincinnati College of Medicine, OH)

J Clin Endocrinol Metab 94:2092-2098, 2009

Context.—Thyroid nodules are common in adults, but only a small fraction of them are malignant. Fine-needle aspiration (FNA) with cytological evaluation is the most reliable tool for cancer diagnosis in thyroid nodules. However, 10–40% of nodules are diagnosed as indeterminate by cytology, making it difficult to optimally manage these patients.

Objective.—The aim of this study was to establish the feasibility and role of testing for tumor-specific mutations in improving the FNA diagnosis of thyroid nodules.

Design.—The prospective study included 470 FNA samples of thyroid nodules from 328 patients. At the time of aspiration, a small portion of the material was collected and tested for *BRAF*, *RAS*, *RET/PTC*, and *PAX8/PPAR*γ mutations. The mutational status was correlated with cytology and either surgical pathology diagnosis or follow-up (mean, 34 months).

Results.—A sufficient amount of nucleic acids were isolated in 98% of samples. Thirty-two mutations were found, including 18 *BRAF*, eight *RAS*, five *RET/PTC*, and one *PAX8/PPAR*γ. The presence of any mutation

TABLE 1.—Performance Characteristics of Cytology and Molecular Analysis in Definitive Diagnosis of Malignancy in FNA Samples from Thyroid Nodules

Diagnostic Modality	Sensitivity	Specificity	PPV	NPV	Accuracy
Cytology (positive for malignancy)	44.0	100	100	92.9	93.3
Molecular analysis (positive for mutation)	62.0	99.7	96.9	95.1	95.2
Cytology (positive) and molecular (positive)	80.0	99.7	97.6	97.4	97.4

Data are expressed as percentage.

was a strong indicator of cancer because 31 (97%) of mutation-positive nodules had a malignant diagnosis after surgery. A combination of cytology and molecular testing showed significant improvement in the diagnostic accuracy and allowed better prediction of malignancy in the nodules with indeterminate cytology.

Conclusions.—These results indicate that molecular testing of thyroid nodules for a panel of mutations can be effectively performed in a clinical setting. It enhances the accuracy of FNA cytology and is of particular value for thyroid nodules with indeterminate cytology (Table 1).

▶ To my knowledge, the study by Nikiforov et al is the first large prospective study aimed at determining the feasibility and diagnostic utility of molecular genetic testing in refining the fine needle aspiration (FNA) diagnosis of thyroid nodules. The authors show that testing for a panel of mutations, including *BRAF*, *RAS*, *RET/PTC*, and *PAX8/PPARγ*, significantly improved the accuracy of the cytological diagnosis, particularly for samples with indeterminate cytology. In this category, the detection of any mutation was highly predictive of malignancy and should provide a strong indication for surgery. Two examples are shown in Fig 3 in the original article; complete results, including sensitivity, specificity, positive and negative predictive value, and accuracy are shown in Table 1. These results are of particular importance for the least worrisome category of indeterminate cytology (ie, follicular lesion of undetermined significance) where the estimated risk of malignancy is only 5% to 10%.[1] These patients would benefit most from molecular testing, which should provide accurate prediction of malignancy, eliminate delay in surgical treatment, and avoid the costs of repeat FNA recommended to those patients.[1] In light of the finding in this study, patients with nodules that yield indeterminate cytology and are positive for mutation would be strong candidates for total thyroidectomy, particularly when *BRAF* or *RET/PTC* mutation is detected. If surgical treatment is considered for nodules with indeterminate cytology that are negative for mutations, a reduced risk of malignancy would seem to suggest lobectomy as an appropriate initial surgical approach. If one would follow this algorithm in managing patients enrolled in this study, the application of the molecular analysis would have decreased the need for a second surgery in 30% of patients with an indeterminate cytology. Because of that, I believe that the results of Nikiforov et al are of major importance for clinical practice. Nonetheless, these results need also to be re-evaluated in other prospective trials.

M. Schott, MD, PhD

Reference

1. Baloch ZW, LiVolsi VA, Asa SL, et al. Diagnostic terminology and morphologic criteria for cytologic diagnosis of thyroid lesions: a synopsis of the National Cancer Institute Thyroid Fine-Needle Aspiration State of the Science Conference. *Diagn Cytopathol.* 2008;36:425-437.

Thyroid Cancer

BRAF^{V600E} Mutation and Outcome of Patients with Papillary Thyroid Carcinoma: A 15-Year Median Follow-Up Study

Elisei R, Ugolini C, Viola D, et al (Univ Hosp of Pisa, Italy; et al)

J Clin Endocrinol Metab 93:3943-3949, 2008

Background.—The BRAF^{V600E} mutation is the most frequent genetic alteration in papillary thyroid carcinoma (PTC). The role of BRAF^{V600E} mutation as a poor prognostic factor has been controversially reported in series with short-term follow-ups. In this study we verified the prognostic value of the BRAF^{V600E} mutation in PTC patients with a long-term follow-up.

Methods.—We studied 102 PTC patients with a median follow-up of 15 yr. The BRAF^{V600E} mutation was analyzed by PCR-single-strand conformational polymorphism and sequencing. The correlation between the presence/absence of the BRAF^{V600E} mutation, clinicopathological features, and outcome of PTC patients were evaluated.

Results.—The BRAF^{V600E} mutation was found in 38 of 102 (37.3%) PTC patients, and was significantly more frequent in patients older than 60 yr ($P = 0.02$), in advanced stages ($P = 0.03$), and in cases with vascular invasion ($P = 0.02$). At univariate analysis the worst outcome for PTC patients was significantly correlated with clinicopathological features (*i.e.* age, tumor size, extrathyroid extension, lymph node and distant metastases, advanced stage, vascular endothelial growth factor expression, and vascular invasion) and the BRAF^{V600E} mutation ($P < 0.002$). However, at multivariate analysis only the BRAF^{V600E} mutation showed an independent correlation with the worst outcome ($P = 0.03$). Moreover, the survival curves of PTC patients showed a lower percentage of survivors in the BRAF^{V600E}-mutated group ($P = 0.015$).

Conclusions.—In this study the BRAF^{V600E} mutation correlated with the worst outcome for PTC patients, who were not only at a higher risk not to be cured but also for death. In particular, the BRAF^{V600E} mutation was demonstrated to be a poor prognostic factor independent from other clinicopathological features.

▶ Thyroid cancer harbors several genetic alterations, some of which have been described only in papillary thyroid carcinoma (PTCs). Some years ago, an activating mutation in BRAF (the gene for the B-type Raf kinase, BRAF) has been described and represents the most common genetic alteration in PTC. BRAF is the most potent activator of the mitogen-activated protein kinase (MAP kinase; MEK) pathway.[1] The aim of this study by Elisei was to investigate the impact of the presence of a BRAF mutation on the outcome of the patients. As demonstrated in Figure 3, there is a significant difference in the outcome of PTC patients who harbor a BRAF mutation compared with those who do not have a mutation. One possible explanation for this strong impact of the BRAF^{V600E} mutation on the outcome may be related to the recent evidence that the mutation correlates with a lower expression of sodium/iodide symporter (NIS) and thyroperoxidase (TPO) mRNA and related proteins,[2,3] and that the $BRAF^{V600E}$ mutation is associated with a higher risk of developing PTC recurrence with a poor ability to take up 131-I. Because the success of the radioiodine 131-I treatment, which represents the most important and effective therapeutic procedure for PTC, depends mainly on the ability of tumoral cells to incorporate 131-I, it is conceivable that tumors with lower expression of both NIS and TPO are more resistant to this treatment. According to this evidence, it might be hypothesized that the role of the $BRAF^{V600E}$ mutation as a poor prognostic factor is related primarily to the dedifferentiation process more than to its correlation with more advanced stages of PTC at diagnosis. This hypothesis needs, however, to be confirmed in future studies.

M. Schott, MD, PhD

References

1. Mercer KE, Pritchard CA. Raf proteins and cancer: B-Raf is identified as a mutational target. *Biochim Biophys Acta.* 2003;1653:25-40.
2. Durante C, Puxeddu E, Ferretti E, et al. BRAF mutations in papillary thyroid carcinomas inhibit genes involved in iodine metabolism. *J Clin Endocrinol Metab.* 2007;92:2840-2843.
3. Romei C, Ciampi R, Faviana P, et al. BRAFV600E mutation, but not RET/PTC rearrangements, is correlated with a lower expression of both thyroperoxidase and sodium iodide symporter genes in papillary thyroid cancer. *Endocr Relat Cancer.* 2008;15:511-520.

Mutant *BRAF*^{T1799A} Can Be Detected in the Blood of Papillary Thyroid Carcinoma Patients and Correlates with Disease Status

Cradic KW, Milosevic D, Rosenberg AM, et al (Mayo Clinic, Rochester, MN; Healtheast Care System, Maplewood, MN)
J Clin Endocrinol Metab 94:5001-5009, 2009

Context.—The *BRAF*^{T1799A} transversion is the most frequent morphotype-specific somatic mutation in papillary thyroid carcinoma (PTC). The ability to detect this mutation in the circulation could aid in diagnosis and follow-up of PTC patients.

Objective.—Our objective was to develop and clinically validate a sensitive and specific assay for the detection of *BRAF*^{T1799A} in blood samples from PTC patients.

Design.—We developed an allele-specific real-time PCR method for the detection of *BRAF*^{T1799A} in blood samples and studied prospectively blood samples from 193 patients with thyroid cancer (173 PTC, 20 non-PTC) attending for routine follow-up. The results of molecular testing were correlated with disease status and thyroglobulin measurements. *BRAF*^{T1799A} status of the original tumor samples was also confirmed, where available.

Results.—The assay had a detection sensitivity of fewer than one heterozygote *BRAF*^{T1799A}-carrying cell per 100,000 diploid cells, without detectable cross-reactivity between wild-type *BRAF* and *BRAF*^{T1799A}. Circulating *BRAF*^{T1799A} was detected in 20 of 173 PTC patients and in none of the 20 non-PTC patients. *BRAF*^{T1799A}-positive samples contained between one in 326 and fewer than one in 100,000 copies of *BRAF*^{T1799A}. Tissue *BRAF* status correlated with blood *BRAF* status, whereas *BRAF*^{T1799A} positivity in blood correlated with the presence of active disease at the time of the blood draw, with eight of the 38 PTC patients with persistent/recurrent disease being positive for circulating *BRAF*^{T1799A} (relative risk vs. circulating BRAF^{T1799A}-negative, 2.55; $P < 0.04$).

Conclusions.—BRAF^{T1799A} can be detected in the blood of PTC patients with residual or metastatic disease and may provide diagnostic information.

▶ A high portion of papillary thyroid carcinomas (PTCs) is characterized by somatic aberrations in the *BRAF* kinase gene. The most frequent mutation is due to an amino acid change (T1799A/p.V600E) and is associated with gain of function.[1,2]

Investigation for the presence of *BRAF*^{T1799A} was used additionally to conventional cytology obtained from biopsies of thyroid nodules for subclassification of PTC patients and detection of metastatic spread of PTC.[2] With the introduction of microsatellite markers for malignant disease, patients with PTC were analyzed for the presence of *BRAF*^{T1799A} in blood and, in a proof of principal analysis, detection of circulating *BRAF*^{T1799A} served to identify PTC.

In their study, Cradic et al developed an allele-specific quantitative polymerase chain reaction (PCR)-based assay for the detection of *BRAF*^{T1799A} mutations in peripheral blood (Fig 2 in the original article). Using this test, they studied the frequency of *BRAF*^{T1799A} mutations and correlated the results with thyroglobulin measurements and disease status.

Their test had a specificity of 100%. Circulating mutant *BRAF* was found in little more than 10% of PTC patients. In those subjects, a correlation to disease status was observed. However, basal and stimulated thyroglobulin measurement had the same sensitivity in identifying patients with persistent disease. Interestingly, patients with circulating *BRAF*^{T1799A} had a more than 2.5-fold higher risk for persistent PTC.

It is disappointing to see that the presence of tumor DNA or tumor cells in the peripheral blood of PTC patients is obviously a usual event when the primarius is positive for *BRAF* mutations. This may also hold true for tumors without *BRAF* mutations.

In summary, besides the gift of a relatively sensitive test, the great advantage of this study is that such a procedure may be beneficial for patients with PTC (positive for mutant *BRAF*) who were treated with partial thyroidectomy could be followed up.

H. S. Willenberg, MD, PhD
M. Schott, MD, PhD

References

1. Xing M. BRAF mutation in papillary thyroid cancer: pathogenic role, molecular bases, and clinical implications. *Endocr Rev.* 2007;28:742-762.
2. Nikiforova MN, Nikiforov YE. Molecular genetics of thyroid cancer: implications for diagnosis, treatment and prognosis. *Expert Rev Mol Diagn.* 2008;8:83-95.

The BRAF^{V600E} Oncogene Induces Transforming Growth Factor β Secretion Leading to Sodium Iodide Symporter Repression and Increased Malignancy in Thyroid Cancer

Riesco-Eizaguirre G, Rodríguez I, De La Vieja A, et al (Instituto de Investigaciones Biomédicas "Alberto Sols" Consejo Superior de Investigaciones Científicas y Universidad Autónoma de Madrid, Spain; et al)
Cancer Res 69:8317-8325, 2009

The activating mutation BRAF^{V600E} is a frequent genetic event in papillary thyroid carcinomas (PTC) that predicts a poor prognosis, leading to loss of sodium/iodide symporter (NIS) expression and subsequent radioiodide-refractory metastatic disease. The molecular basis of such an aggressive behavior induced by BRAF remains unclear. Here, we show a mechanism through which BRAF induces NIS repression and promotes epithelial to mesenchimal transition and invasion based on the operation of an autocrine transforming growth factor (TGF)β loop. BRAF induces secretion of functional TGFβ and blocking TGFβ/Smad signaling at multiple levels rescues BRAF-induced NIS repression. Although this mechanism is MAP/extracellular signal-regulated kinase (ERK) kinase (MEK)-ERK independent, secreted TGFβ cooperates with MEK-ERK signaling in BRAF-induced cell migration, Matrigel invasion, and EMT. Consistent with this process, TGFβ and other key components of TGFβ signaling, such as TβRII and pSmad2, are overexpressed in human PTC, suggesting a widespread activation of this pathway by locally released TGFβ. Moreover, this high TGFβ/Smad activity is associated with PTCinvasion, nodal metastasis, and BRAF status. Interestingly, TGFβ is overexpressed in the invasive front, whereas NIS is preferentially expressed in the central regions of the tumors, suggesting that this negative correlation between TGFβ and NIS occurs locally inside the tumor. Our study describes a novel mechanism of NIS repression in thyroid cancer and provides evidence that TGFβ may play a key role in promoting radioiodide resistance and tumor invasion during PTC progression.

► The BRAF^{V600E} mutation is the most prevalent somatic mutation. This oncogene is the most frequent event in thyroid cancer, particularly in papillary thyroid carcinomas (PTCs). BRAF^{V600E} mutation has been associated with the loss of ability to accumulate iodide and, therefore, with a poorer prognosis. The aim of this study was to investigate the molecular mechanisms behind this phenomenon. The authors could demonstrate that BRAF induces transforming growth factor (TGF)β secretion (Fig 1 in the original article) leading to sodium/iodide symporter (NIS) repression in a (MEK-ERK)-independent manner (Fig 2 in the original article) but cooperating with the MEK-ERK pathway to induce strong tumor invasion, 2 major traits acquired during PTC progression. Fig 5 in the original article demonstrates the expression of TGFβ pathway members and NIS in PTC. Although this potential dual role of TGFβ in promoting resistance to radioiodide treatment and enhancing tumor spread needs further investigation, including the study of the tumor locally, it might be proposed that TGFβ plays a key role in thyroid carcinogenesis and can be considered as a new therapeutic target for thyroid cancer.

M. Schott, MD, PhD

Association of High Iodine Intake with the T1799A *BRAF* Mutation in Papillary Thyroid Cancer

Guan H, Ji M, Bao R, et al (The Johns Hopkins Univ School of Medicine, Baltimore, MD; Chongqing No. 9 People's Hosp, Chongqing, the People's Republic of China; et al)

J Clin Endocrinol Metab 94:1612-1617, 2009

Context.—Epidemiological studies have indicated that high iodine intake might be a risk factor for papillary thyroid cancer (PTC), which commonly harbors the oncogenic T1799A *BRAF* mutation.

Objective.—The objective of the study was to investigate the relationship between *BRAF* mutation in PTC and iodine intake in patients.

Subjects and Methods.—We analyzed and compared the prevalences of the T1799A *BRAF* mutation in classical PTC of 1032 patients from five regions in China that uniquely harbor different iodine contents in natural drinking water, ranging from normal (10–21 μg/liter) to high (104–287 μg/liter). The *BRAF* mutation was identified by direct DNA sequencing.

Results.—The prevalence of *BRAF* mutation was significantly higher in any of the regions with high iodine content than any of the regions with normal iodine content. Overall, *BRAF* mutation was found in 387 of 559 PTC with high iodine content (69%) *vs.* 252 of 473 PTC with normal iodine content (53%), with an odds ratio of 1.97 (95% confidence interval 1.53–2.55) for the association of *BRAF* mutation with high iodine content ($P < 0.0001$). In addition, clinicopathological correlation analysis, the largest one of its type ever, showed that *BRAF* mutation was significantly associated with extrathyroidal invasion, lymph node metastasis, and advanced tumor stages of PTC.

Conclusions.—High iodine intake seems to be a significant risk factor for the occurrence of *BRAF* mutation in thyroid gland and may therefore be a risk factor for the development of PTC. This large study also confirmed the association of *BRAF* mutation with poorer clinicopathological outcomes of PTC.

▶ This study from China describes an association between high iodine intake with T1799A BRAF mutation. Detailed results are shown in Fig 2 in the orginal article. Up to now, there is no known environmental factor known that can cause a BRAF mutation. Frasca et al[1] recently examined the relationship of BRAF mutation in papillary thyroid cancer (PTC) with iodine intake in some regions in Italy. The authors found BRAF mutation in 107 of 270 cases in an iodine-sufficient region (40%) versus 18 of 53 cases of PTC in an iodine-deficient region (34%) ($P = 0.44$). Although the difference in BRAF mutation between the 2 regions was not statistically significant, the trend of a higher prevalence of BRAF mutation in the higher-iodine (normal iodine) region than the lower-iodine (iodine deficient) region is in line with the findings in this study. It is possible that very high iodine intake, seen in this study, had a stronger impact on the occurrence of BRAF mutation. A recent study in an Irish population demonstrated a higher prevalence of BRAF mutation in PTC from the recent decades than that in earlier times, and the authors suspected that the cause might be an environmental factor.[2] It would be interesting to see whether this environmental factor could be increased iodine intake. The molecular mechanisms in which high iodine might promote the development of BRAF mutation in thyroid cells remain to be elucidated. Speculatively, it could involve generation of harmful molecular species from the normal oxidation process of iodide in the thyroid cell that may lead to DNA damage or impairment of DNA repair with consequent formation of BRAF mutation. The demonstration of high iodine intake as a risk factor for the occurrence of BRAF mutation in thyroid cells seems to provide a molecular explanation for the association of increased iodine intake with PTC or a shift of the type of thyroid cancer to PTC observed in many other epidemiological studies. In this context, increased iodine intake, which may occur through iodine supplementation programs, might have contributed, to some extent, to the overall rising incidence of PTC worldwide in recent decades. This impact of iodine intake on the rising incidence of PTC in the general population, however, is likely smaller than that of increased use of screening and diagnostic testing, as suggested by the rising incidence of PTC accompanied by an actually somewhat decreased iodine intake in the United States in recent years.[3] In this case, some decrease in PTC incidence that presumably could occur with decreased iodine intake might have been over-offset by an increase in the incidence of PTC caused by the increased use of screening and diagnostic testing for thyroid cancer. It also appears that the amount of iodine intake from normal sea fish consumption may not be a significant risk for the occurrence of thyroid cancer as a meta-analysis study did not show an overall increase in the incidence of thyroid cancer (mostly PTC) in association with fish consumption.[4] In this analysis, however, a relatively small positive effect of sea fish iodine on the incidence of PTC could be masked by the effect of the increased use of screening and diagnostic testing on PTC incidence that could more profoundly and equally affect all the subjects regardless of their fish-eating backgrounds.

M. Schott, MD, PhD

References

1. Frasca F, Nucera C, Pellegriti G, et al. BRAF(V600E) mutation and the biology of papillary thyroid cancer. *Endocr Relat Cancer.* 2008;15:191-205.
2. Smyth P, Finn S, Cahill S, et al. ret/PTC and BRAF act as distinct molecular, time-dependant triggers in a sporadic Irish cohort of papillary thyroid carcinoma. *Int J Surg Pathol.* 2005;13:1-8.
3. Hollowell JG, Staehling NW, Hannon WH, et al. Iodine nutrition in the United States. Trends and public health implications: iodine excretion data from National Health and Nutrition Examination Surveys I and III (1971-1974 and 1988-1994). *J Clin Endocrinol Metab.* 1998;83:3401-3408.
4. Bosetti C, Kolonel L, Negri E, et al. A pooled analysis of case-control studies of thyroid cancer. VI. Fish and shellfish consumption. *Cancer Causes Control.* 2001;12:375-382.

RAS Mutations Are the Predominant Molecular Alteration in Poorly Differentiated Thyroid Carcinomas and Bear Prognostic Impact

Volante M, Rapa I, Gandhi M, et al (San Luigi Hosp, Orbassano, Italy; Univ of Pittsburgh School of Medicine, PA; et al)

J Clin Endocrinol Metab 94:4735-4741, 2009

Context.—Poorly differentiated carcinomas represent an aggressive group of thyroid tumors with controversial classification placement and poorly understood pathogenesis. Molecular data in this group of tumors are extremely heterogeneous, possibly reflecting different inclusion criteria. Recently homogeneous diagnostic criteria have been proposed by our group (Turin proposal) that need to be complemented by detailed molecular characterization.

Objective.—The objective of the study was to define a comprehensive molecular typing of poorly differentiated thyroid carcinomas classified following homogeneous diagnostic criteria.

Design.—Sixty-five cases of poorly differentiated carcinoma selected following the Turin proposal have been screened for N-, K-, H-RAS, BRAF, RET/PTC1 and 3, and PAX8/PPARγ mutations-rearrangements using alternative techniques and in two different laboratories. Molecular data were compared with clinical pathological parameters and survival by univariate and multivariate analysis.

Results.—RAS mutations in codon 61 were by far the most common genetic alteration in poorly differentiated carcinomas (23% of cases), with all mutation in NRAS except one in the HRAS gene. A single BRAF mutation was found in a poorly differentiated carcinoma with a residual component of a tall cell variant of papillary carcinoma. No KRAS, RET/PTC, or PAX8/PPARγ genetic alteration was detected. In this series, the presence of RAS mutations was a unique negative prognostic parameter at multivariate analysis.

Conclusions.—The present study demonstrates that strictly classified poorly differentiated carcinomas are genetically homogeneous, RAS mutations being the almost exclusive genetic event. Moreover, the detection of RAS mutations might be clinically relevant for the prognostic stratification of these tumors.

▶ In this study, the authors performed molecular analysis of a large homogeneous series of poorly differentiated thyroid carcinomas (n = 65) selected using the strict Turin criteria.[1] The presented data indicate that RAS mutations constitute the most common genetic alteration in these tumors. With regard to specific mutation hot spots, NRAS mutations at codon 61 were by far the most common. These findings are in agreement with previous data in the literature on the occurrence of NRAS mutations, although the reported frequency ranged from about 18% to more than 60%. By contrast, the authors could not confirm the high prevalence of KRAS mutations observed by another group[2,3] because no mutations could be detected in the present series using 2 different methods. Interestingly, RAS mutations did not correlate with specific clinical or pathological parameters, but were strongly associated with poor prognosis (Fig 2 in the original article). This suggests that RAS mutation detection might be clinically relevant for the prognostic stratification of these generally more aggressive thyroid tumors because it allows the separation of those poorly differentiated carcinomas that are particularly prone to more aggressive behavior. From a methodological point of view, both the techniques used in the present article seem to be adequate for RAS mutational screening in poorly differentiated thyroid carcinomas, although light cycler polymerase chain reaction (PCR) methods showed a slightly higher sensitivity. This study also represents the most comprehensive genetic profiling of poorly differentiated thyroid carcinomas diagnosed according to the World Health Organization (WHO) classification under strict selection criteria, which demonstrates that among the most common known genetic alterations in thyroid malignancies, the RAS gene mutations represent the most common genetic event in poorly differentiated carcinomas. Moreover, RAS mutations appear to bear prognostic information, identifying a subset of more aggressive tumors within the group.

M. Schott, MD, PhD

References

1. Volante M, Collini P, Nikiforov YE, et al. Poorly differentiated thyroid carcinoma: the Turin proposal for the use of uniform diagnostic criteria and an algorithmic diagnostic approach. *Am J Surg Pathol.* 2007;31:1256-1264.
2. Garcia-Rostan G, Zhao H, Camp RL, et al. ras mutations are associated with aggressive tumor phenotypes and poor prognosis in thyroid cancer. *J Clin Oncol.* 2003;21:3226-3235.
3. Costa AM, Herrero A, Fresno MF, et al. BRAF mutation associated with other genetic events identifies a subset of aggressive papillary thyroid carcinoma. *Clin Endocrinol (Oxf).* 2008;68:618-634.

Activation of the PI3 Kinase Pathway By Retinoic Acid Mediates Sodium/Iodide Symporter Induction and Iodine Transport in MCF-7 Breat Cancer Cells

Ohashi E, Kogai T, Kagechika H, et al (Univ of California at Los Angeles; Tokyo Med and Dental Univ, Japan)

Cancer Res 69:3443-3450, 2009

Iodide uptake in the thyroid and breast is mediated by the sodium/iodide symporter (NIS). NIS activation is used for radioiodide imaging and therapeutic ablation of thyroid carcinoma. NIS is expressed in >70% of breast cancers but at a level insufficient for radioiodine treatment. All-*trans* retinoic acid (tRA) induces NIS gene expression and functional iodide uptake in human breast cancer cell lines and mouse breast cancer models. tRA usually regulates gene expression by direct interaction of RA receptor (RAR) with a target gene, but it can also act through nongenomic pathways. We report a direct influence of tRA treatment on the phosphoinositide 3-kinase (PI3K) signal transduction pathway that mediates tRA-induced NIS expression in MCF-7 breast cancer cells. MCF-7 cells express all three RAR isoforms, α, β, and γ, and RXRα. We previously identified RARβ and RXRα as important for NIS induction by tRA. Treatment with LY294002, the PI3K inhibitor, or p85α knockdown with siRNA abolished tRA-induced NIS expression. Immunoprecipitation experiments and glutathione *S*-transferase pull-down assay showed a direct interaction between RARβ2, RXRα, and p85α. RA also induced rapid activation of Akt in MCF-7 cells. Treatment with an Akt inhibitor or Akt knockdown with siRNA reduced NIS expression. These findings indicate that RA induction of NIS in MCF-7 cells is mediated by rapid activation of the PI3K pathway and involves direct interaction with RAR and retinoid X receptor. Defining these mechanisms should lead to methods to further enhance NIS expression, as well as retinoid targets that influence growth and differentiation of breast cancer.

▶ Expression of the sodium/iodide symporter (NIS) in the breast serves to transport iodine into the milk. Interestingly, NIS is also expressed in a considerable portion of malignant mammary cells.[1] Research in the past decade aimed at finding a way for establishing radioiodine therapy in breast cancer.[2,3] Because the expression level of NIS is too low to reach therapeutic concentrations of radionuclide in breast cancer tissue, efforts were made to increase NIS expression. One approach led to the discovery that all-*trans* retinoic acid (tRA) upregulates NIS in the breast cancer cell line MCF-7.[4]

In their article, Ohashi et al investigated the molecular mechanisms involved in the tRA-mediated increase in NIS expression. Using a range of molecular techniques, the authors show that binding of tRA to the β2-isoform of the retinoic acid receptor (RAR) forming heterodimers with the α-isoform of the retinoid X receptor (RXR) leads to association of the tRA-RARβ2-RXRα complex with the regulatory subunit p85α of the phosphoinositide-3-kinase

(PI3K). This process is followed by rapid phosphorylation of the Ser-473 residue of Akt with consequent activation of the PI3K/Akt pathway.

These results are interesting for different reasons. Firstly, the observation is that a nuclear receptor, here the RAR-RXR heterodimer, is able to activate the PI3K/Akt pathway. Secondly, the activation of this pathway occurs in a very rapid fashion and was independent of de novo protein synthesis supporting the concept of a direct modulation of Akt activity by tRA. Also, from their data, the authors developed a model that summarizes their findings and the fact that a hitherto unknown transcription factor is involved in the activation of the NIS gene by tRA (Fig 6 in the original article).

Main limitations of this study are the use of only one breast cancer cell model, and the point that long-term effects of tRA on NIS expression were not studied.

H. S. Willenberg, MD, PhD
M. Schott, MD, PhD

References

1. Tazebay UH, Wapnir IL, Levy O, et al. The mammary gland iodide transporter is expressed during lactation and in breast cancer. *Nat Med.* 2000;6:871-878.
2. Kogai T, Kanamoto Y, Li AI, et al. Differential regulation of sodium/iodide symporter gene expression by nuclear receptor ligands in MCF-7 breast cancer cells. *Endocrinology.* 2005;146:3059-3069.
3. Dwyer RM, Bergert ER, O'Connor MK, Gendler SJ, Morris JC. In vivo radioiodide imaging and treatment of breast cancer xenografts after MUC1-driven expression of the sodium iodide symporter. *Clin Cancer Res.* 2005;11:1483-1489.
4. Kogai T, Schultz JJ, Johnson LS, Huang M, Brent GA. Retinoic acid induces sodium/iodide symporter gene expression and radioiodide uptake in the MCF-7 breast cancer cell line. *Proc Natl Acad Sci USA.* 2000;97:8519-8524.

Gene expression profiling associated with the progression to poorly differentiated thyroid carcinomas

Pita JM, Banito A, Cavaco BM, et al (Centro de Investigação de Patobiologia Molecular [CIPM], Lisboa, Portugal)
Br J Cancer 101:1782-1791, 2009

Background.—Poorly differentiated thyroid carcinomas (PDTC) represent a heterogeneous, aggressive entity, presenting features that suggest a progression from well-differentiated carcinomas. To elucidate the mechanisms underlying such progression and identify novel therapeutic targets, we assessed the genome-wide expression in normal and tumour thyroid tissues.

Methods.—Microarray analyses of 24 thyroid carcinomas – 7 classic papillary, 8 follicular variants of papillary (fvPTC), 4 follicular (FTC) and 5 PDTC – were performed and correlated with *RAS*, *BRAF*, *RET/PTC* and *PAX8-PPARG* alterations. Selected genes were validated by quantitative RT–PCR in an independent set of 28 thyroid tumours.

Results.—Unsupervised analyses showed that gene expression similarity was higher between PDTC and fvPTC, particularly for tumours

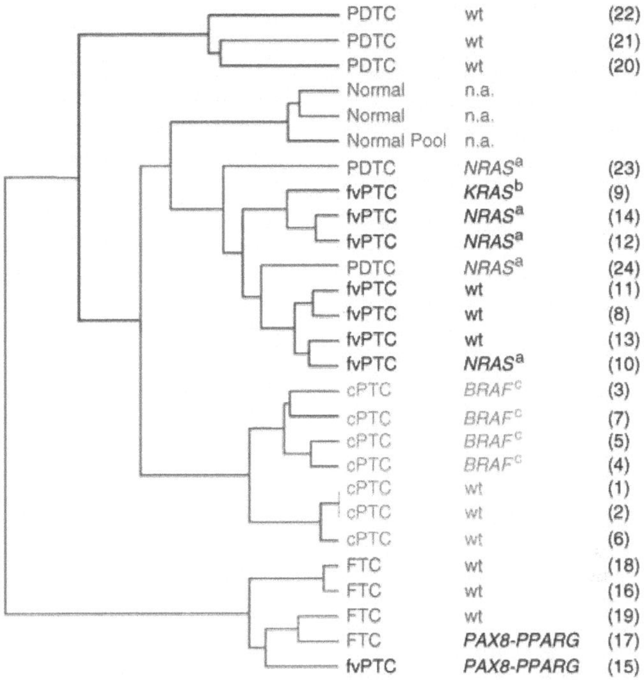

FIGURE 1.—Global gene expression similarity between samples using the unsupervised hierarchical clustering method. In the dendogram, distance separating samples represents the gene expression resemblance between them. The result of mutational analysis for each tumour specimen is shown. Wild-type (wt) label denotes absence of mutation in screened genes; [a]Q61R mutant of *NRAS*; [b]G13R mutant of *KRAS*; [c]V600E mutant of *BRAF*; in parenthesis is indicated the sample number assigned in Supplementary Table 1. cPTC = classic papillary thyroid carcinoma; FTC = follicular thyroid carcinoma; fvPTC = follicular variant of papillary thyroid carcinoma; PDTC = poorly differentiated thyroid carcinoma; n.a. = not applicable. (Courtesy of Pita JM, Banito A, Cavaco BM, et al. Gene expression profiling associated with the progression to poorly differentiated thyroid carcinomas. *Br J Cancer.* 2009;101:1782-1791.)

harbouring *RAS* mutations. Poorly differentiated thyroid carcinomas presented molecular signatures related to cell proliferation, poor prognosis, spindle assembly checkpoint and cell adhesion. Compared with normal tissues, PTC had 307 out of 494 (60%) genes over-expressed, FTC had 137 out of 171 (80%) genes under-expressed, whereas PDTC had 92 out of 107 (86%) genes under-expressed, suggesting that gene downregulation is involved in tumour dedifferentiation. Significant *UHRF1* and *ITIH5* deregulated gene expression in PDTC, relatively to normal tissues, was confirmed by quantitative RT–PCR.

Conclusion.—Our findings suggest that fvPTC are possible precursors of PDTC. Furthermore, *UHRF1* and *ITIH5* have a potential therapeutic/prognostic value for aggressive thyroid tumours.

▶ Patients with well-differentiated thyroid carcinoma (WDTC) usually have a fairly good prognosis. Many patients are monitored clinically, with ultrasound imaging, measurement of secretion of thyroglobulin by residual cells, and idodide scintigraphy. If positive for iodine uptake, they may undergo radioiodide (I-131) therapy for ablation of remaining tissue or even metastasis. Most tumors can be controlled this way for many years. However, some tumors progress to less-differentiated thyroid carcinomas that lose the ability to synthesize thyroglobulin and the capacity for uptake of radiolabeled iodine: poorly differentiated thyroid carcinoma (PDTC). Also, some patients have PDTC at the time of first presentation, and the question is: does PDTC arise from preexisting WDTC or develop de novo?

Using microarray technique for a genome-wide analysis and quantitative polymerase chain reaction (PCR), Pita et al studied the molecular status of 24 thyroid tumors and analyzed the results with respect to the presence of mutations/genetic alterations concerning *BRAF*, *RET/PTC*, *RAS*, and *PAX8-PPARG*.

Interestingly, they found that PDTC exhibits a genetic signature that is similar to papillary thyroid carcinoma (PTC), especially when they are positive for *RAS* mutations and classified as the follicular variant of PTC (fvPTC). When fvPTC had a *PAX8-PPARG* rearrangement, they rather clustered with follicular thyroid carcinomas (Fig 1).

In addition, while the great majority of genes seem to show a lower expression rate in PDTC as compared with normal tissue, activated genes are associated with cell cycle, cell proliferation, and spindle assembly checkpoint. Some genes were reported to be related with a poor prognosis, for example, downregulation of inter-alpha (globulin) inhibitor H5 (*ITIH5*).

The question about whether PDTC arises from pre-existing WDTC or de novo was not answered by the authors, but they showed that fvPTC resemble PDTC providing one argument for such an assumption. One other potential of this study is that genome-wide genetic analysis of malignant tumors has been used to improve diagnosis and prognosis of other tumors,[1] and the authors also found that ubiquitin-like, containing PHD and RING finger domains 1 (UHRF1) was overexpressed. Because the UHRF1 gene product is involved in DNA methylation via DNMT1, it may become a target for therapeutic intervention in patients with PDTC.

H. S. Willenberg, MD, PhD
M. Schott, MD, PhD

Reference

1. Quackenbush J. Microarray analysis and tumor classification. *N Engl J Med.* 2006;354:2463-2472.

Suppressor of Cytokine Signaling 3 Sensitizes Anaplastic Thyroid Cancer to Standard Chemotherapy

Francipane MG, Eterno V, Spina V, et al (Univ of Palermo, Italy; et al)

Cancer Res 69:6141-6148, 2009

We previously showed that cancer cells from papillary, follicular, and anaplastic thyroid carcinomas produce interleukin-4 and interleukin-10, which counteract the cytotoxic activity of conventional chemotherapy through the upregulation of antiapoptotic molecules. Here, we identify Janus kinase/signal transducers and activators of transcription (STAT) and phosphatidyl inositol 3-kinase (PI3K)/AKT as the down-stream pathways through which these cytokines confer resistance to cell death in thyroid cancer. We found that the absence of suppressors of cytokine signaling (SOCS) molecules allows the propagation of the survival signaling. Exogenous expression of SOCS1, SOCS3, and SOCS5 in the highly aggressive anaplastic thyroid cancer cells reduces or abolishes STAT3 and 6 phosphorylation and PI3K/Akt pathway activation resulting in alteration in the balance of proapoptotic and antiapoptotic molecules and sensitization to chemotherapeutic drugs *in vitro*. Likewise, exogenous expression of SOCS3 significantly reduces tumor growth and potently enhances the efficacy of chemotherapy *in vivo*. Our results indicate that SOCS3 regulation of cytokines-prosurvival programs might represent a new strategy to overcome the resistance to chemotherapy-induced cell death of thyroid cancer.

▶ Insensitivity to chemotherapy is a major problem in undifferentiated (anaplastic) thyroid cancer. The resistance to ligand- and chemotherapy-induced cell death is mediated by cytokines, for example, by an autocrine production of interleukin (IL)-4 and IL-10.[1,2] The aim of this article was to investigate the molecular basis of the cytokine-based chemotherapy resistance in thyroid cancer. As demonstrated in Fig 1 in the original article, Janus kinase/signal transducer and activator of transcription (JAK/STAT) and phosphatidyl inositol 3-kinase (PI3K)/Akt pathways are activated in thyroid cancer cells. Importantly, the authors could demonstrate that thyroid cancer cells express low levels of SOCS molecules and express IL-4, IL-10, and their respective receptors (Fig 2 in the original article). In vivo studies also demonstrated that exogenous expression of SOCS3 sensitizes undifferentiated thyroid carcinoma cells to chemotherapy-induced cell death (Fig 6 in the original article). These results suggest that drug resistance in thyroid cancer cells is achieved by the production of cytokines and loss of expression of tumor suppressor genes such as *SOCS*. It is, however, not clear why the 3 *SOCS* genes displayed different abilities in increasing death susceptibility. It is presumable that despite the shared structural similarities, they regulate cytokine signal transduction in different ways. These data provide evidence that exogenous expression of *SOCS* genes may represent another strategy to overcome undifferentiated thyroid cancer refractoriness to chemotherapy. Future in vivo studies should now aim to prove the clinical effectiveness of this approach.

M. Schott, MD, PhD

References

1. Stassi G, Todaro M, Zerilli M, et al. Thyroid cancer resistance to chemotherapeutic drugs via autocrine production of interleukin-4 and interleukin-10. *Cancer Res*. 2003;63:6784-6790.
2. Todaro M, Zerilli M, Ricci-Vitiani L, et al. Autocrine production of interleukin-4 and interleukin-10 is required for survival and growth of thyroid cancer cells. *Cancer Res*. 2006;66:1491-1499.

Prophylactic Lymph Node Dissection for Papillary Thyroid Cancer Less Than 2 cm: Implication for Radioiodine Treatment

Bonnet S, Hartl D, Leboulleux S, et al (Institut Gustave Roussy, Villejuif Cedex, France)

J Clin Endocrinol Metab 94:1162-1167, 2009

Objective.—Prophylactic neck dissection for small papillary carcinoma remains controversial. Radioiodine ablation is not recommended for tumors less than 10 mm and depends on various factors for tumors between 10 and 20 mm. The aim was to determine the effect of lymph node (LN) staging on the indication for treatment with radioiodine.

Patients and Methods.—We conducted a retrospective study of 115 patients presenting with papillary thyroid carcinoma less than 2 cm without ultrasonographically detectable cervical LN treated by total thyroidectomy and complete selective dissection of the central and lateral compartment. Radioiodine treatment was based on definitive pathology (tumor and LN). Follow-up was based on neck ultrasound and thyroglobulin levels.

Results.—LN were found for 41.7% of cases. Radioiodine was not used for 42% of patients with tumors less than 20 mm and no metastatic LN. Fifty-eight percent of patients were treated with radioiodine due to LN metastasis, extracapsular thyroid invasion, or unfavorable histological subtype. LN status affected the indication for radioiodine in 30.5% of cases classified as T1, 12 cases with tumors less than 10 mm but with LN metastases (who received radioiodine), and 13 cases with tumors between 10 and 20 mm but without LN metastases (who did not receive radioiodine). Definitive vocal fold paralysis and hypoparathyroidism each occurred in 0.9% of cases. At 1 yr, ultrasound was normal in all patients, and recombinant human TSH-stimulated thyroglobulin was undetectable for 97% of the patients.

TABLE 3.—Results of LN Dissection Depending on PTC Size

	PTC Size		
	1–10 mm (n = 51)	10–20 mm (n = 64)	1–20 mm (total n = 115)
Absence of LN metastasis: central –, lateral –	34 (66.7%)	33 (51.6%)	67 (58.3%)
Presence of LN metastasis	17 (33.3%)	31 (48.4%)	48 (41.7%)
Central +, lateral +	7/17 (41.2%)	14/31 (45.2%)	21/48 (43.7%)
Central +, lateral –	7/17 (41.2%)	14/31 (45.2%)	21/48 (43.7%)
Central –, lateral +	3/17 (17.6%)	3/31 (9.6%)	6/48 (12.5%)

Conclusion.—Precise LN staging by prophylactic neck dissection for tumors initially staged T1N0 modified the indication for radioiodine ablation for 30% of patients (Table 3).

▶ The aim of this study by Bonnet et al was to determine the effect of lymph node (LN) staging on the indication for radioiodine treatment. One hundred and fifteen patients with 10- to 20-mm papillary thyroid cancers were investigated, all of whom had negative preoperative neck ultrasonography and had prophylactic central- and lateral-compartment LN dissection (details are given in Table 3). In this study, 42% of the patients with tumors < 20 mm without LN metastases were not treated with ^{131}I. However, 58% were treated with ^{131}I because they had LN metastasis, extracapsular thyroid tumor invasion, or an unfavorable histologic subtype. Similar to the study by Hartl et al,[1] after 1 year the neck ultrasonography was normal in all patients, and recombinant human thyroid-stimulating hormone (TSH)-stimulated thyroglobulin was undetectable for 97% of the patients. This study is also of major importance as it shows that precise LN staging by prophylactic neck dissection for tumors initially staged T1N0 modified the indication for radioiodine ablation for about 30% of patients.

M. Schott, MD, PhD
S. Schinner, MD, PhD

Reference

1. Hartl DM, Al GA, Chami L, Leboulleux S, Schlumberger M, Travagli JP. High rate of multifocality and occult lymph node metastases in papillary thyroid carcinoma arising in thyroglossal duct cysts. *Ann Surg Oncol.* 2009;16:2595-2601.

High Rate of Multifocality and Occult Lymph Node Metastases in Papillary Thyroid Carcinoma Arising in Thyroglossal Duct Cysts

Hartl DM, Ghuzlan AA, Chami L, et al (Institut Gustave Roussy, Villejuif, France)

Ann Surg Oncol 16:2595-2601, 2009

Background.—The incidence of cancer in thyroglossal duct cysts (TDC) is low and management is controversial. The objective was to report the rate of multifocality, lymph node metastases, and long-term results for TDC carcinomas in adults.

Materials and Methods.—Files from 1979 to 2008 were reviewed for tumor stage, multifocality in the lobes, lymph node metastases, treatment, and follow-up.

Results.—A total of 18 patients (13 females, 5 males, average age 41.5 years) were treated for papillary carcinoma arising in a TDC. Of these, 15 underwent total thyroidectomy, 1 isthmusectomy and 2 a Sistrunk procedure only. Also, 16 patients underwent neck dissection of the central and/or lateral compartments. Tumors were staged pT1 (n = 15), pT3 (n = 3), pN0 (n = 4), pN1a (n = 3), pN1b (n = 9), Nx (n = 2), M0 (n = 17), and M1 (n = 1, lung metastases). Tumor foci were found in the thyroid lobes in 9 of 16 patients (56%). Lymph node metastases were found in 12 of 16 (75%). Nodes were positive in 6 of 15 central compartment dissections (40%) and in 9 of 15 lateral neck dissections (60%). Metastases to the lateral compartment, with no central compartment metastasis, were found in 6 of 15 patients (40%). Radioiodine was

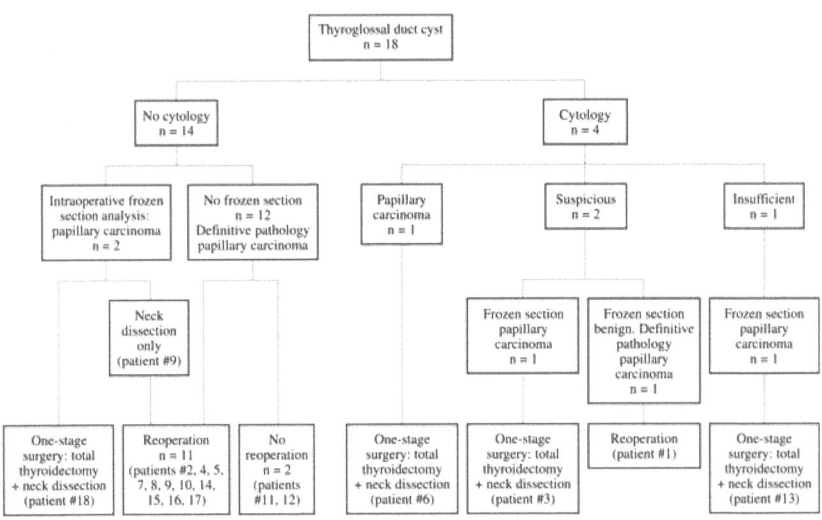

FIGURE 2.—Diagnostic and surgical management of the 18 patients in this series. (With kind permission from Springer Science+Business Media: Hartl DM, Ghuzlan AA, Chami L, et al. High rate of multifocality and occult lymph node metastases in papillary thyroid carcinoma arising in thyroglossal duct cysts. *Ann Surg Oncol.* 2009;16:2595-2601.)

administered to 12 patients. Median follow-up was 12 years (range 1-22 years). All had negative ultrasound. Stimulated Tg levels available for 11 patients were undetectable for 10 and 2 ng/mL for the remaining patient.

Conclusions.—This series shows a high rate of thyroid lobe foci and lymph node metastases but an excellent long-term outcome, characteristics shared with classic papillary carcinoma. Lateral neck metastases seem to be more frequent. These findings are in favor of following the current guidelines for differentiated thyroid cancer in general for the treatment of these rare tumors.

▶ Thyroid cancer occurring in a thyroglossal cyst is an important problem in endocrinology. Many controversial issues swirl around the management of small well-differentiated thyroid carcinomas in this area.[1] The problem is that thyroglossal cysts are very common, yet they rarely contain tumors. However, when they do, there are myriad diagnostic and therapeutic problems. The diagnostic accuracy of fine-needle aspiration biopsy is low, especially in large cystic lesions with a small mural tumor. Moreover, thyroglossal-duct remnants are ubiquitous, comprising more than 75% of midline neck tumors in children, and they are even found in about 7% of adults.[1] Still, only a very small number of people have thyroglossal-duct cancers. Although some report a higher incidence of thyroid cancers,[2] the largest study from California[3] found only 14 thyroid cancers in thyroglossal-duct remnants. Luna-Oritz et al found only 215 cases in the world literature in 2004.

This study shines a bright light on this hazy problem. The study is unique insofar as the surgical approach that was taken in this group of 18 patients. Although the Sistrunk procedure was performed on all of the 18 patients, 15 (83%) also had total thyroidectomy as a secondary procedure, and 1 had an isthmusectomy in addition to the Sistrunk procedure, and 2 had only a Sistrunk procedure. In addition, prophylactic neck dissection in the central compartment with or without lateral-compartment dissection was performed in 16 patients (89%) as part of a surgical protocol used by the authors to optimize tumor staging to facilitate selection of patients for ^{131}I therapy. As a consequence, tumor foci were found in the thyroid in 9 of the 16 patients (56%) who had a total thyroidectomy or in one case, isthmusectomy. In addition to tumor in the thyroglossal-duct remnant, 3 of the 16 patients (19%) were found to have bilateral tumor foci. Lymph-node metastases were found in 12 of the 16 patients (75%) who had prophylactic neck dissections. Lymph-node metastases were found in 6 of 15 central compartment (level VI) dissections (40%) and in 9 of 15 lateral neck dissections (60%). Furthermore, lateral lymph-node metastases were bilateral in 4 patients, on the left side only in 3 patients and on the right side only in 2 patients. A striking finding was skip metastases to the lateral compartments (levels III and IV), without central compartment metastases, which were found in 6 of 15 patients (40%), which is much higher than the usual rate of skip metastases, which was approximately 20% in several large studies.[4,5] Also, level II (subdigastric) lymph nodes were positive in 2 patients, 1 of whom had only 2 isolated level II lymph-node, and the other had levels III and IV lymph-node metastases. Of the 12 patients with lymph-node metastases, 6 (50%) also had tumor foci in the thyroid gland and the other 50% had no thyroid tumors (Fig 2).

A total of 12 patients (67%) were treated with 100 mCi or more of ^{131}I, 11 of whom (92%) had multifocal thyroid tumors with or without lymph-node metastases, and 8 of the 18 patients (44%) were treated with ^{131}I on the basis of lymph-node metastases found as a result of tumors being upstaged to N1a or N1b after prophylactic neck dissection.

Unlike most studies of thyroglossal-duct cancers, the average follow-up was 11 years, with a median of 12 years and a range of 1 to 22. None were lost to follow-up, and no patient had physical evidence of persistent or recurrent disease. All had negative neck ultrasonography and 11 of the 18 patients (61%) had thyrotropin-stimulated serum thyroglobulin measurements, 10 of whom had levels <1 μg/L. Of importance, none of the patients had either temporary or permanent recurrent laryngeal-nerve paralysis or hypoparathyroidism.

The findings of this study are very similar to the study by Bonnet and associates,[6] which was also reviewed. Both studies found that precise lymph-node staging by prophylactic neck dissection for tumors initially staged T1N0 modified the indication for ^{131}I ablation, which was over twice as many patients (67%) with thyroglossal-duct papillary cancers in the Hartl study. Moreover, Hartl and associates point out that prophylactic neck dissection is controversial but that routine central-compartment (level VI) dissection allows staging of the extent of the disease in lymph nodes and is performed by many surgeons to reduce the incidence of reoperation in this region. They also note that prophylactic lateral neck dissection is not part of the current management guidelines for differentiated thyroid cancer. Hartl and associates reach the conclusion that because the rationale for total versus less-than-total thyroidectomy and for elective neck dissection mirrors that for papillary carcinoma arising in the thyroid lobes, we believe that current guidelines for treatment of differentiated thyroid cancer should be followed in treating papillary thyroid cancer arising in thyroglossal duct remnants. This is a well-reasoned conclusion based on important studies that will help further focus the debate over the routine use of prophylactic lymph-node compartment dissection and will facilitate the selection of ^{131}I therapy only in patients with metastases. In my eyes, it is also true that lymph-node level VI compartment dissections must be performed by well trained and highly experienced surgeons.

M. Schott, MD, PhD
S. Schinner, MD, PhD

References

1. Mazzaferri EL. Thyroid cancer in thyroglossal duct remnants: a diagnostic and therapeutic dilemma. *Thyroid*. 2004;14:335-336.
2. Tew S, Reeve TS, Poole AG, Delbridge L. Papillary thyroid carcinoma arising in thyroglossal duct cysts: incidence and management. *Aust N Z J Surg*. 1995;65: 717-718.
3. Doshi SV, Cruz RM, Hilsinger RL Jr. Thyroglossal duct carcinoma: a large case series. *Ann Otol Rhinol Laryngol*. 2001;110:734-738.

4. Machens A, Holzhausen HJ, Dralle H. Skip metastases in thyroid cancer leaping the central lymph node compartment. *Arch Surg*. 2004;139:43-45.
5. Mirallie E, Visset J, Sagan C, Hamy A, Le Bodic MF, Paineau J. Localization of cervical node metastasis of papillary thyroid carcinoma. *World J Surg*. 1999;23: 970-973.
6. Bonnet S, Hartl D, Leboulleux S, et al. Prophylactic lymph node dissection for papillary thyroid cancer less than 2 cm: implications for radioiodine treatment. *J Clin Endocrinol Metab*. 2009;94:1162-1167.

Follow-Up of Low-Risk Differentiated Thyroid Cancer Patients Who Underwent Radioiodine Ablation of Postsurgical Thyroid Remnants after Either Recombinant Human Thyrotropin or Thyroid Hormone Withdrawal

Elisei R, Schlumberger M, Driedger A, et al (Univ of Pisa, Italy; Univ of Paris-Sud XI, France; Univ of Western Ontario, London, Canada; et al)
J Clin Endocrinol Metab 94:4171-4179, 2009

Background.—We previously demonstrated comparable thyroid remnant ablation rates in postoperative low-risk thyroid cancer patients prepared for administration of 3.7GBq ^{131}I (100 mCi) after recombinant human (rh) TSH during T_4 (L-T4) therapy *vs.* withholding L-T4 (euthyroid *vs.* hypothyroid groups). We now compared the outcomes of these patients 3.7 yr later.

Patients and Methods.—Fifty-one of the 63 original patients (28 euthyroid, 23 hypothyroid) participated. Forty-eight received rhTSH and serum thyroglobulin (Tg) sampling. A ^{131}I whole-body scan was performed in 43 patients, and successful ablation was defined by criteria from the previous study. Based on the criterion of uptake less than 0.1% in thyroid bed, 100% (43 of 43) remained ablated. When no visible uptake instead was used, five patients (four euthyroid, one hypothyroid) had minimal visible activity. When the TSH-stimulated Tg criterion was used, only two of 45 (one euthyroid, one hypothyroid) had a stimulated Tg level greater than 2 ng/ml.

Results.—No patient in either group died, and no patient declared disease free had sustained tumor recurrence. Nine (four euthyroid, five hypothyroid) had received additional ^{131}I between the original and current studies due to detectable Tg or imaging evidence of disease; with follow-up, all now had a negative rhTSH-stimulated whole-body scan and seven (three euthyroid, four hypothyroid) had a stimulated serum Tg less than 2 ng/ml.

Conclusions.—In conclusion, after a median 3.7 yr, low-risk thyroid cancer patients prepared for postoperative remnant ablation either with rhTSH or after L-T4 withdrawal were confirmed to have had their thyroid remnants ablated and to have comparable rates of tumor recurrence and persistence (Table 4).

▶ Ablation of postsurgical thyroid tissue is a key element in treatment for selected differentiated epithelial thyroid cancer (DTC) patients. Because

TABLE 4.—Comparison of 8-Month and Current Study Result for Evaluable Patients

	8-Month Postablation Testing in Original Study		3- to 4-yr Postablation Testing in Current Study	
	Hypothyroid Group (n = 30)	Euthyroid Group (n = 33)	Former Hypothyroid Group (n = 21)	Former Euthyroid Group (n = 27)
Patients included in scan analysis/all original patients	28/30	32/33	18/21	25/27
Patients with no visible uptake or less than 0.1%/patients in scan analysis	28/28 (100%)	32/32 (100%)	18/18 (100%)	25/25 (100%)
Patients included in scan analysis/all original patients	28/30	32/33	18/21	25/27
Patients with no visible uptake/patients in scan analysis	24/28 (86%)	24/32 (75%)	17/18 (94%)	21/25 (84%)
Patients with serum Tg measured and no interfering TgAb/all original patients	21/30	24/33	20/21	25/27
Patients with serum Tg less than 2 ng/ml/all patients with Tg analyzed	18/21 (86%)	23/24 (96%)	19/20 (95%)	24/25 (96%)
Patients with serum Tg measured and no interfering TgAb/all original patients	21/30	24/33	20/21	25/27
Patients with serum Tg less than 1 ng/ml/all patients with Tg analyzed	18/21 (86%)	20/24 (83%)	18/20 (90%)	23/25 (92%)

postoperative thyroid remnant ablation requires TSH activation of tissue, the traditional approach of preparation for radioiodine therapy has been to withhold thyroid hormone therapy to induce an endogenous TSH rise.[1] Although this strategy is effective, it causes clinical hypothyroidism with unpleasant symptoms[2] and, in some settings, the need for longer hospitalization compared with patients prepared by recombinant human TSH (rhTSH).[3] In a previous prospective randomized trial,[4] comparable successful postsurgical ^{131}I thyroid remnant ablation rates in 2 groups of low-risk DTC patients who were prepared for administration of 3.7 GBq ^{131}I with either endogenous TSH stimulation induced by 4 or more weeks of thyroid hormone withdrawal or by rhTSH were demonstrated. Successful ablation was achieved in all patients in both groups, based on the primary prospectively defined criterion for thyroid remnant ablation: either no visible uptake or less than 0.1% thyroid bed uptake of the administered ^{131}I activity on imaging performed 8 months after therapy. Up to now, however, no study exists describing the outcome of patients receiving rhTSH. In this study by Elisei et al. there were no differences between the two approaches in eliminating thyroid remnants or in instances of residual disease detected (results summarized in Table 4). These findings confirm that rhTSH is an effective and safe alternative to thyroid hormone withdrawal in preparing low-risk DTC patients for the postsurgical thyroid remnant ablation. This study also confirms that rhTSH-stimulated serum Tg measurement is a highly sensitive indicator of residual disease or normal tissue and one that is superior to radioiodine scanning. Finally, the study confirms the long-term safety of repeated rhTSH exposures.

M. Schott, MD, PhD
S. Schinner, MD, PhD

References

1. Mazzaferri EL, Robyn J. Postsurgical management of differentiated thyroid carcinoma. *Otolaryngol Clin North Am.* 1996;29:637-662.
2. Dow KH, Ferrell BR, Anello C. Quality-of-life changes in patients with thyroid cancer after withdrawal of thyroid hormone therapy. *Thyroid.* 1997;7:613-619.
3. Borget I, Remy H, Chevalier J, et al. Length and cost of hospital stay of radioiodine ablation in thyroid cancer patients: comparison between preparation with thyroid hormone withdrawal and thyrogen. *Eur J Nucl Med Mol Imaging.* 2008;35:1457-1463.
4. Pacini F, Ladenson PW, Schlumberger M, et al. Radioiodine ablation of thyroid remnants after preparation with recombinant human thyrotropin in differentiated thyroid carcinoma: results of an international, randomized, controlled study. *J Clin Endocrinol Metab.* 2006;91:926-932.

PET imaging of medullary thyroid carcinoma in MEN2A transgenic mice using 6-[^{18}F]F-L-DOPA

Pestourie C, Thézé B, Kuhnast B, et al (Service Hospitalier Frédéric Joliot, Orsay Cedex, France)
Eur J Nucl Med Mol Imaging 37:58-66, 2010

Purpose.—6-[^{18}F]Fluoro-3,4-dihydroxy-L-phenylalanine (6-[^{18}F]F-L-DOPA) is increasingly used for PET imaging of neuroendocrine tumours. In this study, we investigated the use of 6-[^{18}F]F-L-DOPA to detect and to monitor the progression of medullary thyroid carcinoma (MTC) in a genetically engineered mouse model of multiple endocrine neoplasia type 2A (MEN2A).

Methods.—Dynamic [^{18}F]FDG and 6-[^{18}F]F-L-DOPA small animal PET scans were acquired during 60 or 90 min in 8- to 20-month-old MEN2A transgenic mice. The kinetics of 6-[^{18}F]F-L-DOPA, standardized uptake values (SUV) at 60 min and tumour volumes were recorded. The detection of MTCs using PET was confirmed by autopsy and histological analysis.

Results.—6-[^{18}F]F-L-DOPA performs better than [^{18}F]FDG for MTC detection in this transgenic mouse model. Uptake kinetics of 6-[^{18}F]F-L-DOPA in MTCs are very different between mice but, in all cases, high contrast could be observed. Furthermore, 6-[^{18}F]F-L-DOPA can detect tumours

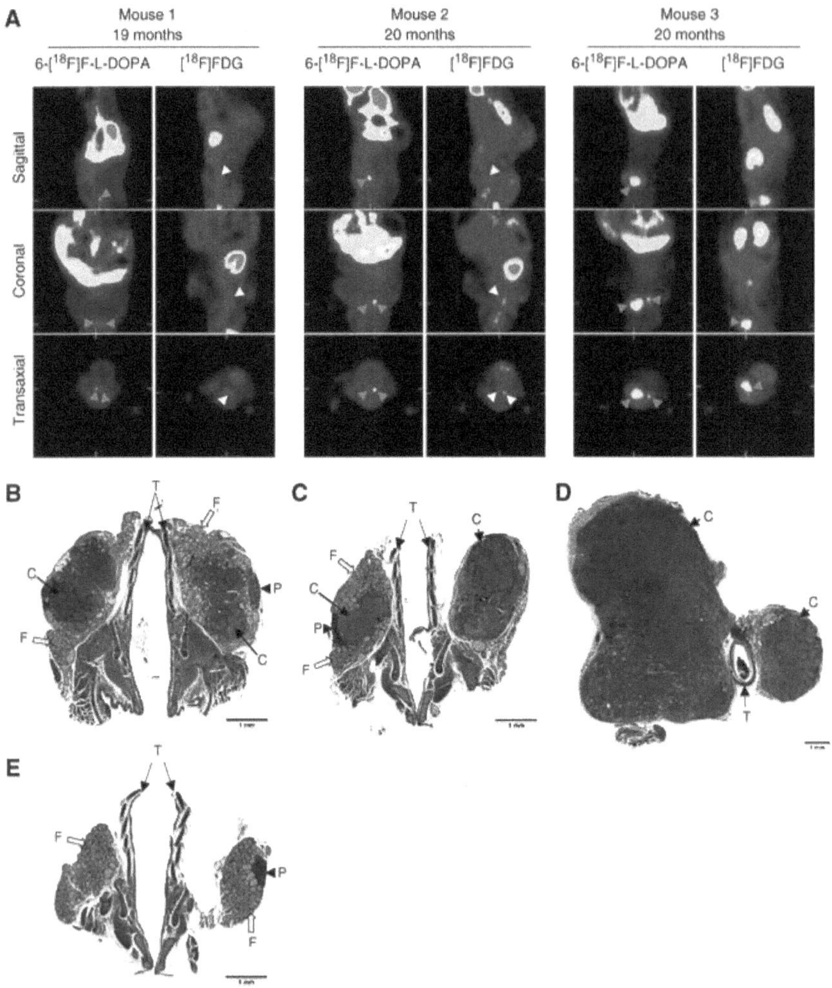

FIGURE 1.—Comparison of 6-[^{18}F]F-L-DOPA vs [^{18}F]FDG MTC labelling in MEN2A transgenic mice. **a** For each mouse, the *left panel* shows 6-[^{18}F]F-L-DOPA labelling and the right panel shows [^{18}F]FDG labelling. *Top to bottom* sagittal, coronal and transaxial section of the mouse, with red arrows indicating the labelled MTC and *white arrows* indicating the [^{18}F]FDG unspecific labelling in the neck. The transaxial section is centred on the thyroid, which appears at the bottom of the images for the two other sections. The images represent the sum of the frame acquired during 1.5 h after i.v. injection of the radiotracer. **b–e** Whole section of thyroid gland in RET-MEN2A transgenic mice after haematoxylin and eosin staining. **b–d** correspond to the thyroid of each of the three mice presented in **a**. **b** corresponds to mouse 1 and is oriented as the coronal PET section, **c** to mouse 2 and is oriented as the coronal PET section and **d** to mouse 3 and is oriented as the transaxial PET section. *F* follicles, *P* parathyroid gland, *T* trachea, *C* carcinoma. Carcinomas are clearly present on these three thyroids. **e** corresponds to a thyroid of a 17-month-old mouse that was labelled neither by 6-[^{18}F]F-L-DOPA nor by [^{18}F]FDG (data not shown): in that case the thyroid had a normal aspect even by histopathological study. The *scale* bar represents 1 mm. For interpretation of the references to color in this figure legend, the reader is referred to web version of this article. (Reprinted from Pestourie C, Thézé B, Kuhnast B, et al. PET imaging of medullary thyroid carcinoma in MEN2A transgenic mice using 6-[^{18}F]F-L-DOPA. *Eur J Nucl Med Mol Imaging.* 2010;37:58-66, with kind permission from Springer Science and Business Media.)

with sizes (1.8 mm^3) that are near the resolution limit of PET, whereas they were undetectable by autopsy at the macroscopic level.

Conclusion.—6-[^{18}F]F-L-DOPA PET imaging can monitor the progression of MTCs in a genetically engineered mouse model (Fig 1).

▶ 6-[^{18}F]Fluoro-3,4-dihydroxy-L-phenylalanine (^{18}F-DOPA) PET is a new functional nuclear medicine procedure that enables metabolic imaging in neuroendocrine tumors. This approach is based on the increased activity of large amino acid transporter (LAT) systems in neuroendocrine tumors such as in MTC.[1] Therefore, in contrast to 2-[18F]Fluoro-2-deoxy-D-glucose (18F-FDG)-PET that uses an increased glucose metabolism to detect metastases, this method is more specific for the neuroendocrine system. Two initial reports some years ago with a very limited number of patients revealed some promising results.[2,3] Within this study the authors demonstrate that ^{18}F-DOPA PET imaging is much more sensitive in detecting MTC in a transgenic mouse model for MTC (with a Ret-Protooncogene mutation). Three extremely impressive examples are shown in Fig 1. Based on that, clinical trial in patients with metastasized MTC should now be performed, for example, in MTC patients with occult metastases.

M. Schott, MD, PhD

References

1. Uchino H, Kanai Y, Kim DK, et al. Transport of amino acid-related compounds mediated by L-type amino acid transporter 1 (LAT1): insights into the mechanisms of substrate recognition. *Mol Pharmacol.* 2002;61:729-737.
2. Hoegerle S, Altehoefer C, Ghanem N, Brink I, Moser E, Nitzsche E. 18F-DOPA positron emission tomography for tumour detection in patients with medullary thyroid carcinoma and elevated calcitonin levels. *Eur J Nucl Med.* 2001;28:64-71.
3. Gourgiotis L, Sarlis NJ, Reynolds JC, VanWaes C, Merino MJ, Pacak K. Localization of medullary thyroid carcinoma metastasis in a multiple endocrine neoplasia type 2A patient by 6-[^{18}F]-fluorodopamine positron emission tomography. *J Clin Endocrinol Metab.* 2003;88:637-641.

Procalcitonin Levels Predict Clinical Course and Progression-Free Survival in Patients With Medullary Thyroid Cancer

Walter MA, Meier C, Radimerski T, et al (Univ Hosp Basel, Switzerland; et al)
Cancer 116:31-40, 2010

Background.—Procalcitonin has been well established as an important marker of sepsis and systemic infection. The authors evaluated the diagnostic and predictive value of calcitonin and its prohormone procalcitonin in medullary thyroid cancer.

Methods.—The authors systematically explored the ability of calcitonin and procalcitonin to identify medullary thyroid cancer and predict the endpoints local recurrence and distant metastases, as well as the progression-free survival. Patients with C-cell hyperplasia; patients after thyroidectomy for differentiated thyroid cancer, goiter, or Graves disease; and

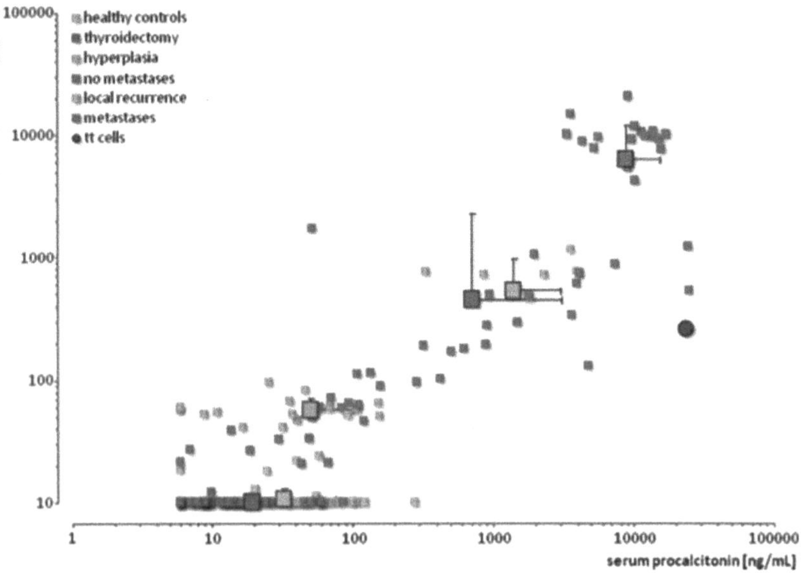

FIGURE 2.—Distribution of calcitonin and procalcitonin (including mean and standard deviation) is shown in the different patient groups. (Reprinted from Walter MA, Meier C, Radimerski T, et al. Procalcitonin levels predict clinical course and progression-free survival in patients with medullary thyroid cancer. *Cancer.* 2010;116:31-40, with permission from Wiley-Liss, Inc.)

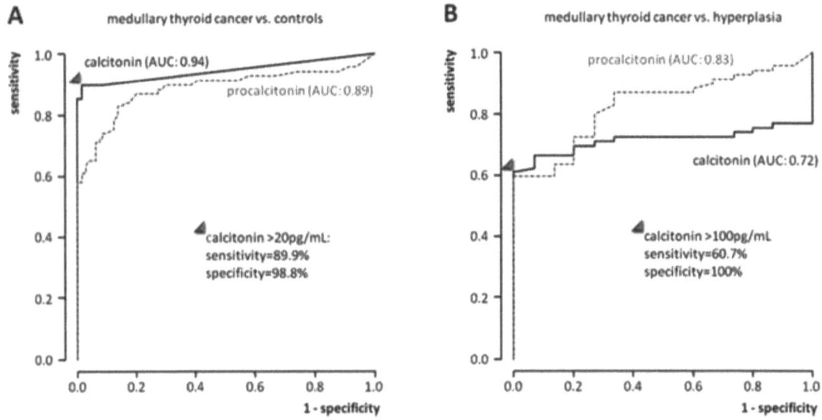

FIGURE 3.—Receiver operating characteristic curves demonstrate the diagnostic value of calcitonin and procalcitonin for differentiating medullary thyroid cancer from (A) controls or (B) patients with C-cell hyperplasia, respectively. Diagonal segments are produced by ties. AUC indicates area under the curve. (Reprinted from Walter MA, Meier C, Radimerski T, et al. Procalcitonin levels predict clinical course and progression-free survival in patients with medullary thyroid cancer. *Cancer.* 2010;116: 31-40, with permission from Wiley-Liss, Inc.)

healthy subjects served as controls. The study was performed in accordance with the Reporting Recommendations for Tumor Marker Prognostic Studies of the National Cancer Institute.

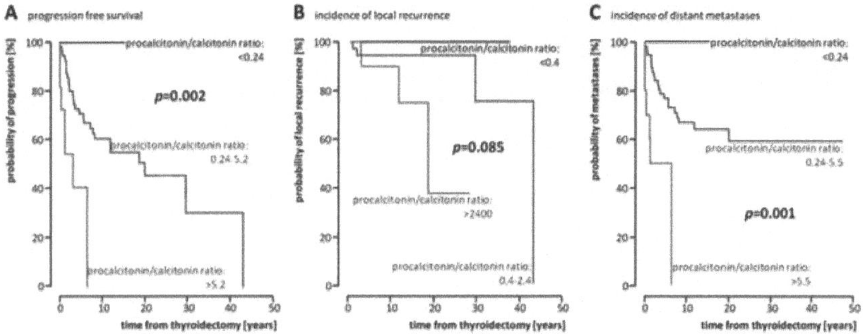

FIGURE 5.—Kaplan-Meier plots demonstrate (A) progression-free survival, (B) incidence of local disease recurrence, and (C) incidence of distant metastases in groups with different procalcitonin:calcitonin ratios. *P* values were derived using the Mantel-Cox log-rank test. (Reprinted from Walter MA, Meier C, Radimerski T, et al. Procalcitonin levels predict clinical course and progression-free survival in patients with medullary thyroid cancer. *Cancer.* 2010;116:31-40, with permission from Wiley-Liss, Inc.)

Results.—Sixtynine medullary thyroid cancer patients and 96 controls were included (median observed interval: 10.9 years [range, 1.4-47.5 years]; 981.8 patient-years). The 1-year, 5-year, 10-year, and 20-year recurrence rates were 9%, 34%, 45%, and 56%, respectively. Calcitonin had a higher diagnostic accuracy for detecting medullary thyroid cancer than procalcitonin (area under the curve [AUC], 0.94; 95% confidence interval [95% CI], 0.90-0.99 vs AUC, 0.89; 95% CI, 0.83-0.95 [*P* =.038]). The procalcitonin:calcitonin ratio predicted disease progression (AUC, 0.63; 95% CI, 0.51-0.75 [*P* =.036]) and progression-free survival (hazards ratio, 1.49; 95% CI, 1.09-2.04 [*P* =.013]).

Conclusions.—The results of the current study indicate a superior diagnostic accuracy of calcitonin and an independent predictive value of the procalcitonin: calcitonin ratio. These findings may lead to improved diagnostic and therapeutic strategies for medullary thyroid cancer patients (Figs 2, 3 and 5).

▶ Medullary thyroid carcinoma (MTC) is a malignant tumor of the thyroid C cells, accounting for about 3% of thyroid cancers. Most MTCs overproduce the main C cell secretory product, calcitonin (CT). CT is considered a sensitive and a specific marker for MTC and is, therefore, used for the diagnosis and the follow-up of MTC. Serial measurements of CT are useful for quantification of tumor mass and disease progression, with doubling times of less than 2 years being associated with a poorer prognosis. Carcinoembryonic antigen (CEA) is also used for monitoring MTC patients. CEA, although a nonspecific and insensitive marker for the detection of early MTC, is a useful follow-up marker, with increases being a possible predictor of disease progression. One of the shortcomings of CT is that modest increases in serum CT concentrations might be observed in C-cell hyperplasia, other neuroendocrine tumors, etc. A possible alternative tumor marker that is largely free of these and other problems is the precursor of CT, procalcitonin (PCT). Expression of PCT in healthy individuals is limited to thyroid C cells, and it is found at low concentrations in the circulation. Unlike CT, PCT has a concentration-independent and highly predictable in vivo half-life of 20 to 24 h, and it displays excellent in vitro stability in serum or plasma. The aim of this study was to validate PCT as an MTC tumor marker. As shown in Fig 2, there is a clear correlation between CT and PCT in different patient groups. Receiver operating characteristic curves, however, demonstrate that the diagnostic sensitivity for the diagnosis of MTC is higher for CT than for PCT (Fig 3). Importantly, however, the procalcitonin/calcitonin ratio will help predict the progression-free survival and the incidence of local disease recurrence and distant metastases (Fig 5). This may also help for a more personalized disease prediction.

M. Schott, MD, PhD

Phase II Study of Safety and Efficacy of Motesanib in Patients With Progressive or Symptomatic, Advanced of Metastatic Medullary Thyroid Cancer

Schlumberger MJ, Elisei R, Bastholt L, et al (Univ Paris Sud, Villejuif, France; Centre Léon Bérard, Lyon, France; Univ of Pisa, Italy; et al)
J Clin Oncol 27:3794-3801, 2009

Purpose.—This phase II study investigated the efficacy and tolerability of motesanib, an investigational, highly selective inhibitor of vascular endothelial growth factor receptors 1, 2, and 3; platelet-derived growth factor receptor; and Kit in advanced medullary thyroid cancer (MTC).

Patients and Methods.—Patients with locally advanced or metastatic, progressive or symptomatic MTC received motesanib 125 mg/d orally for up to 48 weeks or until unacceptable toxicity or disease progression. The primary end point was objective response by independent review. Other end points included duration of response, progression-free survival, safety, pharmacokinetics, and changes in tumor markers.

Results.—Of 91 enrolled patients who received motesanib, two (2%) achieved objective response (95% CI, 0.3% to 7.7%); their duration of response was 32 weeks (censored) and 21 weeks (disease progressed). Eighty-one percent of patients had stable disease (48% had durable stable disease ≥ 24 weeks), 8% had disease progression as best response, and 9% were not evaluated; 76% experienced a decrease from baseline in target lesion measurement. Median progression-free survival was 48 weeks (95% CI, 43 to 56 weeks). Among patients with tumor marker analysis, 69 (83%) of 83 and 63 (75%) of 84 had decreased serum calcitonin and carcinoembryonic antigen during treatment, respectively, compared with baseline. The most common treatment-related adverse events were diarrhea (41%), fatigue (41%), hypothyroidism (29%), hypertension (27%), and anorexia (27%). In pharmacokinetic analyses, motesanib trough concentrations were lower compared with differentiated thyroid cancer patients from the same study.

Conclusion.—Although the objective response rate was low, a significant proportion of MTC patients (81%) achieved stable disease while receiving motesanib.

▶ Medullary thyroid carcinoma (MTC) arises from the C-cells of the thyroid gland. The treatment paradigm for MTC is now shifting. Previously, patients with advanced progressive disease were relegated to receiving traditional parenteral chemotherapies, which have many toxic side effects and low response rates.[1] With evolving insight into the pathways that promote tumorigenesis and metastatic spread and apoptosis inhibition, multiple new agents have been created to target refractory thyroid cancers.[2] These targeted molecular therapies were initially received with much enthusiasm with the hope that one may offer a cure for MTC. While there have been no complete responses seen with the various agents tested, not all optimism is lost. Such new therapy modality may represent a treatment with vascular endothelial growth factor (VEGF) inhibitors. VEGF is a potent angiogenesis stimulator. As prerequisite, an increased VEGF expression has already been demonstrated in differentiated thyroid cancers (DTC). This was associated with increased growth, progression, and invasiveness of the tumor and with decreased recurrence-free survival.[3] For this reason, an inhibitor of angiogenesis may be effective when initial therapy fails. Motesanib diphosphate is an oral inhibitor of the tyrosine kinases of VEGF receptors (VEGFRs) 1, 2, and 3; platelet-derived growth-factor receptor; and KIT. The study of Schlumberger et al describes a high rate (81%) of stable disease in patients with metastasized MTC (Fig 1 in the original article). These findings are encouraging in that VEGFR inhibitors appear to be effective cytostatic agents for patients with progressive MTC.

Because disease stabilization is considered an acceptable end point in patients with thyroid cancer, the current methodology of determining objective responses in clinical trials may not be ideal. Further, the existing Response Evaluation Criteria in Solid Tumors (RECIST) do not consider some clinically meaningful end points that translate into reductions in tumor burden. For example, patients with bone metastases or bilateral subcentimeter pulmonary metastases are deemed to have nonmeasurable lesions by RECIST, and a significant proportion of patients with thyroid cancer may fall into this category. Reductions in the size of such tumors will not be represented with the existing RECIST. In the study by Schlumberger et al, 76% of the patients had significant reductions in tumor burden but were categorized as stable disease by RECIST. Other indications of improving clinical course include tumor markers and symptom control; RECIST does not capture these clinical parameters.

It is also important to discuss that plasma concentrations may also influence the outcome of patients. Plasma concentrations of motesanib were consistently lower in the patients with MTC than their DTC counterparts on a parallel study.[3] It is not known whether the higher objective response rate (14%) in patients with differentiated tumors is attributable to this discrepancy in serum concentrations. The authors have speculated that the higher incidence of diarrhea in patients with MTC at study entry may be responsible for a reduction in the absorbed dose of motesanib. It would certainly be valuable to know whether higher doses of motesanib would result in improved response rates. Additional studies may be needed to answer this question.

M. Schott, MD, PhD

References

1. Droz JP, Rougier P, Goddefroy V, Schlumberger M, Gardet P, Parmentier C. [Chemotherapy for medullary cancer of the thyroid. Phase II trials with adriamycin and cis-platinum administered as monochemotherapy]. *Bull Cancer.* 1984;71:195-199 [in French].
2. Sherman SI. Advances in chemotherapy of differentiated epithelial and medullary thyroid cancers. *J Clin Endocrinol Metab.* 2009;94:1493-1499.
3. Sherman SI, Wirth LJ, Droz JP, et al. Motesanib diphosphate in progressive differentiated thyroid cancer. *N Engl J Med.* 2008;359:31-42.

Galectin-3 Targeted Therapy with a Small Molecule Inhibitor Activates Apoptosis and Enhances Both Chemosensitivity and Radiosensitivity in Papillary Thyroid Cancer

Lin C-I, Whang EE, Donner DB, et al (Brigham and Women's Hosp, Boston, MA; Univ of California at San Francisco; et al)
Mol Cancer Res 7:1655-1662, 2009

Although most patients with papillary thyroid cancer (PTC) have favorable outcomes, some have advanced PTC that is refractory to external beam radiation and systemic chemotherapy. Galectin-3 (Gal-3) is a β-galactoside-binding protein with antiapoptotic activity that is consistently overexpressed in PTC. The purpose of this study is to determine if Gal-3 inhibition promotes apoptosis, chemosensitivity, and radiosensitivity in PTC. PTC cell lines (8505-C and TPC-1) and human *ex vivo* PTC were treated with a highly specific small molecule inhibitor of Gal-3 (Td131_1). Apoptotic activity was determined by flow cytometric analysis as well as caspase-3 and PARP cleavage. The minimum inhibitory concentrations of Td131_1 and doxorubicin were determined, and their combined effects were measured to test for synergistic activity. The effects of Td131_1 on radiosensitivity were determined by a clonogenic assay. Td131_1 promoted apoptosis, improved radiosensitivity, and synergistically enhanced chemosensitivity to doxorubicin in PTC cell lines. In PTC *ex vivo*, Td131_1 treatment alone induced the cleavage of caspase-3 and PARP. Td131_1 and doxorubicin together activated apoptosis in PTC *ex vivo* to a greater degree than their combined individual effects. Td131_1 activated apoptosis and had synergistic activity with doxorubicin in PTC. We conclude that Gal-3 targeted therapy is a promising therapeutic strategy for advanced PTC that is refractory to surgery and radioactive iodine therapy.

▶ Galectin-3 (Gal-3) is a β-galactoside–binding protein that is consistently overexpressed in papillary thyroid cancer (PTC).[1] Gal-3 has potent antiapoptotic effects and promotes chemoresistance to doxorubicin in PTC.[1] High Gal-3 expression is associated with unfavorable tumor characteristics in PTC, such as tumor invasion.[2] Because the principal mechanism of action of doxorubicin and external beam radiation therapy involves the activation of apoptosis, Gal-3 targeted therapy is a rational strategy to improve the efficacy of both modalities. Because a previous study found that Gal-3 inhibition in vivo resulted in minimal overt toxicity,[3] the authors believed that combination therapy that includes Gal-3 inhibition is a promising strategy for patients with advanced cancers, such as PTC. Here they could demonstrate that a treatment with Td131_1 (a binding protein to Galectin-3) has a direct effect on tumor cell growth (Fig 2 in the original article) as well as on chemosensitivity (Fig 4 in the original article) and radioresistance (Fig 7 in the original article). This substance may, therefore, represent a new molecule for the treatment of poorly differentiated thyroid cancer. This needs, however, to be proven in a clinical setting.

M. Schott, MD, PhD

References

1. Lin CI, Whang EE, Abramson MA, et al. Galectin-3 regulates apoptosis and doxorubicin chemoresistance in papillary thyroid cancer cells. *Biochem Biophys Res Commun.* 2009;379:626-631.
2. Savin S, Cvejic D, Isic T, Paunovic I, Tatic S, Havelka M. Thyroid peroxidase and galectin-3 immunostaining in differentiated thyroid carcinoma with clinicopathologic correlation. *Hum Pathol.* 2008;39:1656-1663.
3. John CM, Leffler H, Kahl-Knutsson B, Svensson I, Jarvis GA. Truncated galectin-3 inhibits tumor growth and metastasis in orthotopic nude mouse model of human breast cancer. *Clin Cancer Res.* 2003;9:2374-2383.

Phase I Clinical Trials in 56 Patients with Thyroid Cancer: The M. D. Anderson Cancer Center Experience

Tsimberidou AM, Vaklavas C, Wen S, et al (Univ of Texas M. D. Anderson Cancer Ctr; The Univ of Texas Med School at Houston)
J Clin Endocrinol Metab 94:4423-4432, 2009

Introduction.—Thyroid cancer is the most common endocrine malignancy. The outcomes of patients with relapsed thyroid cancer treated on early-phase clinical trials have not been systematically analyzed.

Patients and Methods.—We reviewed the records of consecutive patients with metastatic thyroid cancer referred to the Phase I Clinical Trials Program from March 2006 to April 2008. Best response was assessed by Response Evaluation Criteria in Solid Tumors.

Results.—Fifty-six patients were identified. The median age was 55 yr (range 35–79 yr). Of 49 patients evaluable for response, nine (18.4%) had a partial response, and 16 (32.7%) had stable disease for 6 months or longer. The median progression-free survival was 1.12 yr. With a median follow-up of 15.6 months, the 1-yr survival rate was 81%. In univariate analysis, factors predicting shorter survival were anaplastic histology ($P = 0.0002$) and albumin levels less than 3.5 g/dl ($P = 0.05$). Among 26 patients with tumor decreases, none died (median follow-up 1.3 yr), whereas 52% of patients with any tumor increase died by 1 yr ($P = 0.0001$). The median time to failure in our phase I clinical trials was 11.5 months vs. 4.1 months for the previous treatment ($P = 0.04$).

Conclusion.—Patients with advanced thyroid cancer treated on phase I clinical trials had high rates of partial response and prolonged stable disease. Time to failure was significantly longer on the first phase I trial compared with the prior conventional treatment. Patients with any tumor decrease had significantly longer survival than those with any tumor increase.

▶ In recent years, the discoveries of signalling pathways and mutational analysis have introduced targeted therapies for treating thyroid carcinoma. Elucidating the molecular pathways involved in thyroid carcinogenesis has led to the development of novel targeted therapeutic approaches. Within the last couple of years, some very interesting studies have been published on the use of new substances (mainly tyrosine kinase inhibitors) for the treatment of metastatic thyroid cancer. In this article, the authors summarized the data of phase 1 studies performed at The University of Texas M. D. Anderson Cancer Center. A number of different agents were applied (Table 2 in the original article). Clinical data (by Response Evaluation Criteria in Solid Tumors [RECIST] criteria) are shown in Fig 1 in the original article. It is important to note that there is 1 patient with an anaplastic thyroid cancer beautifully responding to such a new therapy. These results also demonstrate that patients with advanced thyroid cancer treated in phase 1 clinical trials of predominantly targeted agents had high rates of durable partial response and prolonged stable disease. Of interest, time to failure on their first phase 1 trial was significantly longer than that of their last systemic medical treatment. These observations suggest that such patients benefit from enrolling in early clinical trials and refute the belief that any apparent benefit may be due to a favorable natural history of the subpopulation treated. It might be postulated that molecular profiling and selection of personalized targeted therapies are likely to further optimize the clinical outcomes of patients with metastasized thyroid cancer.

M. Schott, MD, PhD

Amino Acid-Modified Calcitonin Immunization Induces Tumor Epitope-Specific Immunity in a Transgenic Mouse Model for Medullary Thyroid Carcinoma

Wuttke M, Papewalis C, Meyer Y, et al (Univ Hosp Duesseldorf, Germany)
Endocrinology 149:5627-5634, 2008

Up to now, no relevant tumor antigen has been identified in medullary thyroid carcinoma (MTC). The aim of the present study was to prove the concept of an immunization with an amino acid-modified calcitonin (CT) for the treatment of MTC in a transgenic mouse model. Amino acid-modified (human) CT has been chosen for vaccination because of its higher binding affinity to the murine H2-K^b-MHC molecule. Mice were immunized over 6 months with monthly injections of amino acid-modified CT-pulsed dendritic cells. For enumeration of tumor epitope-specific $CD8^+$ cytotoxic T cells, tetramer analyses were performed. CT peptide-treated mice revealed a mean 0.73 ± 0.45 and 0.91 ± 0.59% positive cells, depending on the two tetramers tested, whereas no increase was seen in control protein-immunized mice (0.08–0.12% tetramer-positive cells). Importantly, the subset of CT-specific $CD8^+$ T cells also showed a high expression of interferon-γ. In line with these results, CT-immunized mice also showed an intratumor infiltration with $CD8^+$ T lymphocytes. Importantly, we also found a diminished tumor outgrowth of −57% and a decrease of the serum CT levels (2.0 ± 0.1 pg/ml) compared with control protein-immunized Ret/Cal mice (3.0 ± 0.4 pg/ml). In summary, we show that amino acid-modified CT is recognized from the immune system leading to a specific antitumor immune response and a diminished tumor outgrowth in transgenic MTC mice. The results are of potential importance because they might be applicable to patients with metastatic spread of a MTC.

▶ In the past the same group already proved the concept that calcitonin can be recognized from the immune system and that immunization strategies with calcitonin as target molecule may lead to clinical effects in some cases.[1,2] The authors now used an innovative approach to increase the immunogenicity of tumor antigens, here shown for calcitonin in medullary thyroid carcinoma (MTC). This approach has already been described to be successful in other non-endocrine malignancies.[3-5] Based on a computer-based mathematical epitope prediction program (SYFPEITHI) for calculating high binding affinities of certain peptides to a given MHC molecule, they have chosen human calcitonin for immunization with antigen-presenting dendritic cells. Based on tetramer analyses they could demonstrate a large increase of epitope-specific $CD8^+$T cells (Fig 3 in the original article). These cells were able to directly lyse MTC cells in vitro. Importantly, the authors found a tumor infiltration with $CD8^+$T lymphocytes and a diminished tumor outgrowth together with a decline of serum calcitonin levels (Fig 5 & 6 in the original article).

The results demonstrated are in line with previous data from another group who immunized patients with parathyroid carcinoma with amino acid-modified parathyroid hormone peptides.[6,7] These data may not only represent a basis for future vaccination trials in polypeptide secreting neuroendocrine malignancies such as MTC, but also for other endocrine cancers such as poorly differentiated thyroid cancers where upcoming tumor antigens might be modified in their structure to increase their immunogenicity.

S. Schinner, MD, PhD

References

1. Schott M, Seissler J, Lettmann M, et al. Immunotherapy for medullary thyroid carcinoma by dendritic cell vaccination. *J Clin Endocrinol Metab.* 2001;86: 4965-4969.
2. Schott M, Feldkamp J, Klucken M, et al. Calcitonin-specific antitumor immunity in medullary thyroid carcinoma following dendritic cell vaccination. *Cancer Immunol Immunother.* 2002;51:663-668.
3. Rubio V, Stuge TB, Singh N, et al. Ex vivo identification, isolation and analysis of tumor-cytolytic T cells. *Nat Med.* 2003;9:1377-1382.
4. Gold JS, Ferrone CR, Guevara-Patino JA, et al. A single heteroclitic epitope determines cancer immunity after xenogeneic DNA immunization against a tumor differentiation antigen. *J Immunol.* 2003;170:5188-5194.
5. Zirlik KM, Zahrieh D, Neuberg D, et al. Cytotoxic T cells generated against heteroclitic peptides kill primary tumor cells independent of the binding affinity of the native tumor antigen peptide. *Blood.* 2006;108:3865-3870.
6. Bradwell AR, Harvey TC, Yancy CW, et al. Control of hypercalcaemia of parathyroid carcinoma by immunisation. *Lancet.* 1999;353:370-373.
7. Betea D, Bradwell AR, Harvey TC, et al. Hormonal and biochemical normalization and tumor shrinkage induced by anti-parathyroid hormone immunotherapy in a patient with metastatic parathyroid carcinoma. *J Clin Endocrinol Metab.* 2004;89:3413-3420.

Long-term prognosis of medullary thyroid carcinoma

Rendl G, Manzl M, Hitzl W, et al (Paracelsus Private Med Univ Salzburg, Austria)
Clin Endocrinol 69:497-505, 2008

Objective.—The clinical course of patients with medullary thyroid carcinoma (MTC) is variable, even in the subgroup of patients after surgery with curative intent and postoperatively persistent elevated calcitonin levels. This study aimed to evaluate the long-term prognosis of survival in patients with MTC.

Patients.—Long-term survival was analysed in 32 patients with MTC being treated in an endocrine centre over a 40-year period. Patients were classified as having sporadic MTC, familial MTC (FMTC), multiple endocrine neoplasia (MEN) IIA or MEN IIB.

Results.—Seventeen patients had sporadic MTC (53·1%), eight had MEN IIA (25%) and three had MEN IIB (9·4%); the remaining four patients (12·5%) had not undergone genetic analysis until now. The overall average age at diagnosis was 42·0 years, and the median follow-up time was 9·5 years (range 0·5–39 years). Mortality due to progressive MTC was 15·6%. The 5-year survival rate was 96% (95% CI 89–100), the 10-year survival rate 91% (95% CI 79–100), and the 15-year survival rate 85% (95% CI 78–100). The estimated mean survival time after initial diagnosis was 31 years (95% CI 26·7–37·0). There is a significant difference in survival time between patients achieving complete remission compared with patients with biochemical persistent disease ($P = 0{\cdot}038$) or metastasis ($P = 0{\cdot}0003$). In five patients, advanced imaging with

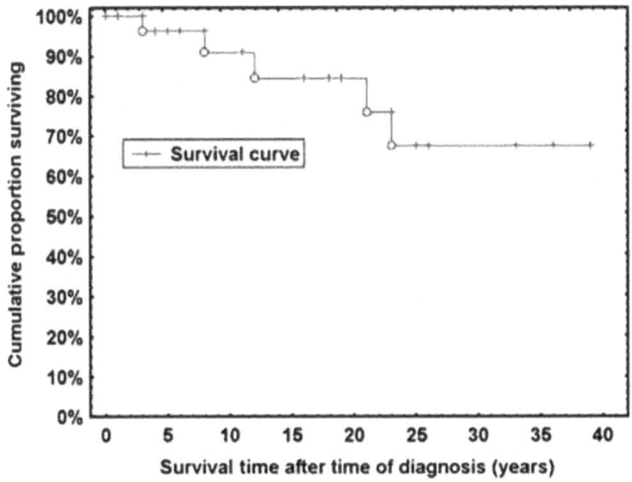

FIGURE 1.—Kaplan–Meier plot of cumulative proportion of patients surviving after initial diagnosis (terminal event = patient was alive or dead). Five-year, 10-year and 15-year survival rates were 96%, 91% and 85%, respectively. (Reprinted from Rendl G, Manzl M, Hitzl W, et al. Long-term prognosis of medullary thyroid carcinoma. *Clin Endocrinol.* 2008;69:497-505, with permission from Wiley-Blackwell.)

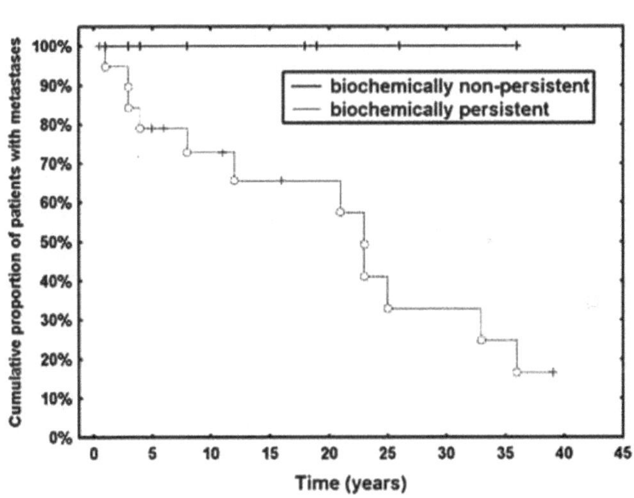

FIGURE 2.—Kaplan–Meier plot of cumulative proportion of patients with metastases in biochemically persistent and nonpersistent patients (terminal event = metastases were present/absent), $P = 0{\cdot}038$. (Reprinted from Rendl G, Manzl M, Hitzl W, et al. Long-term prognosis of medullary thyroid carcinoma. *Clin Endocrinol.* 2008;69:497-505, with permission from Wiley-Blackwell.)

positron emission tomography/computed tomography (PET/CT) identified additional sites of tumour load. Eight more lymph node metastases were found in four patients and one local tumour recurrence in one patient by PET/CT.

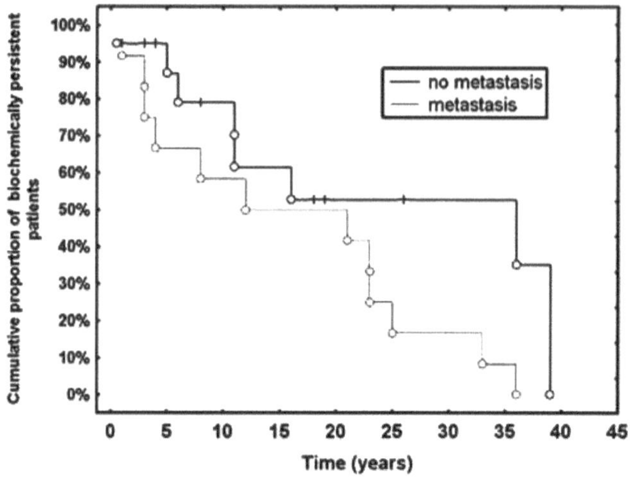

FIGURE 3.—Kaplan–Meier plot of cumulative proportion of biochemically persistent patients in patients with and without metastases (terminal event = patient was biochemically persistent/nonpersistent), $P = 0{\cdot}0003$. (Reprinted from Rendl G, Manzl M, Hitzl W, et al. Long-term prognosis of medullary thyroid carcinoma. *Clin Endocrinol.* 2008;69:497-505, with permission from Wiley-Blackwell.)

Conclusion.—The overall prognosis of MTC is favourable, even if the rate of biochemical cure is lower in MTC than in differentiated types of thyroid cancer. This is also true for patients with biochemically persistent disease. Whether the identification of further tumour sites by advanced imaging procedures such as PET/CT translates into a better prognosis in patients with persistently elevated calcitonin levels remains to be investigated.

▶ Medullary thyroid carcinoma (MTC) is a rare tumor derived from the parafollicular calcitonin (CT) secreting cells of the thyroid, explaining the key role of CT as a specific and sensitive marker of this cancer. MTC occurs in the sporadic form in about 70% to 80% of cases, while the remaining 20% to 30% are due to inherited forms,[1] including either isolated (familial MTC) or part of multiple endocrine neoplasia syndromes. Former studies demonstrated that prognosis of MTC is relatively good with a 10-yr survival rate ranging from 47% to 78%[2] and even better in patients with CT, doubling time of more than 2 years. Within the past decade the prognosis has improved mainly because of earlier diagnosis and improvement in surgical procedures. Nevertheless, more than 50% of nonprophylactic thyroidectomized patients are not cured after surgery. In these cases, residual tumor cells can be detected by measuring serum CT alone or in combination with pentagastrin stimulation. In patients with metastatic spread, CT doubling time is an independent predictor of survival.[3]

The aim of this study by Rendl was to investigate the long-term prognosis of MTC patients in a single center over a 40 year period. Fig 1 shows the overall survival and in Fig 2 a discrimination between patients with persistent and nonpersistent disease is shown. Fig 3 shows the survival of patients depending on the presence of morphologically detectable metastases. This study shows that the overall survival of patients with MTC is favorable. Therefore, the question arises whether extensive nuclear imaging procedures should be used regularly in clinical practice, or rather applied selectively based on patient history or an increase (doubling time) in CT level. These questions have not yet been addressed in prospective studies.

M. Schott, MD, PhD

References

1. Vitale G, Caraglia M, Ciccarelli A, et al. Current approaches and perspectives in the therapy of medullary thyroid carcinoma. *Cancer.* 2001;91:1797-1808.
2. Samaan NA, Schultz PN, Hickey RC. Medullary thyroid carcinoma: prognosis of familial versus nonfamilial disease and the role of radiotherapy. *Horm Metab Res Suppl.* 1989;21:21-25.
3. Barbet J, Campion L, Kraeber-Bodere F, Chatal JF. Prognostic impact of serum calcitonin and carcinoembryonic antigen doubling-times in patients with medullary thyroid carcinoma. *J Clin Endocrinol Metab.* 2005;90:6077-6084.

Miscellaneous

Small-molecule agonists for the thyrotropin receptor stimulate thyroid function in human thyrocytes and mice

Neumann S, Huang W, Titus S, et al (Natl Inst of Diabetes and Digestive and Kidney Diseases, Bethesda, MD; Natl Insts of Health Chemical Genomics Ctr, Bethesda, MD; et al)

Proc Natl Acad Sci U S A 106:12471-12476, 2009

Seven-transmembrane-spanning receptors (7TMRs) are prominent drug targets. However, small-molecule ligands for 7-transmembrane-spanning receptors for which the natural ligands are large, heterodimeric glycoprotein hormones, like thyroid-stimulating hormone (TSH; thyrotropin), have only recently been reported, and none are approved for human use. We have used quantitative high-throughput screening to identify a small-molecule TSH receptor (TSHR) agonist that was modified to produce a second agonist with increased potency. We show that these agonists are highly selective for human TSHR versus other glycoprotein hormone receptors and interact with the receptor's serpentine domain. A binding pocket within the transmembrane domain was defined by docking into a TSHR homology model and was supported by site-directed mutagenesis. In primary cultures of human thyrocytes, both TSH and the agonists increase mRNA levels for thyroglobulin, thyroperoxidase, sodium iodide symporter, and deiodinase type 2, and deiodinase type 2 enzyme activity. Moreover, oral administration of the agonist stimulated thyroid function in mice, resulting in increased serum thyroxine and thyroidal radioiodide uptake. Thus, we discovered a small molecule that activates human TSHR in vitro, is orally active in mice, and could be a lead for development of

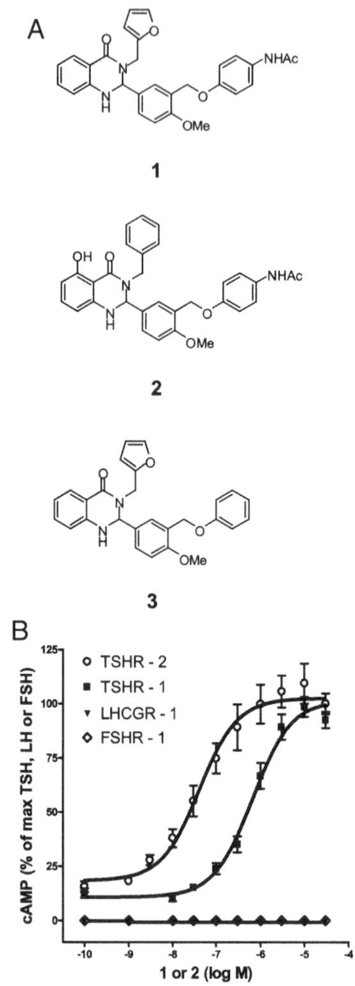

FIGURE 1.—Structures, selectivity, and potencies of compounds 1, 2, and 3. (*A*) Chemical structure of compound **1**: (*N*-(4-(5-(3-(furan-2-ylmethyl)-4-oxo-1,2,3,4-tetrahydroquinazolin-2-yl)-2-methoxybenzyloxy)-phenyl)acetamide) [NCGC00168126–01]. Chemical structure of compound **2**: (*N*-(4-(5-(3-benzyl-5-hydroxy-4-oxo-1,2,3,4-tetrahydroquinazolin-2-yl)-2-methoxybenzyloxy)-phenyl)acetamide) [NCGC00161870–01]. Chemical structure of compound 3: 3-(furan-2-ylmethyl)-2-(4-methoxy-3-(phenoxymethyl)phenyl)-2,3-dihydroquinazolin-4(1*H*)-one [NCGC00165237–01]. (*B*) Cells stably expressing TSHRs, LHCGRs, or FSHRs were exposed to the noted concentrations of compounds **1** and **2** or to a maximally effective concentration of the cognate ligand, TSH (540 nM), LH (34 nM), or FSH (34 nM), respectively, in the presence of 1 mM isobutylmethylxanthine as described in *Materials and Methods*. After 60 min, the cells were lysed and cAMP levels were measured by ELISA. The data from 3 independent experiments with duplicate samples are shown as the percent of stimulation by the cognate hormone. (Reprinted from Neumann S, Huang W, Titus S, et al. Small-molecule agonists for the thyrotropin receptor stimulate thyroid function in human thyrocytes and mice. *Proc Natl Acad Sci U S A*. 2009;106:12471-12476.)

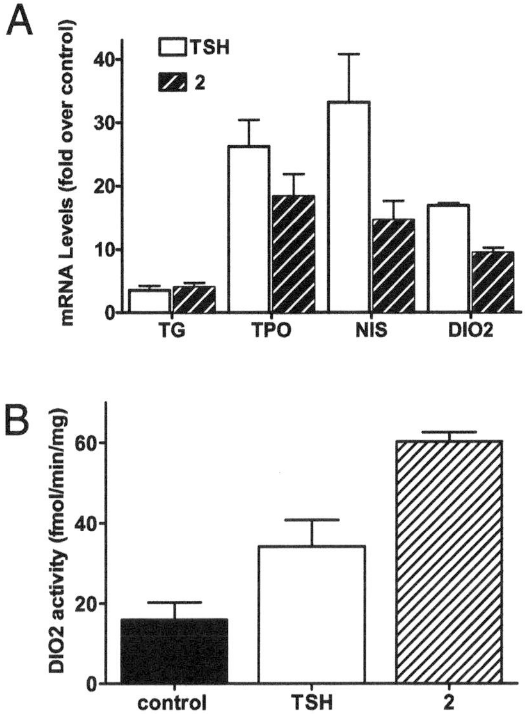

FIGURE 3.—Stimulation of the expression of the mRNAs for TG, TPO, NIS, and DIO2, and DIO2 protein by TSH or compound 2 in primary cultures of human thyrocytes. (*A*) Thyrocytes were incubated in media containing 2% FBS and TSH (18 nM) or compound 2 (30 μM) as described in *Materials and Methods*. After 24 h, the cells were lysed and the levels of the mRNAs were measured and normalized to GAPDH mRNA. The mRNA levels are presented as fold stimulation over control. The data from 3 independent experiments with duplicate samples are shown. (*B*) DIO2 enzymatic activity is presented as rates of thyroxine deiodination. The data from 3 independent experiments with duplicate samples are shown. (Reprinted from Neumann S, Huang W, Titus S, et al. Small-molecule agonists for the thyrotropin receptor stimulate thyroid function in human thyrocytes and mice. *Proc Natl Acad Sci U S A*. 2009;106:12471-12476.)

drugs to use in place of recombinant human TSH in patients with thyroid cancer (Figs 1, 3 and 4).

▶ Recombinant human thyroid-stimulating hormone (rhTSH) is currently prescribed primarily as an adjunct for monitoring patients who are taking thyroid hormones after undergoing ablative surgery for thyroid cancer. rhTSH stimulates uptake of iodide and release of thyroglobulin (TG) from any residual thyroid cancer and thereby increases the sensitivity of measurements of radioiodine uptake or serum TG levels in these patients. However, rhTSH is difficult to produce, which leads to its high cost, and it must be administered by injection. A small-molecule TSH receptor (TSHR) agonist would be worthwhile because it could produce the same beneficial effects as rhTSH but at a lower cost and with greater ease of oral administration and may therefore be available for use in a larger patient population. The aim of this study was therefore to

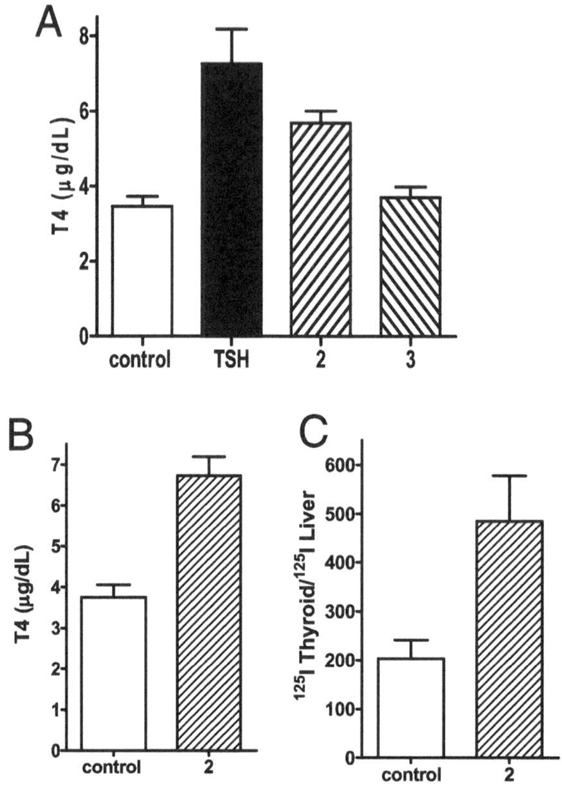

FIGURE 4.—Stimulation by compound **2** of thyroxine (T4) secretion and thyroidal radioiodide uptake in mice. (*A*) Mice were given vehicle (PEG300, control), TSH (32 μg), compound **2** (0.5 mg), or the inactive analogue compound 3 (0.5 mg) by i.p. injection. Blood was withdrawn 2 h later and T4 was measured in the serum. The data from 2 independent experiments with 3 mice each are shown. (*B*) Vehicle (control) or compound **2** (2.5 mg) was given by esophageal gavage and serum T4 was measured 2 h later. The data from 4 independent experiments with 3 mice each are shown. (C) Vehicle (control) or compound **2** (2.5 mg) was given by esophageal gavage on d 1 and 2. On d 3, $Na^{125}I$ (20 μCi) was administered by esophageal gavage and the mice were killed 2 h later. The thyroid glands and small pieces of liver were excised and counted for ^{125}I radioactivity. The data are presented as the ratio of radioactivity in the thyroid/liver. The data from 2 independent experiments with 2 and 4 mice each are shown. (Reprinted from Neumann S, Huang W, Titus S, et al. Small-molecule agonists for the thyrotropin receptor stimulate thyroid function in human thyrocytes and mice. *Proc Natl Acad Sci U S A.* 2009;106:12471-12476.)

identify and describe a new small-molecule TSHR agonist. The molecule described here is an agonist for a 7-transmembrane-spanning receptor like the TSHR. The structure and the ability to stimulate cAMP is shown in Fig 1. Importantly, the authors could demonstrate that binding of this compound to the TSHR results in an increase of TG, thyroperoxidase (TPO), and sodium iodide symporter (NIS) mRNA levels (Fig 3), as well as an increase of T4 in mice after administration (Fig 4). These results provide proof of principle for the effectiveness of small-molecule agonists for TSHR in human and murine cells expressing TSHRs endogenously. Although the full efficacy and high selectivity of the new agonists described in this article are promising, chemical optimization of these new scaffolds supported by molecular modeling need to be performed in an effort to further improve their potencies and therapeutic potential.

M. Schott, MD, PhD

Morphological Ultrasound Microimaging of Thyroid in Living Mice

Mancini M, Vergara E, Salvatore G, et al (Università "Federico II", Naples, Italy; Università "Parthenope" Naples, Italy; et al)

Endocrinology 150:4810-4815, 2009

The objective of the study was to explore high-frequency ultrasound (HFUS) for noninvasive microimaging of thyroid in living mice. Thyroid examination was performed by HFUS in 10 normal C57BL/6 mice, eight mice treated by propylthiouracil, and 22 Tg-TRK-T1 transgenic mice. The dimension of the gland and the presence of nodules were evaluated. Nodules were classified as malignant (hypoechogenicity, poorly defined margins, internal microcalcification, irregular shapes, and extra glandular extension) or not, and the findings were compared with histological data. Thyroid images were successfully obtained in all the animals analyzed. Normal thyroid reached a volume of 4.92 μl (range 2.11–4.92 μl). Mice with propylthiouracil-induced goiter showed diffuse thyroid enlargement (median volume 6.67 μl, range 4.09–8.82 μl). In 19 of 22 Tg-TRK-T1 mice (86%), HFUS identified a nodular process (the smallest detected nodule had a diameter of 0.46 mm). Eleven nodules were classified as malignant and eight as benign. Compared with histological analysis, HFUS showed a sensitivity of 100% in the detection of thyroid nodules and a specificity of 60% (two of the nodules identified by HFUS were not confirmed at the histology). The specificity and sensitivity of HFUS in predicting the malignancy of the thyroid nodules were 83 and 91%, respectively. Thus, HFUS is an accurate imaging modality that can potentially replace more invasive techniques, and, therefore, it represents a significant advancement in phenotypic assessment of mouse models of thyroid cancer.

► Current imaging techniques do not allow evaluation of the thyroid gland in living mice. Thus, necroscopy followed by histology is still the gold standard for the study of mouse models of thyroid disease. The visualization, at microscopic resolution (microimaging), of the thyroid in living animals would represent a significant advance to study thyroid tumor development and the effects of experimental therapies. Within the last few years, several noninvasive methods, such as computed tomography, magnetic resonance, and ultrasound were developed to evaluate the presence and the growth of tumors in living mice.[1,2] These methods have been limited to resolution of the order of millimeters. High-frequency ultrasound (HFUS; 20-100 MHz) is a novel imaging methodology that extends the visualization to microscopic resolution (of the order of 100 μm). The aim of this study was to evaluate this new technique in mouse models. The authors were able to precisely evaluate the dimension and morphology of mouse thyroid glands (Fig 1 in the original article) as well as to distinguish benign from malignant nodules with high sensitivity and specificity (Fig 3 in the original article). Therefore, this technique is of major importance in mouse studies. However, HFUS imaging also has limitations and disadvantages. According to the authors it requires a well-trained and skilled operator to obtain accurate, repeatable, and high-quality images.

M. Schott, MD, PhD

References

1. Raman V, Pathak AP, Glunde K, Artemov D, Bhujwalla ZM. Magnetic resonance imaging and spectroscopy of transgenic models of cancer. *NMR Biomed.* 2007;20: 186-199.
2. Liang H, Yang Y, Yang K, Wu Y, Boone JM, Cherry SR. A microPET/CT system for in vivo small animal imaging. *Phys Med Biol.* 2007;52:3881-3894.

Genetic Predisposition to Elevated Serum Thyrotropin is Associated with Exceptional Longevity

Atzmon G, Barzilai N, Surks MI, et al (Albert Einstein College of Medicine, Bronx, NY)

J Clin Endocrinol Metab 94:4768-4775, 2009

Context.—Exceptional longevity is associated with raised serum TSH.

Objective.—The aim of this study was to examine whether offspring of people with exceptional longevity have elevated serum TSH and whether specific single nucleotide polymorphisms (SNPs) in the *TSH*-B gene and *TSH* receptor (*TSHR*) gene are associated with this phenotype.

Design/Setting/Patients.—We measured serum TSH and free T_4 in Ashkenazi Jewish centenarians (n = 232; median age, 97 yr), their offspring (n = 366; median age, 69 yr), and age-matched controls without familial longevity (n = 163; median age, 70 yr). We determined TSH heritability, its distribution, and association with SNPs in the TSH-B and TSHR genes.

Results.—Offspring had higher median serum TSH [1.68 mIU/liter (97.5% confidence interval, 0.65 to 4.79 mIU/liter)], compared to controls [1.50 mIU/liter (97.5% confidence interval, 0.63 to 3.93 mIU/liter); $P = 0.02$], with estimated heritability of 0.33 ($P = 0.004$). Allele frequency of two SNPs in the promoter/enhancer region of *TSHR* gene, associated with increased serum TSH, was higher in centenarians and their offspring compared to controls (rs10149689 G allele frequency, 0.57 and 0.53 *vs.* 0.48; $P = 0.001$ and $P = 0.08$; odds ratio, 1.56 and 1.22, respectively; and rs12050077 A allele frequency, 0.57 and 0.53 *vs.* 0.46; $P = 0.0001$ and $P = 0.01$; odds ratio, 1.68 and 1.32, respectively). Linkage disequilibrium between the two SNPs was high ($r^2 = 0.95$), suggesting interaction between them. Furthermore, GA haplotype frequency was significantly higher among centenarians and offspring compared to controls (0.57 and 0.53 *vs.* 0.46; $P = 0.0001$ and $P = 0.01$, respectively).

Conclusions.—A heritable phenotype characterized by raised serum TSH is associated with human longevity. Carriers of rs12050077 and rs10149689 SNPs in the *TSHR* have higher serum TSH, possibly contributing to decreased thyroid function and longevity.

▶ The data presented by Atzmon et al show that offspring of the centenarian group have raised serum thyroid-stimulating hormone (TSH) concentrations compared with age-matched controls. Furthermore, offspring of the centenarian group who had elevated serum TSH levels also had higher TSH concentrations suggesting a heritable trait. After searching for genetic markers that could be associated with, and possibly responsible for, the raised serum TSH in centenarians and their offspring, the authors demonstrated for the first time that 2 single nucleotide polymorphisms (SNPs) (rs10149689 and rs12050077 of the thyroid-stimulating hormone receptor [TSHR]), located between enhancer regions and close to the promoter region, were significantly associated with raised TSH concentrations in the Ashkenazi Jewish centenarians and their offspring compared with controls, and showed strong linkage disequilibrium (Fig 5 in the original article). These results raise the possibility that these genetic changes exert an effect on TSHR gene expression that leads to increased TSH and may be, at least in part, transmitted from individuals with exceptional longevity to their offspring.

There are different reasons for the concordance between TSH levels and longevity. Thyroid hormone has profound impact on metabolic rate and body temperature by various mechanisms, including modulating mitochondrial activity, membrane composition and ion permeability, and substrate cycling.[1] The relationship between longevity and hypothyroidism is considered to be due to lower levels of reactive oxygen species production and oxidative stress in response to changes in both obligate and facultative thermogenesis.[2]

A limitation of our study is that, at present, our findings and conclusions are restricted to the Ashkenazi Jewish population and cannot be generalized to other populations. Clearly, genetic studies in non-Ashkenazi populations in North America would be of great interest in this regard. Others have reported on serum TSH in individuals of exceptional longevity, some showing increased concentrations[3] and others showing decreased concentrations. None have reported on genetic changes as in the present work. Therefore, the authors suggest that those reported studies be interpreted cautiously because the study populations were small, have different genetic backgrounds from our study groups, and live in areas of variable iodine supply. Another limitation is that, because of lack of availability of serum in some individuals, the authors could not examine the relationship between free T_4 (FT4) and TSH in the entire control and offspring groups.

M. Schott, MD, PhD

References

1. Harper ME, Seifert EL. Thyroid hormone effects on mitochondrial energetics. *Thyroid.* 2008;18:145-156.
2. Hulbert AJ, Pamplona R, Buffenstein R, Buttemer WA. Life and death: metabolic rate, membrane composition, and life span of animals. *Physiol Rev.* 2007;87: 1175-1213.
3. Ravaglia G, Forti P, Maioli F, et al. Blood micronutrient and thyroid hormone concentrations in the oldest-old. *J Clin Endocrinol Metab.* 2000;85:2260-2265.

Gaining ligand selectivity in thyroid hormone receptors via entropy

Martínez L, Nascimento AS, Nunes FM, et al (Universidade Estadual de Campinas, Brazil; Universidade de São Paulo, Brazil; et al)
Proc Natl Acad Sci 106:20717-20722, 2009

Nuclear receptors are important targets for pharmaceuticals, but similarities between family members cause difficulties in obtaining highly selective compounds. Synthetic ligands that are selective for thyroid hormone (TH) receptor β (TRβ) vs. TRα reduce cholesterol and fat without effects on heart rate; thus, it is important to understand TRβ-selective binding. Binding of 3 selective ligands (GC-1, KB141, and GC-24) is characterized at the atomic level; preferential binding depends on a nonconserved residue (Asn-331β) in the TRβ ligand-binding cavity (LBC), and GC-24 gains extra selectivity from insertion of a bulky side group into an extension of the LBC that only opens up with this ligand. Here we report that the natural TH 3,5,3′-triodothyroacetic acid (Triac) exhibits a previously unrecognized mechanism of TRα selectivity. TR x-ray structures reveal better fit of ligand with the TRα LBC. The TRβ LBC, however, expands relative to TRα in the presence of Triac (549 Å^3 vs. 461 Å^3), and molecular dynamics simulations reveal that water occupies the extra space. Increased solvation compensates for weaker interactions of ligand with TRβ and permits greater flexibility of the Triac carboxylate group in TRβ than in TRα. We propose that this effect results in lower entropic restraint and decreases free energy of interactions between Triac and TRβ, explaining subtype-selective binding. Similar effects could potentially be exploited in nuclear receptor drug design (Figs 2 and 5).

▶ Two genes encode the receptors for thyroid hormone (TR), including *NR1A1* for the α-isoform (TRα) and *NR1A2* for the β1-3-isoforms (TRβ). TRα and TRβ are expressed in a tissue-specific manner. There is an interest in discovering ligands specific for one or the other TR subtype because differential activation thereof may result in favorable metabolic changes. While the TRβ mediates the cholesterin and fat-lowering effects of TH, TRα confers the action of TH on the heart.

The authors report in their article that the natural TH 3,5,3′-triodothyroacetic acid (Triac) harbors a mechanism of TRβ selectivity (Fig 2). Preferential binding

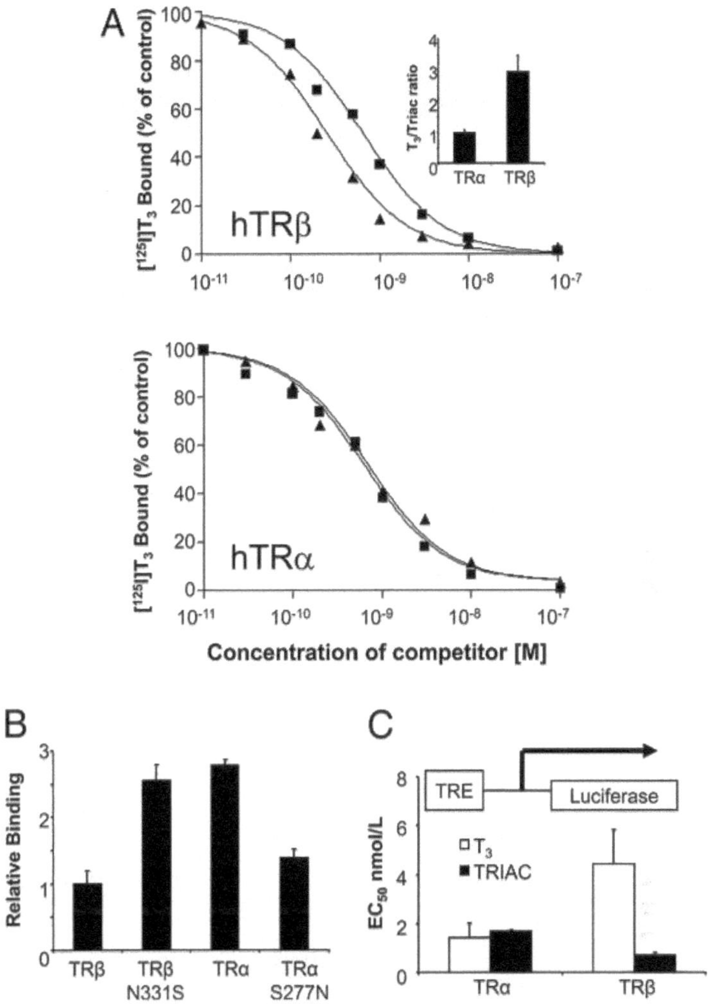

FIGURE 2.—TR subtype-selective binding and activity of Triac. (*A*) Competition curves with TR*β* and TR*α* obtained with T_3 (squares) and Triac (triangles). *Inset*: Ratios of T_3/Triac binding for both TRs from several experiments ($n = 3$). (*B*) Relative KI values from Triac competition curves ($n = 4$) with TRs and TR mutants were compared with TR*β*, arbitrarily set to 1. (C) Average EC_{50} values from luciferase assays using extracts of TR*α*- and TR*β*-expressing cells transfected with a TRE-responsive reporter (DR-4) and treated with ligand ($n = 3$). (Reprinted from Martínez L, Nascimento AS, Nunes FM, et al. Gaining ligand selectivity in thyroid hormone receptors via entropy. *Proc Natl Acad Sci.* 2009;106:20717-20722.)

of Triac to TRβ has been known for quite a while.[1,2] This was confirmed again using a TR element-driven reporter, showing that T3 is 2.5-fold selective for TRα and Triac 3-fold selective for TRβ in vitro. However, analysis of crystal structures with high resolution x-ray and computation of molecular interactions revealed that Triac fits better into the ligand-binding cavity of TRα, forms more hydrogen bonds, and has stronger energetic interaction with TRα than TRβ.

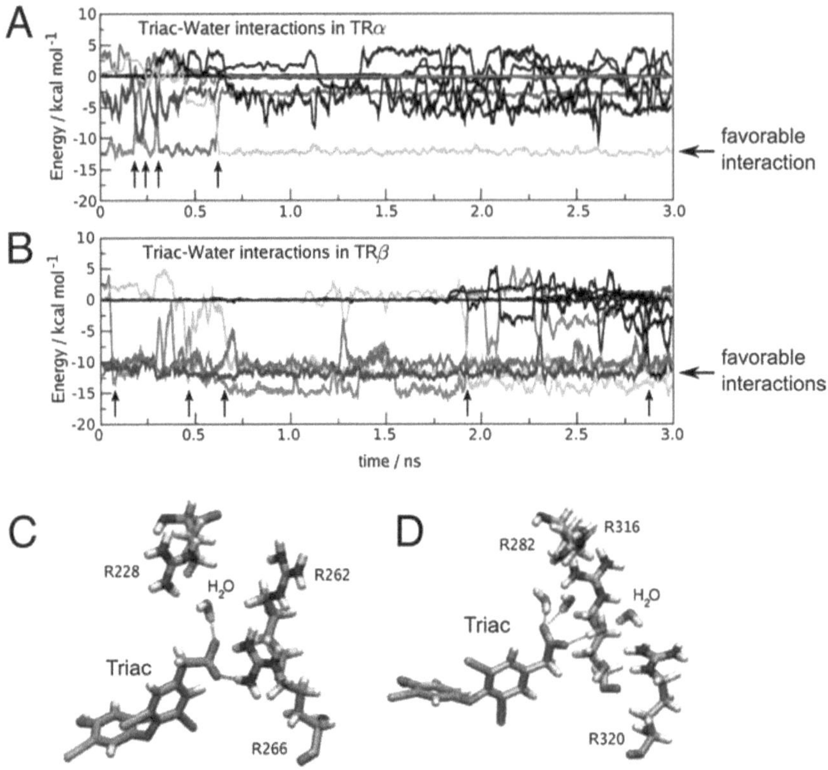

FIGURE 5.—Triac makes more water contacts in TRβ. Interaction energy profiles of most favorable interacting water molecules obtained from MD simulation (*A*) hTRα and (*B*) hTRβ. Each colored trace represents interaction energies of different water molecules with Triac as a function of time. Arrows indicate water exchange events. Representative views of key amino acids in the hTRα (*C*) and hTRβ (*D*) LBCs and nearby space in the LBC from the simulation, showing higher hydration level in TRβ and that highly favorable interacting waters lie close to the Triac carboxylate. Waters are represented by white/red stick figures, and hydrogen bond interactions with Triac are represented by dotted lines. Note that there are more waters close to the Triac molecule in TRβ than in TRα. (Reprinted from Martínez L, Nascimento AS, Nunes FM, et al. Gaining ligand selectivity in thyroid hormone receptors via entropy. *Proc Natl Acad Sci.* 2009;106:20717-20722.)

However, Triac is more restricted in TRα, and molecular dynamics stimulations suggest that water molecules compensate for interaction energies between Triac and TRβ (Fig 5). This observation could be made because the authors tried to simulate soluble conditions using new human TRα- and human TRβ-Triac structures and a shell of water and ions.

This study shows that best molecular fit does not necessarily mean best molecular interaction. Thus, it may be reasonable in the future to design drugs slightly smaller than predicted from the size of the binding pocket because molecules of a drug may need more freedom of mobility and the help of small molecules (such as water) to gain a higher selectivity for binding.

H. S. Willenberg, MD, PhD
M. Schott, MD, PhD

References

1. Schueler PA, Schwartz HL, Strait KA, Mariash CN, Oppenheimer JH. Binding of 3,5,3'-triiodothyronine (T3) and its analogs to the in vitro translational products of c-erbA protooncogenes: differences in the affinity of the alpha- and beta-forms for the acetic acid analog and failure of the human testis and kidney alpha-2 products to bind T3. *Mol Endocrinol.* 1990;4:227-234.
2. Wagner RL, Huber BR, Shiau AK, et al. Hormone selectivity in thyroid hormone receptors. *Mol Endocrinol.* 2001;15:398-410.

Activation of Dual Oxidases Duox1 and Duox2: differential regulation mediated by camp-dependent protein kinase and protein kinase C-dependent phosphorylation

Rigutto S, Hoste C, Grasberger H, et al (Université Libre de Bruxelles, Belgium; Univ of Chicago, IL)
J Biol Chem 284:6725-6734, 2009

Dual oxidases were initially identified as NADPH oxidases producing H_2O_2 necessary for thyroid hormone biosynthesis. The crucial role of Duox2 has been demonstrated in patients suffering from partial iodide organification defect caused by bi-allelic mutations in the *DUOX2* gene. However, the Duox1 function in thyroid remains elusive. We optimized a functional assay by co-expressing Duox1 or Duox2 with their respective maturation factors, DuoxA1 and DuoxA2, to compare their intrinsic enzymatic activities under stimulation of the major signaling pathways active in the thyroid in relation to their membrane expression. We showed that basal activity of both Duox isoenzymes depends on calcium and functional EF-hand motifs. However, the two oxidases are differentially regulated by activation of intracellular signaling cascades. Duox1 but not Duox2 activity is stimulated by forskolin ($EC_{50} = 0.1$ μM) via protein kinase A-mediated Duox1 phosphorylation on serine 955. In contrast, phorbol esters induce Duox2 phosphorylation via protein kinase C activation associated with high H_2O_2 generation (phorbol 12-myristate 13-acetate $EC_{50} = 0.8$ nM). These results were confirmed in human thyroid cells, suggesting that Duox1 is also involved in thyroid hormonogenesis. Our data provide, for the first time, detailed insights into the mechanisms controlling the activation of Duox1–2 proteins and reveal additional phosphorylation-mediated regulation.

▶ Dual oxidases (Duox1 and Duox2) are necessary for the synthesis of thyroid hormones. Patients with a defective Duox2 enzyme activity exhibit partial iodide organification defects. Duox enzymes are calcium-dependent membrane-associated proteins with an NADPH oxidase activity and provide H_2O_2 for thyroid hormone synthesis.

Rigutto et al studied the generation of H_2O_2 by and regulation of Duox proteins using several molecular approaches. They found a linear relationship between peroxide generation and Duox expression and association of Duox to the membrane, independent of isoform 1 or 2. Also, for the generation of peroxide, the expression of both Duox and Duox activator was necessary.

However, they found different mechanisms of activation for Duox1 and Duox2. Both isoforms respond to the phosphatidylinositol-bisphosphate cascade activation by ionomycin with an emphasis on Duox1, as shown with ionomycin (Fig 2 in the original article). Adenylate cyclase agonism enhanced H_2O_2 generation by Duox1 but not by Duox2. Three potential phosphorylation sites were identified in the Duox1 enzyme. PKC pathway activity increased Duox2 more readily than Duox1, and was additive to the ionomycin effect. Mutation of calcium-binding sites permitted Duox to associate to the cell membrane but prevented peroxide generation, even under stimulatory conditions suggesting that the regulation of Duox occurs in a calcium-dependent way.

In summary, both enzymes seem to play a role in thyroid hormone synthesis. They are regulated differentially. The implicated signaling pathways suggest that TSH is a major stimulator of Duox expression.

H. S. Willenberg, MD, PhD
M. Schott, MD, PhD

A thyroid hormone receptor mutation that dissociates thyroid hormone regulation of gene expression in vivo

Machado DS, Sabet A, Santiago LA, et al (Johns Hopkins Univ School of Medicine, Baltimore, MD; et al)

Proc Natl Acad Sci U S A 106:9441-9446, 2009

Resistance to thyroid hormone (RTH) is most often due to point mutations in the β-isoform of the thyroid hormone (TH) receptor (TR-β). The majority of mutations involve the ligand-binding domain, where they block TH binding and receptor function on both stimulatory and inhibitory TH response elements. In contrast, a few mutations in the ligand-binding domain are reported to maintain TH binding and yet cause RTH in certain tissues. We introduced one such naturally occurring human RTH mutation (R429Q) into the germline of mice at the TR-β locus. R429Q knock-in (KI) mice demonstrated elevated serum TH and inappropriately normal thyroid-stimulating hormone (TSH) levels, consistent with hypothalamic–pituitary RTH. In contrast, 3 hepatic genes positively regulated by TH (*Dio1, Gpd1, and Thrsp*) were increased in R429Q KI animals. Mice were then rendered hypothyroid, followed by graded T_3 replacement. Hypothyroid R429Q KI mice displayed elevated TSH subunit mRNA levels, and T_3 treatment failed to normally suppress these levels. T_3 treatment, however, stimulated pituitary *Gh* levels to a greater degree in R429Q KI than in control mice. *Gsta*, a hepatic gene negatively regulated by TH, was not suppressed in R429Q KI mice after T_3 treatment, but hepatic *Dio1* and *Thrsp* mRNA levels increased in response to TH. Cardiac myosin heavy chain isoform gene expression also showed a specific defect in TH inhibition. In summary, the R429Q mutation is associated with selective impairment of TH-mediated gene repression, suggesting that the affected domain, necessary for TR homodimerization and corepressor binding, has a critical role in negative gene regulation by TH.

▶ Two forms of resistance to thyroid hormone (RTH) are clinically recognized: a generalized form (GRTH) and a central form (CRTH). However, the existence of CRTH as a distinct clinical entity remains controversial for 3 reasons: (1) the clinical characterization of affected patients is many times incomplete, (2) unaffected and affected patients in the same family have been found to harbor the same thyroid hormone receptor (TR)-β mutation, and (3) in vivo validation of CRTH in a model system is lacking. The authors of this study successfully generated a transgenic mouse model of CRTH. Analysis of gene regulation in R429Q mice revealed that this TR-β mutation dissociates positive and negative gene regulations by thyroid hormone (TH) rather than differentially affecting gene regulation on an anatomic basis (central vs peripheral) (Figs 2 and 3 in the original article). Specifically, mice harboring the R429Q mutation demonstrate a selective defect in TH-mediated negative regulation of hepatic (Gsta), cardiac (Mhy7), and pituitary (Cga and Tshb) genes, and preserved TH action on both peripheral and central genes that are positively regulated by TH (Fig 4 in the original article). This is in contrast to other TR-β mutant mouse models of GRTH, all of which demonstrate defects in both positive and negative gene regulations by TH. The ability to dissociate these pathways in vivo with a single TR-β mutation indicates that the thyroid hormone receptor contains a distinct domain that mediates TH inhibition. Further studies will be required to determine the specific mechanism by which a mutation affecting this region, which is critical for TR homodimer formation and corepressor binding, results in selective disruption of T3-mediated gene repression.

M. Schott, MD, PhD

5 Calcium and Bone Metabolism

Introduction

Multiple clinical advances were made in the area of calcium and bone metabolism over the last year. Most of the studies reviewed are major clinical trials published regarding the clinically important area of osteoporosis, with others discussing aspects of metabolic bone disease, and mineral and vitamin D metabolism. These studies highlight major advances in the understanding of the pathophysiology and treatment of calcium and bone disorders, and together will impact clinical practice significantly. This chapter describes a sampling of many of the most important papers published in this field over the last year.

The first section reviews major new contributions to the epidemiology and pathophysiology of osteoporosis. The first article compares the prevalence of low bone mineral density (BMD) at the femoral neck and total hip in a population-based study of US adults in 2005 and 2006, compared with previous prevalence estimates in NHANES III from 1988 to 1994. The study shows that age-adjusted prevalence of low hip BMD decreased by 7% in women and 3% in men over this interval, but the total number of affected individuals increased due to aging of the population. The second article reports that older men with the highest level of bone turnover markers in the population-based MrOS study had more rapid total hip bone loss than older men with lower levels of bone turnover markers, but these men did not have increased risk of hip or nonvertebral fractures after adjustment for baseline hip bone density. These findings imply that measurement of markers of bone turnover in older men does not improve the ability to predict future fractures beyond the prediction obtained by measurement of hip BMD alone. Also investigated is an article that addresses low bone mass and high bone turnover in postmenopausal women infected with HIV.

The second section emphasizes current issues in osteoporosis therapy. The first two articles help clarify the reported association between use of thiazolidenedione (TZD) medications to treat type 2 diabetes mellitus and minimally traumatic distal limb fractures, and the probable mechanisms that result in these fractures. The first paper confirms that distal limb fractures occur more commonly in postmenopausal women treated with TZD medications, but not in older men. The second study evaluates markers of bone turnover in subjects treated with rosiglitazone, metformin, or glyburide in the ADOPT study, and reports that markers of bone resorption in postmenopausal women increased in subjects taking rosiglitazone, whereas markers of bone formation decreased in all subjects, regardless of the drug taken. These findings suggest that decreased bone formation and increased bone resorption contribute to increased fracture risk with rosiglitazone.

The third article reports that markers of bone turnover decreased significantly in subjects treated with zoledronic acid once a year for 3 years as part of the HORIZON fracture reduction trial. Each infusion reduced markers of bone turnover into the premenopausal normal range for the following year, including the bone formation marker serum P1NP, but fracture risk did not increase despite prolonged suppression of bone formation. These findings suggest that marked suppression of bone formation over several years does not necessarily lead to fractures, as has been reported to occur with long-term suppression of bone formation by some bisphosphonate medications. The next article compares BMD treatment effects of zoledronic acid compared with risedronate in subjects with glucocorticoid-induced osteoporosis. The study showed that zoledronic acid was noninferior, and possibly superior, to risedronate in subjects receiving glucocorticoid therapy. Another article explores the possible mechanisms why zoledronic acid, when given within 90 days of a hip fracture, not only reduced subsequent clinical fractures by 35%, but also reduced mortality by 28% in subjects in the HORIZON secondary hip fracture prevention trial. The study suggests that only 8% of the mortality reduction seen in this trial was due to fracture reduction, whereas zoledronic acid significantly reduced both the risk of pneumonias and cardiac arrhythmias beginning 1 year after the initial dose was given.

The next article reports that teriparatide is more effective than alendronate in increasing BMD and reducing radiographic vertebral fractures in subjects with glucocorticoid-induced osteoporosis. The significance of this study is limited by the fairly high study discontinuation rate of 44%, but this rate was attributed to the nature of the diseases being treated with glucocorticoid therapy. An article that follows assessed BMD, markers of bone turnover, and serum calcium levels in postmenopausal women with osteoporosis who were previously treated with alendronate or raloxifene for at least 18 months; the women were then randomized to receive teriparatide alone or teriparatide in addition to their previous therapy. Subjects who switched to teriparatide alone had greater increases in their bone turnover markers, but those who added teriparatide to their previous alendronate or raloxifene had greater increases in BMD. The next article evaluates bone loss occurring over 12 months upon discontinuation of teriparatide after treatment for 2 years in a small number of postmenopausal women and eugonadal men. The women and men both had similar increases in BMD during treatment, but the postmenopausal women lost bone density more rapidly at the lumbar spine and hip after discontinuation than the men. These findings suggest that postmenopausal women require more rapid institution of antiresorptive therapy after stopping teriparatide than men. The next study describes changes in bone histomorphometry in subjects treated with teriparatide or strontium ranelate over 6 months. Strontium ranelate has been reported to both stimulate bone formation and inhibit bone resorption in rodents, but this histomorphometric study demonstrates that strontium acts primarily as a modest antiresorptive agent in humans, without any significant anabolic effect.

The next article reports that lasofoxifene, a new selective estrogen receptor modulator (SERM), reduces both vertebral and nonvertebral fractures, estrogen receptor-positive breast cancer, coronary heart disease, and strokes compared with placebo in postmenopausal women with osteoporosis. Lasofoxifene also increased venous thromboembolic events but did not increase endometrial cancer or mortality. The last study demonstrates lack of significant pain relief after vertebroplasty for vertebral fractures. This randomized controlled study compared pain relief after vertebroplasty with a sham vertebroplasty procedure and found that improvement in back pain intensity, pain-related disability, and quality of life after vertebral fractures were similar in subjects treated with vertebroplasty or the sham procedure.

The third section emphasizes a novel therapy for osteoporosis. The first article reports that denosumab, a fully human monoclonal antibody to receptor activator of nuclear factor-κB ligand (RANKL), reduces new vertebral fractures by 68%, hip fractures by 40%, and nonvertebral fractures by 20%, compared with placebo, in a pivotal phase III fracture reduction trial in postmenopausal women with osteoporosis. This new drug is currently undergoing FDA review for approval for treatment of postmenopausal osteoporosis. The second article reports that denosumab improves lumbar spine, total hip, femoral neck, and wrist BMD over 3 years, and it reduces vertebral fractures by 62% compared with placebo in men receiving androgen deprivation therapy for prostate cancer. The next article shows that denosumab improves lumbar spine, total hip, femoral neck, wrist, and total body BMD in women receiving adjuvant aromatase inhibitors for nonmetastatic breast cancer, but denosumab did not reduce fractures compared with placebo.

The fourth section describes recent advances in our understanding of osteoporosis in other settings. The first article reports that adolescent girls with anorexia nervosa have increased bone marrow fat in their peripheral skeleton, suggesting that mesenchymal stem cells preferentially differentiate into adipocytes rather than osteoblasts in this disorder. This change in differentiation is thought to lead to reduced bone formation in young women affected with this disorder. The second article reports that HIV-infected postmenopausal Hispanic and African American women have lower BMD, higher prevalence of low BMD, and increased bone turnover compared to non-infected age-, body mass index (BMI), and ethnicity-matched women. The last article reports that serum dickkopf-1 (Dkk-1), an inhibitor of the canonical Wnt signaling pathway in osteoblasts, is increased in patients with thalassemia-induced osteoporosis, leading to low BMD due to decreased bone formation. Dkk-1 has been shown to inhibit bone formation in postmenopausal osteoporosis and contribute to development of skeletal lytic lesions in multiple myeloma and breast cancer. The study also shows that zoledronic acid reduced serum Dkk-1 levels over 12 months and that this correlated with increased BMD in the study subjects.

The fifth section describes new findings in mineral and vitamin D metabolism. The first article reports for the first time that circulating fibroblast growth factor-23 (FGF-23) in patients with end-stage renal disease treated by peritoneal dialysis is intact and biologically active. Patients with end-stage renal disease accumulate fragments of C-terminal PTH, which is thought to have reduced biological activity. This study shows that FGF-23, a hormone that regulates phosphorus metabolism by stimulating expression of sodium-dependent phosphate transporters in the proximal renal tubule, is not metabolized to inactive fragments of C-terminal FGF-23 in end-stage renal disease. The second article provides bone histomorphometric evidence that serum 25-hydroxyvitamin D levels above 30 ng/mL are not associated with bone mineralization defects in 675 iliac crest bone biopsies taken at autopsy. However, the study was not able to clearly identify a lower threshold of serum 25-hydroxyvitamin D below which mineralization defects did occur.

The final section reviews current issues in metabolic bone disease. The first article reports for the first time that the calcimimetic compound cinacalcet may be an effective medical treatment for primary hyperparathyroidism for as long as 5.5 years in patients in whom parathyroidectomy is contraindicated, or those who have failed previous surgery. This drug binds to the extracellular calcium sensing receptor on parathyroid cells and increases their sensitivity to extracellular calcium, thereby reducing parathyroid hormone (PTH) secretion. The study shows for the first time that cinacalcet is able to maintain serum calcium in the normal range, suppress PTH secretion toward normal, and prevent bone loss over long-term treatment. The second article shows that cinacalcet effectively decreases serum calcium and PTH levels in patients with more severe intractable primary hyperparathyroidism in an open-label study over up to 152 weeks of treatment. The next study shows that patients with Paget's disease of bone had similar long-term outcomes regardless of whether they were treated only when symptoms developed, or intensively without regard to symptoms. Subjects were treated when symptomatic with oral risedronate or other oral bisphosphonates, or intensively with intravenous bisphosphonates without regard to symptoms, over 3 years. Both approaches to treatment affected outcomes similarly, including overall pain, pagetic bone pain, bone fractures, requirement for orthopedic surgery, hearing loss, or quality of life. The next article reports that 40 patients who were clinically diagnosed with pseudohypoparathyroidism type Ia, with skeletal features of Albright hereditary osteodystrophy and resistance to multiple hormones but no detectable GNAS mutations, had an unexpected high prevalence of GNAS cluster imprinting defects. Patients with pseudohypoparathyroidism type Ia classically have GNAS mutations and no detectable GNAS cluster imprinting defects, whereas patients with pseudohypoparathyroidism type Ib normally have GNAS cluster imprinting defects but not GNAS mutations. These findings suggest that a new molecular classification system for pseudohypoparathyroidism type I is needed.

Bart L. Clarke, MD

Epidemiology and Pathophysiology of Osteoporosis

Prevalence and Trends in Low Femur Bone Density Among Older US Adults: NHANES 2005–2006 Compared With NHANES III

Looker AC, Melton LJ III, Harris TB, et al (Ctrs for Disease Control and Prevention, Hyattsville, MD; Mayo Clinic, Rochester, MN; Natl Inst on Aging, Bethesda, MD; et al)

J Bone Miner Res 25:64-71, 2010

Hip fracture incidence appears to be declining in the United States, but changes in bone mineral density (BMD) of the population have not been evaluated. We used femur BMD data from the National Health and Nutrition Examination Survey (NHANES) 2005–2006 to estimate the prevalence of low femoral BMD in adults age 50 years and older and compared it with estimates from NHANES III (1988–1994). Dual-energy X-ray absorptiometry systems (pencil-beam geometry in NHANES III, fan-beam geometry in NHANES 2005–2006) were used to measure femur BMD, and World Health Organization (WHO) definitions of low BMD were used to categorize skeletal status. In 2005–2006, 49% of older US women had osteopenia and 10% had osteoporosis at the femur neck. In men, 30% had femur neck osteopenia and 2% had femur neck osteoporosis. An estimated 5.3 million older men and women had osteoporosis at the femur neck, and 34.5 million more had osteopenia in 2005–2006. When compared with NHANES III, the age-adjusted prevalence of femur neck osteoporosis in NHANES 2005–2006 was lower in men (by 3 percentage units) and women (by 7 percentage units) overall and among non-Hispanic whites. Changes in body mass index or osteoporosis medication use between surveys did not fully explain the decline in osteoporosis. Owing to the increase in the number of older adults in the US population, however, more older adults had low femur neck BMD (osteoporosis + osteopenia) in 2005–2006 than in 1988–1994. Thus, despite the decline in prevalence, the estimated number of affected older adults in 2005–2006 remained high.

▶ Two recent national- and community-based studies have shown that hip fracture rates are declining in the United States,[1,2] but the cause for the decline is not known. It has not been determined whether bone mineral density (BMD) is improving, whether treatments for osteoporosis are reducing the incidence of fractures, or whether other factors are playing a role. The most recent study of osteoporosis prevalence rates representative of the US population was based on femur BMD data collected by the third National Health and Nutrition Examination Survey (NHANES III, 1988-1994).[3] Total body and regional BMD data from NHANES 1999-2004 have also been published,[4] but these data do not provide femoral neck osteoporosis estimates as proposed by the WHO[5] or total hip osteoporosis estimates as proposed by Healthy People 2010.[6] The continuous NHANES began collecting proximal femur dual-energy X-ray absorptiometry (DXA) BMD measurements in 2005. This NHANES study allows for comparison of osteoporosis prevalence in representative samples of the non-institutionalized US population measured at 2 different times, so that changes in population BMD over time can be assessed.

This study assessed the prevalence of low BMD at the femoral neck and total hip in US adults older than 50 years in 2005-2006, compared the prevalence of low total hip BMD in 2005-2006 with target prevalence goals identified for the population in Healthy People 2010, and contrasted the prevalence of low BMD at the femoral neck and total hip in 2005-2006 with those reported in NHANES III. The study showed that 49% of US women older than 50 years had osteopenia and 10% had osteoporosis at the femoral neck, whereas 30% of men had osteopenia and 2% had osteoporosis, using WHO criteria. Projections from these findings indicate that 5.3 million women and men met criteria for femoral neck osteoporosis, and 34.5 million met criteria for femoral neck osteopenia in 2005-2006. Comparison with NHANES III data showed that age-adjusted prevalence of osteoporosis had decreased by 7% in women and by 3% in men, overall and in non-Hispanic whites by 2005-2006, but increases in body mass index (BMI) or use of osteoporosis medications between the surveys did not explain the decreased osteoporosis prevalence. The increase in the number of older adults in the US population between 1984 and 2006 led to an increase in the overall number of adults with low femoral neck BMD. The authors concluded that despite the mild decrease in prevalence, the number of affected adults with low BMD increased between the 2 survey periods.

These findings are important because they confirm that low BMD and osteoporosis are not becoming less prevalent over time. NHANES III projected that 5.3 million adults met criteria for osteoporosis and 26.3 million met criteria for osteopenia from 1988-1994. Increasing BMI in the population between the surveys affects only a small proportion of the total population of older women, and only 16% of the affected population was treated with osteoporosis medication in 2005-2006, compared with 10% in 1988-1994. Changes in DXA BMD technology do not explain the difference in prevalence seen between the 2 studies, even though NHANES III used Hologic pencil-beam technology and NHANES 2005-2006 used Hologic fan-beam instruments. Ethnic differences in femur BMD were similar between the 2 surveys, with non-Hispanic blacks having the highest BMD and non-Hispanic whites having the lowest BMD. In spite of decreasing prevalence of femoral low BMD or osteoporosis, total annual health care expenditures are expected to rise from $17 billion in 2005 to $25 billion in 2025.

B. L. Clarke, MD

References

1. Melton LJ, Kearns AE, Atkinson EJ, et al. Secular trends in hip fracture incidence and recurrence. *Osteoporos Int.* 2009;20:687-694.
2. Gehlbach SH, Avrunin JS, Puleo E. Trends in hospital care for hip fractures. *Osteoporos Int.* 2007;18:585-591.
3. Looker AC, Orwoll ES, Johnston CC, et al. Prevalence of low femoral bone density in older U.S. adults from NHANES III. *J Bone Miner Res.* 1997;12: 1761-1768.
4. Looker AC, Melton LJ, Harris T, Borrud L, Shepherd J, McGowan J. Age, gender, and race/ethnic differences in total body and subregional bone density. *Osteoporos Int.* 2009;20:1141-1149.
5. Kanis JA, McCloskey EV, Johansson H, Oden A, Melton LJ 3rd, Khaltaev N. A standard for the description of osteoporosis. *Bone.* 2008;42:467-475.
6. U.S. Department of Health and Human Services. Arthritis, osteoporosis and back conditions. In: Healthy People 2010. 2nd ed. Washington: U.S. Government Printing Office; 2000:17-18.

Biochemical Markers of Bone Turnover, Hip Bone Loss, and Fracture in Older Men: The MrOS Study

Bauer DC, Garnero P, Harrison SL, et al (Univ of California, San Francisco; INSERM Unit 664 and CCBR-Synarc, Lyon, France; San Francisco Coordinating Ctr, CA; et al)
J Bone Miner Res 24:2032-2038, 2009

We used data from the Osteoporotic Fractures in Men (MrOS) study to test the hypothesis that men with higher levels of bone turnover would have accelerated bone loss and an elevated risk of fracture. MrOS enrolled 5995 subjects >65 yr; hip BMD was measured at baseline and after a mean follow-up of 4.6 yr. Nonspine fractures were documented during a mean follow-up of 5.0 yr. Using fasting serum collected at baseline and stored at −190°C, bone turnover measurements (type I collagen N-propeptide [PINP]; β C-terminal cross-linked telopeptide of type I collagen [βCTX]; and TRACP5b) were obtained on 384 men with nonspine fracture (including 72 hip fractures) and 947 men selected at random. Among randomly selected men, total hip bone loss was 0.5%/yr among those in the highest quartile of PINP (>44.3 ng/ml) and 0.3%/yr among those in the lower three quartiles ($p = 0.01$). Fracture risk was elevated among men in the highest quartile of PINP (hip fracture relative hazard = 2.13; 95% CI: 1.23, 3.68; nonspine relative hazard = 1.57, 95% CI: 1.21, 2.05) or βCTX (hip fracture relative hazard = 1.76, 95 CI: 1.04, 2.98; nonspine relative hazard = 1.29, 95% CI: 0.99, 1.69) but not TRACP5b. Further adjustment for baseline hip BMD eliminated all associations between bone turnover and fracture. We conclude that higher levels of bone turnover are associated with greater hip bone loss in older men,

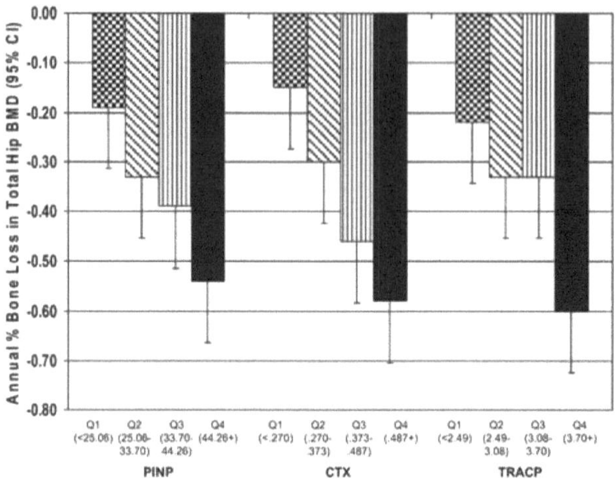

FIGURE 1.—Total hip bone loss over 4.6 yr of follow-up ($N = 682$) by quartile of baseline bone turnover marker, adjusted for age and clinic. For each marker, P trend <0.01. (Reprinted from Bauer DC, Garnero P, Harrison SL, et al. Biochemical markers of bone turnover, hip bone loss, and fracture in older men: the MrOS study. *J Bone Miner Res.* 2009;24:2032-2038, with permission from the American Society for Bone and Mineral Research.)

but increased turnover is not independently associated with the risk of hip or nonspine fracture (Fig 1).

▶ Osteoporosis affects predominantly not only postmenopausal women but also men.[1] The pathophysiology of bone loss and low-trauma fractures in men is presumed to be similar to the pathophysiology in postmenopausal women, but this has not been fully studied to date. Gonadal sex steroids, cytokines, and other biological factors likely play a role in causation of bone loss in men,[2-4] as in women, and it is also likely that these factors affect skeletal health in men, at least in part, by affecting bone turnover.

Bone turnover is usually assessed by iliac crest bone histomorphometry, but bone turnover markers are also used to estimate bone resorption and bone formation.[5] In early postmenopausal women, increased bone turnover is associated with rapid bone loss, but the association is not strong enough in most studies to predict rates of bone loss. A number of studies have shown that increased markers of bone turnover, particularly increased urinary resorption markers, predict fracture risk independent of bone mineral density (BMD).[6,7] Few prospective studies have evaluated the association of bone turnover markers with bone loss and fractures in men. One recent study showed a modest association,[8] and another study no association,[9] between bone turnover markers and fracture risk.

This study reports that bone turnover markers are associated with hip bone loss, but not hip or nonvertebral fractures, in a subset of the 5995 community dwelling men older than 65 years enrolled in the Osteoporosis in Men study (MrOS). Baseline serum type I collagen N-propeptide (PINP), β C-terminal cross-linked telopeptide of type I collagen (βCTX), and tartrate-resistant acid phosphatase 5b (TRACP5b) were measured in 384 men with nonvertebral fractures and 947 men without fractures randomly selected from the cohort and followed for 5 years. Total hip bone loss and hip and nonvertebral fracture risk were increased in men with the highest levels of serum P1NP and βCTX but not TRACP5b. However, adjustment for baseline hip BMD removed all associations between bone turnover and fracture. The authors concluded that increased bone turnover is associated with higher rates of hip bone loss in older men and not associated with increased risk of hip or nonvertebral fracture.

These findings do not support the use of bone turnover markers to assess fracture risk in older men if hip BMD is available. The study showed that increased bone turnover is associated with increased bone loss and fractures in older men, but after accounting for baseline hip BMD an independent effect of bone turnover markers on fractures did not persist. The findings imply that the association between P1NP and βCTX and fracture risk was due to lower BMD in men with higher bone turnover markers. Perhaps novel biomarkers will predict fractures better, but this study showed that the bone turnover markers that were evaluated failed to predict fractures independent of BMD in older men.

B. L. Clarke, MD

References

1. Ebeling PR. Clinical practice. Osteoporosis in men. *N Engl J Med.* 2008;358: 1474-1482.
2. Mellstrom D, Johnell O, Ljunggren O, et al. Free testosterone is an independent predictor of BMD and prevalent fractures in elderly men: MrOS in Sweden. *J Bone Miner Res.* 2006;21:529-535.
3. Riggs BL, Khosla S, Melton LJ III. A unitary model for involutional osteoporosis: estrogen deficiency causes both type I and type II osteoporosis in postmenopausal women and contributes to bone loss in aging man. *J Bone Miner Res.* 1998;13: 763-773.
4. Szulc P, Uusi-Rasi K, Claustrat B, Marchand F, Beck TJ, Delmas PD. Role of sex steroids in the regulation of bone morphology in men. The MINOS study. *Osteoporos Int.* 2004;15:909-917.
5. Szulc P, Delmas PD. Biochemical markers of bone turnover: potential use in the investigation and management of postmenopausal osteoporosis. *Osteoporos Int.* 2008;19:1683-1704.
6. Garnero P, Sornay-Rendu E, Claustrat B, Delmas PD. Biochemical markers of bone turnover, endogenous hormones and the risk of fractures in postmenopausal women: the OFELY Study. *J Bone Miner Res.* 2000;15:1526-1536.
7. Gerdheim P, Ivaska KK, Alatalo SL, et al. Biochemical markers of bone metabolism and prediction of fracture in elderly women. *J Bone Miner Res.* 2007;19: 386-393.
8. Meier C, Nguyen TV, Center JR, Seibel MJ, Eisman JA. Bone resorption and osteoporotic fractures in elderly men: the dubbo osteoporosis epidemiology study. *J Bone Miner Res.* 2005;20:579-587.
9. Szulc P, Montella A, Delmas PD. High bone turnover is associated with accelerated bone loss but not with increased fracture risk in men aged 50 and over: the prospective MINOS study. *Ann Rheum Dis.* 2008;67:1249-1255.

Low Bone Mass and High Bone Turnover in Postmenopausal Human Immunodeficiency Virus-Infected Women

Yin MT, McMahon DJ, Ferris DC, et al (Columbia Univ Med Ctr, NY; Bronx-Lebanon Hosp Ctr, NY; et al)
J Clin Endocrinol Metab 95:620-629, 2010

Context.—Low bone mineral density (BMD) is commonly reported in young men and women with HIV infection, and fracture rates may be higher. With effective antiretroviral therapy (ART), the HIV population is aging. However, little is known about the skeletal status of postmenopausal women.

Objective.—We aimed to assess the effects of HIV infection and ART on BMD and bone turnover in postmenopausal minority women.

Design, Setting, and Patients.—A prospective cohort study was performed in 92 HIV+ and 95 HIV− postmenopausal Hispanic and African-American women.

Main Outcome Measures.—We measured BMD by dual-energy x-ray absorptiometry, fracture prevalence, serum levels of inflammatory cytokines (TNFα, IL-6), bone turnover markers, calciotropic hormones, and estrone.

Results.—HIV+ women were younger (56 ± 1 *vs.* 60 ± 1 yr; $P < 0.01$) and had lower BMI (28 ± 1 *vs.* 30 ± 1 kg/m^2; $P < 0.01$) and estrone levels. Prevalence of T scores below −1.0 was greater in HIV+ women at the spine (78 *vs.* 64%; $P < 0.05$), total hip (45 *vs.* 29%; $P < 0.05$), and femoral neck (64 *vs.*46%; $P < 0.05$), and Z scores adjusted for BMI were lower in HIV+ women at the same sites. Serum TNFα, N-telopeptide, and C-telopeptide were significantly higher in HIV+ than HIV− women, particularly those receiving ART. HIV+ status was independently and negatively associated with spine and hip BMD after adjustment for age, ethnicity, BMI, and alcohol.

Conclusion.—The lower BMD, higher prevalence of low BMD, and higher levels of bone turnover markers detected in HIV+ postmenopausal minority women could place them at high risk for future fractures.

▶ It is well known that human immunodeficiency virus (HIV) infection is associated with low bone mineral density (BMD) in younger adults[1,2] and that this group may also be at increased risk of fracture.[3] Advances in antiretroviral therapy (ART) in recent years have led to prolonged survival of patients with HIV infection. By 2015, more than 50% of HIV-infected patients will be older than 50 years.[4] Relatively little is known about BMD or fracture risk in older patients with HIV infection.

Lower BMD in HIV-infected individuals is attributed to multiple causes. Low BMD is correlated with decreased body weight in these patients as it is in noninfected individuals. HIV infection itself and several drugs used for ART are thought to directly adversely affect the skeleton. Bone density decreases by 2% to 6% within the first 2 years of starting various ART drugs[5,6] but then appears to stabilize in patients on established ART.[7,8] Age-related bone loss independent of HIV infection and comorbid illnesses associated with HIV infection, such as accelerated renal disease, also play a role in causing lower BMD in HIV-infected patients.

This prospective cohort study in 92 HIV+ and 95 HIV– postmenopausal Hispanic and African American women showed that HIV-infected minority women were younger, had lower body mass index (BMI), and had lower estrone levels (24 vs 29 pg/mL) than noninfected women. More HIV+ women had low BMD or osteoporosis at the lumbar spine, total hip, and femoral neck. Z scores adjusted for BMI were lower in HIV-infected women than noninfected women at the same skeletal sites. Markers of bone turnover and tumor necrosis factor-alpha (TNF-α) were higher in HIV+ women than HIV– women, especially in those on ART. Women with HIV infection had lower spine and hip BMD after adjustment for age, ethnicity, BMI, and alcohol.

The authors concluded that HIV-infected postmenopausal Hispanic and African American women have lower BMD, higher prevalence of low BMD, and increased bone turnover compared with noninfected women. The younger age, lower BMI, and lower estrone levels in the HIV-infected women confound the study results somewhat, but these findings are nonetheless important because this is the first study to focus on BMD and bone turnover in postmenopausal minority women with HIV infection.

B. L. Clarke, MD

References

1. Dolan SE, Huang JS, Killilea KM, Sullivan MP, Aliabadi N, Grinspoon S. Reduced bone density in HIV-infected women. *AIDS.* 2004;18:475-483.
2. Teichman J, Stephan E, Lange U, et al. Osteopenia in HIV-infected women prior to highly active antiretroviral therapy. *J Infect.* 2003;46:221-227.
3. Triant VA, Brown TT, Lee H, Grinspoon SK. Fracture prevalence among human immunodeficiency virus (HIV)-infected versus non-HIV-infected patients in a large U.S. healthcare system. *J Clin Endocrinol Metab.* 2008;93:3499-3504.
4. Luther VP, Wilkin AM. HIV infection in older adults. *Clin Geriatr Med.* 2007;23: 567-583. vii.
5. Brown TT, McComsey GA, King MS, Qaqish RB, Bernstein BM, da Silva BA. Loss of bone mineral density after antiretroviral therapy initiation, independent of antiretroviral regimen. *J Acquir Immune Defic Syndr.* 2009;51:554-561.
6. Duvivier C, Kolta A, Assoumou L, et al. Greater decrease in bone mineral density with protease inhibitor regimens compared with non-nucleoside reverse transcriptase inhibitor regimens in HIV-1 infected naïve patients. *AIDS.* 2009;23:817-824.
7. Mondy K, Yarasheski K, Powderly WG, et al. Longitudinal evolution of bone mineral density and bone markers in human immunodeficiency virus-infected individuals. *Clin Infect Dis.* 2003;35:482-490.
8. Dolan SE, Kanter JR, Grinspoon S. Longitudinal analysis of bone density in human immunodeficiency virus-infected women. *J Clin Endocrinol Metab.* 2006;91:2938-2945.

Current Issues in Osteoporosis Therapy

Thiazolidenedione Use and the Longitudinal Risk of Fractures in Patients with Type 2 Diabetes Mellitus

Habib ZA, Havstad SL, Wells K, et al (Henry Ford Hosp, Detroit, MI)
J Clin Endocrinol Metab 95:592-600, 2010

Context.—Thiazolidinedione (TZD) use has recently been associated with an increased risk of fractures.

Objective.—The aim of this study was to determine the time-dependent relationship between TZD use and fracture risk.

Design.—We conducted a retrospective cohort study in a large health system in southeast Michigan.

Patients.—Patients who received care from the health system were included if they were at least 18 yr of age, had a diagnosis of diabetes, and had at least one prescription for an oral diabetes medication. These criteria identified 19,070 individuals (9,620 women and 9,450 men).

Intervention.—This study compared patients treated with TZDs to patients without TZD treatment. Cox proportional hazard models were used to assess the relationship between exposure and outcomes.

Main Outcome Measures.—The primary outcome was the time to fracture. Secondary analyses examined the risk of fractures in subgroups defined by sex and age.

Results.—TZD use was associated with an increased risk of fracture in the cohort overall [adjusted hazard ratio (aHR), 1.35; 95% confidence interval (CI), 1.05–1.71] and in women (aHR, 1.57; 95% CI, 1.16–2.14), but not in men (aHR, 1.05; 95% CI, 0.70–1.58). Women more than 65 yr of age appeared to be at greatest risk for fracture (aHR, 1.72; 95% CI, 1.17–2.52). Among women, the increased fracture risk was not apparent until after 1 yr of TZD treatment.

Conclusions.—TZD use was associated with an increased risk for fractures in women, particularly at ages above 65 yr. Clinicians should be aware of this association when considering TZD therapy so as to appropriately manage and counsel their patients.

▶ Thiazolidenediones (TZDs) are effective in improving insulin resistance in patients with type 2 diabetes mellitus.[1] This category of drug is among the most commonly prescribed oral agent for treatment of type 2 diabetes mellitus in the United States. Several studies have reported an increased risk of bone loss and fractures in diabetic subjects taking TZDs.[2-6] The risk of bone loss and fractures associated with TZD use appears to be independent of the effect of the more rapid bone loss and increased fracture risk associated with type 2 diabetes mellitus.[7-9] Insulin use itself has been reported to be associated with increased fracture risk in patients with diabetes.[10] Other factors, including decreased visual acuity and peripheral neuropathy due to diabetes, may increase fall risk, and diabetic nephropathy also increases bone loss and fractures. Most studies reporting increased fracture risk associated with TZD use in type 2 diabetes are based on adverse event reports in large randomized controlled trials, small observational studies, a single case-control study, and one meta-analysis. One randomized controlled trial evaluated the effect of rosiglitazone on markers of bone turnover, but not fractures. Another longitudinal observational study evaluated fracture risk due to TZDs in older adults compared with other oral agent therapies. This study reports an increased risk of fracture in 9620 women, but not 9450 men, aged 18 years or older, who had type 2 diabetes mellitus followed for at least 7 years. The adjusted hazard ratio for fracture for women treated with TZDs was 1.35 (95% CI, 1.05-1.71). Postmenopausal women over age 65 years were at greatest risk of fracture, with an adjusted hazard ratio of 1.72 (95% CI, 1.17-2.52). The increased risk of fracture in these women took 1 year of TZD treatment to become evident (Fig 2 in the original article). Fractures seen in the women in this cohort were primarily in the upper and distal lower extremities, as reported in other clinical studies. These findings provide additional support that TZDs may increase fracture risk in older postmenopausal women. The mechanisms by which TZDs affect fracture risk are still not completely elucidated, although available bone marker data suggest that TZDs acting as PPARγ agonists stimulate the differentiation of bone marrow mesenchymal stem cells into adipocytes and not osteoblasts. In addition, TZDs appear to suppress osteoblast function and bone formation while stimulating osteoclast differentiation. Further studies are needed to clarify the mechanisms of bone loss associated with TZD use, and whether fracture risk is increased throughout the skeleton and not just the upper and distal lower extremities.

B. L. Clarke, MD

References

1. Yki-Järvinen H. Thiazolidenediones. *N Engl J Med.* 2004;351:1106-1118.
2. Schwartz AV, Sellmeyer DE, Vittinghoff E, et al. Thiazolidenedione use and bone loss in older diabetic patients. *J Clin Endocrinol Metab.* 2006;91:3349-3354.
3. Kahn SE, Haffner SM, Heise MA, et al. ADOPT Study Group. Glycemic durability of rosiglitazone, metformin, or glyburide monotherapy. *N Engl J Med.* 2006;355:2427-2443.
4. Dormandy J, Bhattacharya M, van Troostenburg de Bruyn AR, PRO active investigators. Safety and tolerability of pioglitazone in high-risk patients with type 2 diabetes: an overview of data from PROactive. *Drug Saf.* 2009;32:187-202.
5. Home PD, Pocock SJ, Beck-Nielsen H, et al. RECORD Study Team. Rosiglitazone evaluated for cardiovascular outcomes in oral agent combination therapy for type 2 diabetes (RECORD): a multicenter, randomised, open-label trial. *Lancet.* 2009;373:2125-2135.
6. Loke YK, Singh S, Furberg CD. Long-term use of thiazolidenediones and fractures in type 2 diabetes mellitus: a meta-analysis. *CMAJ.* 2009;180:32-39.
7. Schwartz AV, Sellmeyer DE, Strotmeyer ES, et al. Health ABC Study. Diabetes and bone loss at the hip in older black and white adults. *J Bone Miner Res.* 2005;20:596-603.
8. Bonds DE, Larson JC, Schwartz AV, et al. Risk of fracture in women with type 2 diabetes mellitus: the Women's Health Initiative Observational Study. *J Clin Endocrinol Metab.* 2006;91:3404-3410.
9. Leslie WD, Lix LM, Prior HJ, Derksen S, Metge C, O'Neil J. Biphasic fracture risk in diabetes: a population-based study. *Bone.* 2007;40:1595-1601.

10. Ivers RQ, Cumming RG, Mitchell P, Peduto AJ, Blue Mountains Eye Study. Diabetes and risk of fracture: the Blue Mountains Eye Study. *Diabetes Care*. 2001; 24:1198-1203.

Effect of Rosiglitazone, Metformin, and Glyburide on Bone Biomarkers in Patients with Type 2 Diabetes

Zinman B, Haffner SM, Herman WH, et al (Mount Sinai Hosp and Univ of Toronto, Ontario, Canada; Univ of Texas Health Science Ctr at San Antonio; Univ of Michigan, Ann Arbor; et al)

J Clin Endocrinol Metab 95:134-142, 2010

Context.—An increase in bone fractures has been observed in women taking thiazolidinediones.

Objective.—The objective of the study was to examine whether changes in circulating bone biomarkers provide insight into the underlying mechanisms responsible for the increase in bone fractures in female participants randomized to rosiglitazone in A Diabetes Outcome Progression Trial (ADOPT).

Research Design and Methods.—Paired stored baseline and 12-month serum samples were available from 1605 participants (689 women, 916 men) in ADOPT, a long-term clinical trial comparing the effects of rosiglitazone, glyburide, and metformin on glycemic control in patients with type 2 diabetes.

Results.—This subset was well matched to the total ADOPT study population. In women a marker of osteoclast activity, C-terminal telopeptide (for type 1 collagen), increased by 6.1% with rosiglitazone compared with reductions of 1.3% ($P = 0.03$ *vs.* rosiglitazone) and 3.3% ($P = 0.002$ *vs.* rosiglitazone) with metformin and glyburide, respectively. In men, C-terminal telopeptide was unchanged on rosiglitazone (−1.0%) and fell on metformin (−12.7%; $P < 0.001$) and glyburide (−4.3%, $P = \text{NS}$). Markers of osteoblast activity, procollagen type 1 N-propeptide (P1NP) and bone alkaline phosphatase, were reduced for women and men in almost all treatment groups, with the greatest changes in the metformin group (P1NP in females, −14.4%; P1NP in males, −19.3%), intermediate for rosiglitazone (P1NP in females,−4.4%; P1NP in males,−14.4%), and smallest for glyburide (P1NP in males, +0.2%; bone alkaline phosphatase in females, −11.6%).

Conclusions.—Commonly measured bone biomarkers suggest that changes in bone resorption may be partly responsible for the increased risk of fracture in women taking thiazolidinediones.

▶ Postmenopausal women with type 2 diabetes mellitus who take thiazolidenediones (TZDs) have been reported to be at increased risk of fracture, independent of the fracture risk associated with their diabetes. The fact that TZDs increase fracture risk was reported in A Diabetes Outcome Progression Trial (ADOPT).[1] ADOPT was a randomized, double-blind, prospective, controlled clinical trial comparing the effects of the TZDs rosiglitazone, metformin, and glyburide on glucose control in recently diagnosed drug-naïve type 2 diabetic patients.[2] Rosiglitazone was not only shown to cause more durable blood glucose control than metformin or glyburide, as assessed by fasting glucose and hemoglobin A1c levels, but was also shown to be associated with increased risk of upper and lower limb peripheral fractures in postmenopausal women.[2] Rosiglitazone was not associated with vertebral or hip fractures in postmenopausal women, however, and not associated with fractures in men. Shortly after the results of ADOPT were released, pioglitazone was also reported to be associated with increased fracture risk.[3]

The mechanisms by which TZDs might cause limb fractures are not well understood. Cell culture studies have demonstrated that TZDs stimulate differentiation of mesenchymal progenitor cells into adipocytes rather than osteoblasts[4] and that they may decrease osteoblast differentiation by reducing IGF-1 levels in bone.[5] Rodent studies have shown that TZDs cause bone loss in most studies by reducing bone formation[6] but in some studies by increasing bone resorption.[7] Previous studies of markers of bone turnover in postmenopausal women have shown that TZDs suppress bone formation, without changing bone resorption.[8,9]

This study evaluated paired baseline and 12-month serum markers of bone turnover in a subset of 689 postmenopausal women and 916 men in ADOPT. Serum C-terminal telopeptide of type I collagen (CTX), a marker of bone resorption, increased in the women receiving rosiglitazone but remained stable in men. This marker decreased mildly in women, and more significantly in men, receiving metformin or glyburide. Serum procollagen type 1 aminoN-terminal propeptide (P1NP) and bone alkaline phosphatase, markers of bone formation, decreased in both women and men regardless of the drug received, with the greatest decreases seen in subjects receiving metformin.

These findings suggest that rosiglitazone may affect bone remodeling by both decreasing bone formation and stimulating bone resorption. Limitations of this study include lack of a placebo arm, measurements made only on samples collected during the first year of this 4-year study, lack of systematic collection of samples, and lack of bone density information. Differences in fractures between the 3 study drugs did not occur until after the first year.[2] Nevertheless, this is the largest study to evaluate the effects of TZDs on bone metabolism. Further controlled long-term studies evaluating markers of bone turnover, bone mineral density, and fractures will be required to clearly establish the mechanisms behind TZD-induced fractures.

B. L. Clarke, MD

References

1. Kahn SE, Haffner SM, Heise MA, et al. ADOPT Study Group. Glycemic durability of rosiglitazone, metformin, or glyburide monotherapy. *N Engl J Med.* 2006;355: 2427-2443.
2. Kahn SE, Zinman B, Lachin JM, et al. Diabetes Outcome Progression Trial (ADOPT) Study Group. Rosiglitazone-associated fractures in type 2 diabetes: an analysis from A Diabetes Outcome Progression Trial (ADOPT). *Diabetes Care.* 2008;31:845-851.

3. Takeda Pharmaceuticals. Observation of an increased incidence of fractures in female patients who received long-term treatment with ACTOS (pioglitazone HCl) tablets for type 2 diabetes mellitus (letter to health care providers), 2007.
4. Ali AA, Weinstein RS, Stewart SA, Parfitt AM, Manolagas SC, Jilka RL. Rosiglitazone causes bone loss in mice by suppressing osteoblast differentiation and bone formation. *Endocrinology.* 2005;146:1226-1235.
5. Lecka-Czernik B, Ackert-Bicknell C, Adamo ML, et al. Activation of peroxisome proliferator-activated receptor γ (PPARγ) by rosiglitazone suppresses components of the insulin-like growth factor regulatory system in vitro and in vivo. *Endocrinology.* 2007;148:903-911.
6. Grey A. Skeletal consequences of thiazolidinedione therapy. *Osteoporos Int.* 2008; 19:129-137.
7. Lazarenko OP, Rzonka SO, Hogue WR, et al. Rosiglitazone induces decreases in bone mass and strength that are reminiscent of age bone. *Endocrinology.* 2007; 75:2669-2680.
8. Grey A, Bolland M, Gamble G, et al. The peroxisome proliferator-activated receptor- rosiglitazone decreases bone formation and bone mineral density in healthy postmenopausal women: a randomized, controlled trial. *J Clin Endocrinol Metab.* 2007;92:1305-1310.
9. Berberoglu Z, Gursoy A, Bayraktar N, et al. Rosiglitazone decreases serum bone specific alkaline phosphatase activity in postmenopausal diabetic women. *J Clin Endocrinol Metab.* 2007;92:3523-3530.

Effects of Yearly Zoledronic Acid 5 mg on Bone Turnover Markers and Relation of PINP With Fracture Reduction in Postmenopausal Women With Osteoporosis

Delmas PD, Munoz F, Black DM, et al (INSERM Res Unit 831 and Univ of Lyon, France; Univ of California, San Francisco; et al)
J Bone Miner Res 24:1544-1551, 2009

In patients with osteoporosis treated with antiresorptive agents, reduction in bone turnover explains much of the observed fracture risk reduction. Lower levels of bone turnover markers (BTMs) appear to be associated with a lower risk of fracture in bisphosphonate-treated patients. BTMs were measured in a subset of subjects in the HORIZON Pivotal Fracture Trial. Annual infusions of zoledronic acid 5 mg significantly reduced BTMs: median decrease of 50% for β-C-terminal telopeptides of type 1 collagen (β-CTX), 30% for bone alkaline phosphatase (ALP), and 56% for procollagen type 1 amino-terminal propeptide (PINP). The mean level of BTMs decreased in treated patients but remained within the premenopausal range before the next injection. The percentage of zoledronic acid–treated patients with values below the premenopausal reference range at all time points was 1.7%, 17.8%, and 19% for bone ALP, CTX, and PINP, respectively. The third injection of zoledronic acid resulted in 60% reduction of β-CTX within 9–11 days, followed by a gradual increase, indicating the persistence of osteoclastic bone resorption. The association between changes in BTMs and fracture incidence was assessed in 1132 patients who had PINP measurements at baseline and 1 yr. There was no association between low PINP levels at 1 yr and increased fracture incidence. In summary, (1) annual injections of zoledronic acid reduced BTMs in the premenopausal range, with a significant response persisting after the third infusion; and (2) low levels of PINP were not associated with increased fracture risk.

▶ Zoledronic acid is a potent, long-lasting, and intravenous bisphosphonate used to treat postmenopausal osteoporosis and prevent fractures.[1,2] Bisphosphonates and other antiresorptive drugs significantly reduce bone resorption and formation, and this reduction in bone turnover explains much of the fracture reduction seen with these agents, independent of changes in bone mineral density.[3-5] Concern has been raised that suppression of bone formation for several years with antiresorptive agents might increase fracture risk.[6-8]

In this analysis of the Health Outcomes and Reduced Incidence with Zoledronic Acid Once Yearly (HORIZON) Pivotal Fracture Reduction Trial, markers of bone turnover were measured in subjects treated with zoledronic acid 5 mg intravenously once a year for 3 years. In treated subjects, serum β-C-terminal telopeptides of type 1 collagen (β-CTX) levels were maximally reduced by 50%, serum bone alkaline phosphatase by 30%, and serum procollagen type 1 amino-terminal propeptide (PINP) by 56%, but levels remained within the premenopausal normal range before the next infusion. In patients treated with zoledronic acid, 1.7% had serum β-CTX telopeptide levels below the premenopausal reference range, whereas 17.8% had serum bone alkaline phosphatase levels below this range, and 19% had serum PINP levels below the premenopausal reference range. The third yearly infusion of zoledronic acid caused 60% reduction in serum β-CTX within about 10 days, with gradual increase in serum β-CTX toward baseline over the next 6 months, indicating recovery of normal osteoclast bone resorption after each infusion. In a subset of 1132 subjects, serum PINP was measured at baseline and at 1 year, but there was no association between serum PINP at 1 year and increased fracture incidence.

This study showed that annual infusion of zoledronic acid to treat postmenopausal osteoporosis caused markers of bone turnover to decrease into the premenopausal reference range, with a significant effect still present with the third infusion. In addition, low levels of serum PINP did not increase fracture risk. While zoledronic acid is a potent long-lasting agent, its suppression of bone turnover appears to wane within 1 year. This study also provided no evidence that suppression of bone formation over 3 years resulted in increased fracture risk.

B. L. Clarke, MD

References

1. Black DM, Cummings SR, Karpf DB, et al. Once-yearly zoledronic acid for treatment of postmenopausal osteoporosis. *New Engl J Med.* 2007;356:1809-1822.
2. Lyles KW, Colon-Emeric CS, Magaziner JS, et al. Zoledronic acid and clinical fractures and mortality after hip fracture. *New Engl J Med.* 2007;357:1799-1809.
3. Cummings SR, Karpf DB, Harris F, et al. Improvement in spine bone density and reduction in risk of vertebral fractures during treatment with antiresorptive drugs. *Am J Med.* 2002;112:281-289.
4. Delmas PD, Seeman E. Changes in bone mineral density explain little of the reduction in vertebral or nonvertebral fracture risk with anti-resorptive therapy. *Bone.* 2004;34:599-604.

5. Sarkar S, Mitlak BH, Wong M, Stock JL, Black DM, Harper KD. Relationships between bone mineral density and incident vertebral fracture risk with raloxifene therapy. *J Bone Miner Res.* 2002;17:1-10.
6. Odvina CV, Zerwekh JE, Rao DS, Maalouf N, Gottschalk FA, Pak CY. Severely suppressed bone turnover: a potential complication of alendronate therapy. *J Clin Endocrinol Metab.* 2005;90:1294-1301.
7. Goh SK, Yang KY, Koh JS, et al. Subtrochanteric insufficiency fractures in patients on alendronate therapy: a caution. *J Bone Joint Surg Br.*. 2007;89:349-353.
8. Lenart BA, Lorich DG, Lane JM. Atypical fractures of the femoral diaphysis in postmenopausal women taking alendronate. *New Engl J Med.* 2008;358: 1304-1306.

Zoledronic acid and risedronate in the prevention and treatment of glucocorticoid-induced osteoporosis (HORIZON): a multicentre, double-blind, double-dummy, randomised controlled trial

Reid DM, for the HORIZON investigators (Univ of Aberdeen, UK; et al)

Lancet 373:1253-1263, 2009

Background.—Persistent use of glucocorticoid drugs is associated with bone loss and increased fracture risk. Concurrent oral bisphosphonates increase bone mineral density and reduce frequency of vertebral fractures, but are associated with poor compliance and adherence. We aimed to assess whether one intravenous infusion of zoledronic acid was non-inferior to daily oral risedronate for prevention and treatment of glucocorticoid-induced osteoporosis.

Methods.—This 1-year randomised, double-blind, double-dummy, non-inferiority study of 54 centres in 12 European countries, Australia, Hong Kong, Israel, and the USA, tested the effectiveness of 5 mg intravenous infusion of zoledronic acid versus 5 mg oral risedronate for prevention and treatment of glucocorticoid-induced osteoporosis. 833 patients were randomised 1:1 to receive zoledronic acid (n=416) or risedronate (n=417). Patients were stratified by sex, and allocated to prevention or treatment subgroups dependent on duration of glucocorticoid use immediately preceding the study. The treatment subgroup consisted of those treated for more than 3 months (272 patients on zoledronic acid and 273 on risedronate), and the prevention subgroup of those treated for less than 3 months (144 patients on each drug). 62 patients did not complete the study because of adverse events, withdrawal of consent, loss to follow-up, death, misrandomisation, or protocol deviation. The primary endpoint was percentage change from baseline in lumbar spine bone mineral density. Drug efficacy was assessed on a modified intention-to-treat basis and safety was assessed on an intention-to-treat basis. This trial is registered with ClinicalTrials.gov, number NCT00100620.

Findings.—Zoledronic acid was non-inferior and superior to risedronate for increase of lumbar spine bone mineral density in both the treatment (least-squares mean 4·06% [SE 0·28] *vs* 2·71% [SE 0·28], mean difference 1·36% [95% CI 0·67–2·05], p=0·0001) and prevention (2·60% [0·45] *vs* 0·64% [0·46], 1·96% [1·04–2·88], p<0·0001)

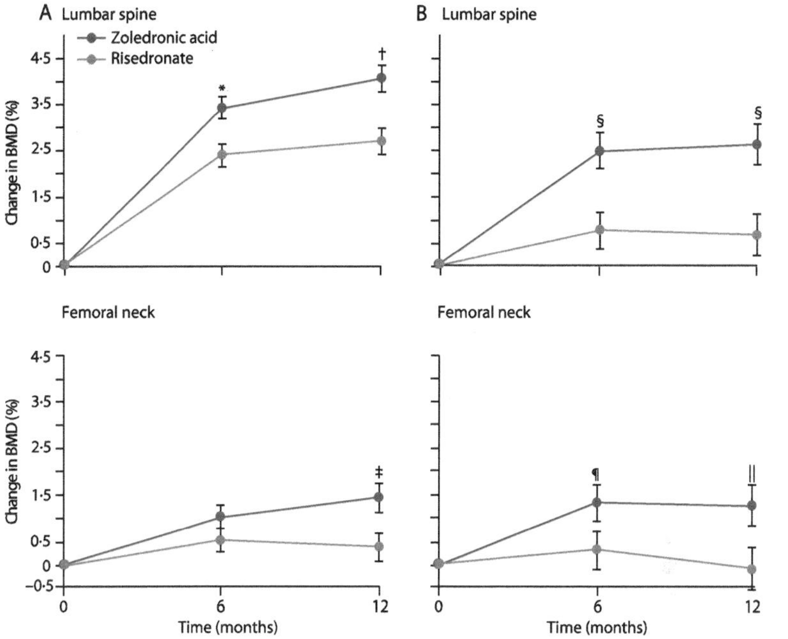

FIGURE 2.—Change in mean bone mineral density of lumbar spine and femoral neck for (A) treatment and (B) prevention subgroups (modified intention-to-treat group). Data are least-squares mean. Error bars=95% CI. BMD=bone mineral density. p values compare change in bone mineral density relative to baseline between drug groups, calculated from a three-way analysis of variance with adjustment for drug group, study region, and sex. *p=0·0005. †p=0·0001. ‡p=0·0050. §p<0·0001. ¶p=0·0156. ||p=0·0049. (Reprinted from Reid DM, for the HORIZON investigators. Zoledronic acid and risedronate in the prevention and treatment of glucocorticoid-induced osteoporosis (HORIZON): a multicentre, double-blind, double-dummy, randomised controlled trial. *Lancet.* 2009;373:1253-1263, with permission from Elsevier.)

subgroups at 12 months. Adverse events were more frequent in patients given zoledronic acid than in those on risedronate, largely as a result of transient symptoms during the first 3 days after infusion. Serious adverse events were worsening rheumatoid arthritis for the treatment subgroup and pyrexia for the prevention subgroup.

Interpretation.—A single 5 mg intravenous infusion of zoledronic acid is non-inferior, possibly more effective, and more acceptable to patients than is 5 mg of oral risedronate daily for prevention and treatment of bone loss that is associated with glucocorticoid use (Fig 2).

▶ Persistent use of glucocorticoid therapy may suppress bone formation and result in increased bone loss and fractures.[1-3] Most studies have shown that the magnitude of the bone loss and increased fracture risk depends on the dose and duration of therapy with glucocorticoids.[4] Oral alendronate and risedronate have been shown to prevent bone loss in patients taking oral glucocorticoid therapy,[5-7] but these placebo-controlled studies were not powered to show fracture reduction.

Zoledronic acid is a potent, long-lasting, intravenous bisphosphonate used to treat postmenopausal osteoporosis and prevent fractures in subjects not taking glucocorticoids.[8,9] This noninferiority study evaluated the effectiveness of zoledronic acid 5 mg given intravenously once a year to risedronate 5 mg orally each day for 1 year for the prevention and treatment of glucocorticoid-induced osteoporosis. The study randomized 833 subjects to receive zoledronic acid or risedronate, and further stratified participants by duration of glucocorticoid therapy. Subjects treated for more than 3 months with glucocorticoids were considered part of the treatment group, whereas subjects taking glucocorticoids for less than 3 months were categorized as part of the prevention group. Zoledronic acid was found to be noninferior and superior to risedronate with regard to lumbar spine bone density increase in both the treatment and prevention groups at 1 year (Fig 2). Adverse events were more common in the zoledronic acid group because of transient symptoms during the first 3 days after the infusion.

This study concluded that once yearly zoledronic acid is noninferior, and possibly more effective, than risedronate in the prevention and treatment of glucocorticoid-induced bone loss. Different bisphosphonates effectively prevent bone loss in subjects treated with glucocorticoids, but studies to date have not been powered to show fracture prevention. This is the first study to compare the effects of two different bisphosphonate therapies head-to-head in patients treated with glucocorticoid-induced osteoporosis.

B. L. Clarke, MD

References

1. von Staa TP, Leufkens HG, Abenhaim L, Zhang B, Cooper C. Use of oral corticosteroids and risk of fractures. *J Bone Miner Res.* 2000;15:993-1000.
2. Von Staa TP, Leufkens HG, Abenhaim L, Zhang B, Cooper C. Oral corticosteroids and fracture risk: relationship to daily and cumulative doses. *Rheumatology (Oxf).* 2000;39:1383-1389.
3. Von Staa TP, Leufkens HG, Cooper C. The epidemiology of corticosteroid-induced osteoporosis: a meta-analysis. *Osteoporos Int.* 2002;13:777-787.
4. American College of Rheumatology Ad Hoc Committee on Glucocorticoid-Induced Osteoporosis. Recommendations for the prevention and treatment of glucocorticoid-induced osteoporosis: 2001 update. *Arthritis Rheum.* 2001;44: 1496-1503.
5. Cohen S, Levy RM, Keller M, et al. Risedronate therapy prevents corticosteroid-induced bone loss: a twelve-month, multicenter, randomized, double-blind, placebo-controlled, parallel-group study. *Arthritis Rheum.* 1999;42:2309-2318.
6. Reid DM, Hughes RA, Laan RF, et al. Efficacy and safety of daily risedronate in the treatment of corticosteroid-induced osteoporosis in men and women: a randomized trial. European Corticosteroid-Induced Osteoporosis Treatment Study. *J Bone Miner Res.* 2000;15:1006-1013.
7. Saag KG, Emkey R, Schnitzer TJ, et al. Alendronate for the prevention and treatment of glucocorticoid-induced osteoporosis. Glucocorticoid-Induced Osteoporosis Intervention Study Group. *N Engl J Med.* 1998;339:292-299.
8. Black DM, Cummings SR, Karpf DB, et al. HORIZON Pivotal Fracture Trial. Once-yearly zoledronic acid for treatment of postmenopausal osteoporosis. *N Engl J Med.* 2007;356:1809-1822.
9. Lyles KW, Colon-Emeric CS, Magaziner JS, et al. HORIZON Recurrent Fracture Trial. Zoledronic acid and clinical fractures and mortality after hip fracture. *N Engl J Med.* 2007;357:1799-1809.

Effects of Teriparatide in Postmenopausal Women with Osteoporosis on Prior Alendronate or Raloxifene: Differences between Stopping and Continuing the Antiresorptive Agent

Cosman F, Wermers RA, Recknor C, et al (Helen Hayes Hosp, West Haverstraw, NY; Mayo Clinic, Rochester, MN; United Osteoporosis Ctrs, Gainesville, GA; et al)

J Clin Endocrinol Metab 94:3772-3780, 2009

Objective.—The aim of the study was to assess adding *vs.* switching to teriparatide 20μg/d in patients on alendronate or raloxifene.

Design.—We conducted a randomized, open-label trial.

Patients and Interventions.—Postmenopausal women with osteoporosis on alendronate or raloxifene for at least 18 months added teriparatide (Add groups) or switched to teriparatide (Switch groups) for 18 months.

Main Outcome Measures.—We measured bone turnover markers (BTM) and bone mineral density (BMD).

Results.—In the alendronate stratum, increases in BTM were smaller in the Add *vs.* Switch group [6-month PINP (64 *vs.* 401%); bone ALP (15 *vs.* 71%); βCTX (27 *vs.* 250%); all $P < 0.001$]. However, at 6 months, total hip BMD increased more in the Add *vs.* Switch group (1.4 *vs.* −0.8%; $P = 0.002$). In the Add *vs.* Switch group, 18-month BMD increments were higher in lumbar spine (8.4 *vs.* 4.8%; $P = 0.003$) and total hip (3.2 *vs.* 0.9%; $P = 0.02$), but not in femoral neck (2.7 *vs.* 2.3%; $P = 0.75$). In the raloxifene stratum, increases in BTM were also smaller in the Add *vs.* Switch group [6-month PINP (131 *vs.* 259%; $P < 0.001$), bone ALP (31 *vs.* 44%; $P = 0.035$), and βCTX (67 *vs.* 144%; $P = 0.001$)]. At 6 months, total hip BMD increase was greater in the Add *vs.* Switch group (1.8 *vs.* 0.5%; $P = 0.028$). At 18 months, increases in lumbar spine (9.2 *vs.* 8.1%), total hip (2.8 *vs.* 1.8%), and femoral neck (3.8 *vs.* 2.2%) were not significantly different between groups.

Conclusions.—In women with osteoporosis treated with antiresorptives, greater bone turnover increases were achieved by switching to teriparatide, whereas greater BMD increases were achieved by adding teriparatide.

▶ Treatment of postmenopausal osteoporosis with the anabolic agent teriparatide (human recombinant parathyroid hormone 1-34) stimulates bone formation and bone resorption, improves cortical and trabecular microarchitecture, improves bone mineral density (BMD), and decreases fractures.[1-4] This agent is approved for the treatment of osteoporosis in postmenopausal women and men at high risk of fracture, or those who have not responded or been able to tolerate other therapies.

There have been fewer studies of the effect of parathyroid hormone in combination with other antiresorptive agents. In postmenopausal osteoporotic women who had not previously been treated for osteoporosis, parathyroid hormone (PTH) 1-84 in combination with alendronate caused similar increases in lumbar spine BMD, but greater increases in total hip and radius BMD, than

PTH 1-84 alone.[5] Similar findings were reported in postmenopausal osteoporotic women not previously treated for osteoporosis who were treated with the combination of teriparatide and raloxifene.[6]

The effect of teriparatide in patients who were previously treated with other osteoporotic drugs is less well understood. This study compared the BMD, bone turnover marker, and calcemic responses to teriparatide over 18 months in 198 postmenopausal osteoporotic women previously treated with alendronate 70 mg/wk or raloxifene 60 mg/d for at least 18 months. Subjects were randomized to continue their previous treatment and add teriparatide 20 μg/d, or to switch from their previous agent to teriparatide 20 μg/d. Subjects who added teriparatide to their previous antiresorptive therapy had greater increases in lumbar spine and hip BMD when previously treated with alendronate, and in hip BMD when previously treated with raloxifene. Subjects who switched to teriparatide had greater increases in their bone turnover markers than those who continued their previous therapy in combination with teriparatide.

This study demonstrated that postmenopausal osteoporotic women previously treated with alendronate or raloxifene for at least 18 months, who added teriparatide for another 18 months, had significant further improvement in BMD at their lumbar spine and hip. Postmenopausal women previously treated with alendronate or raloxifene for at least 18 months, who switched to teriparatide for another 18 months, had mildly increased lumbar spine BMD, but stable hip BMD. In spite of these changes in BMD, the changes in markers of turnover were greater when subjects switched to teriparatide. These findings demonstrate the complexity of skeletal response that may be seen in patients treated sequentially with monotherapy followed by combination therapy, or who are switched to new monotherapy after previous monotherapy with a different agent, and give insight into the variations in response that might be seen with different permutations and combinations of osteoporosis therapies.

B. L. Clarke, MD

References

1. Neer RM, Arnaud CD, Zanchetta JR, et al. Effect of parathyroid hormone (1-34) on fractures and bone mineral density in postmenopausal women with osteoporosis. *N Engl J Med.* 2001;344:1434-1441.
2. Lindsay R, Zhou H, Cosman F, Nieves J, Dempster DW, Hodsman AB. Effects of a one-month treatment with PTH (1-34) on bone formation on cancellous, endocortical, and periosteal surfaces of the human ilium. *J Bone Miner Res.* 2007;22: 495-502.
3. McClung MR, San Martin J, Miller PD, et al. Opposite bone remodeling effects of teriparatide and alendronate in increasing bone mass. *Arch Int Med.* 2005;165: 1762-1768.
4. Jiang Y, Zhao JJ, Mitlak BH, Wang O, Genant HK, Eriksen EF. Recombinant human parathyroid hormone (1-34) [teriparatide] improves both cortical and cancellous bone structure. *J Bone Miner Res.* 2003;18:1932-1941.
5. Black DM, Greenspan SL, Ensrud KE, et al. PaTH Study Investigators. The effects of parathyroid hormone and alendronate alone or in combination in postmenopausal osteoporosis. *N Engl J Med.* 2003;349:1207-1215.

6. Deal C, Omizo M, Schwartz EN, et al. Combination teriparatide and raloxifene therapy for postmenopausal osteoporosis: results from a 6-month double-blind placebo-controlled trial. *J Bone Miner Res.* 2005;20:1905-1911.

Effects of Teriparatide Treatment and Discontinuation in Postmenopausal Women and Eugonadal Men with Osteoporosis

Leder BZ, Neer RM, Wyland JJ, et al (Massachusetts General Hosp, Boston)
J Clin Endocrinol Metab 94:2915-2921, 2009

Context.—In postmenopausal women, bone mineral density (BMD) declines after teriparatide therapy is stopped. The pattern of BMD loss after teriparatide therapy is stopped in men is less clear.

Objective.—The aim of the study was to determine whether the pattern of teriparatide-induced bone accrual and post-teriparatide bone loss differs between postmenopausal women and eugonadal men.

Design.—We conducted a prospective cohort substudy.

Patients.—The study included 14 postmenopausal women and 17 eugonadal men, ages 46–85 yr, with lumbar spine or femoral neck BMD T-scores below −2.

Intervention.—Teriparatide (37 μg sc daily) was administered for 24 months, followed by 12 months off therapy.

Main Outcome Measures.—We measured BMD at various anatomic sites by dual-energy x-ray absorptiometry, trabecular spine BMD by quantitative computed tomography, and bone turnover markers during the treatment and observation periods. The response to teriparatide administration and discontinuation was compared between females and males.

Results.—BMD of the spine, femoral neck, total hip, and trabecular spine increased similarly during the treatment period in men and women, whereas BMD at the radius was stable in men but decreased by 8.1 ± 3.3% in women ($P < 0.0001$). After teriparatide was stopped, BMD at the posterior-anterior spine decreased by 7.1 ± 3.8% in women and by 4.1 ± 3.5% in men ($P = 0.036$). BMD at the total hip and femoral neck decreased by 3.8 ± 3.9 and 3.1 ± 4.3%, respectively, in women but remained stable in men ($P < 0.05$ for both sites). BMD at the distal radius remained stable in men but increased in women by 1.6 ± 3.1% ($P = 0.069$).

Conclusions.—Teriparatide appears to increase BMD similarly in postmenopausal women and eugonadalmen with osteoporosis. After teriparatide is stopped, the decline in BMD is greater in women than in men. If confirmed in larger cohorts, these findings would suggest that the indication for immediate antiresorptive therapy after teriparatide may not be as urgent in men as in women.

▶ Teriparatide (human recombinant parathyroid hormone 1-34) is approved for treatment of osteoporosis in postmenopausal women and in men at high risk of fracture, or those who have not responded or been able to tolerate other therapies. Unlike other therapies for osteoporosis, however, regulatory agencies have approved teriparatide for use for up to 2 years in the United States and for up to 18 months in the European Union. Although long-acting bisphosphonate therapies accumulate in the skeleton and prevent osteoclastic resorption and bone loss for many months after therapy is discontinued,[1,2] teriparatide's effects on the skeleton wear off rapidly after therapy is stopped. Previous studies have shown that stopping teriparatide or parathyroid hormone 1-84 in postmenopausal women results in rapid bone loss within 6 to 12 months.[3] An uncontrolled study suggests that bone loss also occurs in men, similar to that seen in postmenopausal women, after teriparatide is stopped.[4]

This small prospective cohort study compared bone loss after discontinuation of teriparatide in 14 postmenopausal women and 17 eugonadal men aged 46 to 85 years with lumbar spine or femoral neck bone mineral density (BMD) T-scores less than −2.0. Subjects received teriparatide 37 μg/day by subcutaneous injection for 24 months, after which BMD loss was followed for another 12 months. The teriparatide used in this study was manufactured by Bachem, Inc (Torrance, CA), and not Lilly and Co, Inc. BMD increased similarly in both women and men over the 24 months of therapy, but women lost more BMD at the lumbar spine and hip than men after discontinuation of therapy. Men lost a small amount of lumbar spine BMD but did not lose hip BMD.

These findings suggest that postmenopausal women and eugonadal men gain an equivalent amount of bone density on teriparatide therapy but that postmenopausal women lose BMD faster than men after stopping teriparatide therapy. The cause for the apparent more rapid loss in postmenopausal women is not clear, but the findings suggest that eugonadal men may not require rapid institution of antiresorptive therapy after stopping teriparatide, as currently recommended for postmenopausal women. These findings require confirmation in larger studies.

B. L. Clarke, MD

References

1. Black DM, Schwartz AV, Ensrud KE, et al. Effects of continuing or stopping alendronate after 5 years of treatment: the Fracture Intervention Trial Long-term Extension (FLEX): a randomized trial. *JAMA*. 2006;296:2927-2938.
2. Ensrud KE, Barrett-Connor EL, Schwartz A, et al. Randomized trial of effect of alendronate continuation versus discontinuation in women with low BMD: results from the Fracture Intervention Trial long-term extension. *J Bone Miner Res*. 2004; 19:1259-1269.
3. Black DM, Bilezikian JP, Ensrud KE, et al. One year of alendronate after one year of parathyroid hormone (1-84) for osteoporosis. *New Engl J Med*. 2005;353: 555-565.
4. Kaufman JM, Orwoll E, Goemaere S, et al. Teriparatide effects on vertebral fractures and bone mineral density in men with osteoporosis: treatment and discontinuation of therapy. *Osteoporos Int*. 2005;16:510-516.

Effects of Teriparatide Versus Alendronate for Treating Glucocorticoid-Induced Osteoporosis: Thirty-Six–Month Results of a Randomized, Double-Blind, Controlled Trial

Saag KG, Zanchetta JR, Devogelaer J-P, et al (Univ of Alabama at Birmingham, UK; Universidad del Salvador, Buenos Aires, Argentina; Université Catholique de Louvain, Brussels, Belgium; et al)

Arthritis Rheum 60:3346-3355, 2009

Objective.—To compare the bone anabolic drug teriparatide (20 μg/day) with the antiresorptive drug alendronate (10 mg/day) for treating glucocorticoid-induced osteoporosis (OP).

Methods.—This was a 36-month, randomized, double-blind, controlled trial in 428 subjects with OP (ages 22–89 years) who had received ≥5 mg/day of prednisone equivalent for ≥3 months preceding screening. Measures included changes in lumbar spine and hip bone mineral density (BMD), changes in bone biomarkers, fracture incidence, and safety.

Results.—Increases in BMD from baseline were significantly greater in the teriparatide group than in the alendronate group, and at 36 months were 11.0% versus 5.3% for lumbar spine, 5.2% versus 2.7% for total hip, and 6.3% versus 3.4% for femoral neck ($P < 0.001$ for all). In the teriparatide group, median percent increases from baseline in N-terminal type I procollagen propeptide (PINP) and osteocalcin (OC) levels were significant from 1 to 36 months ($P < 0.01$), and increases in levels of C-terminal telopeptide of type I collagen (CTX) were significant from 1 to 6 months ($P < 0.01$). In the alendronate group, median percent decreases in PINP, OC, and CTX were significant by 6 months and remained below baseline through 36 months ($P < 0.001$). Fewer subjects had vertebral fractures in the teriparatide group than in the alendronate group (3 [1.7%] of 173 versus 13 [7.7%] of 169; $P = 0.007$), with most occurring during the first 18 months. There was no significant difference between groups in the incidence of nonvertebral fractures (16 [7.5%] of 214 subjects taking teriparatide versus 15 [7.0%] of 214 subjects taking alendronate; $P = 0.843$). More subjects in the teriparatide group (21%) versus the alendronate group (7%) had elevated predose serum calcium concentrations ($P < 0.001$).

Conclusion.—Our findings indicate that subjects with glucocorticoid-induced OP treated with teriparatide for 36 months had greater increases in BMD and fewer new vertebral fractures than subjects treated with alendronate (Fig 2).

▶ Acute glucocorticoid therapy may cause transiently increased bone resorption, but long-term use of oral or intravenous glucocorticoid therapy may suppress bone formation and maintain normal bone resorption, with resultant increased bone mineral density (BMD) loss and fractures.[1,2] Glucocorticoids not only chronically suppress osteoblast activity, but also decrease intestinal calcium absorption, increase urinary calcium excretion, and decrease pituitary gonadotropin secretion. Decreased intestinal calcium absorption and increased

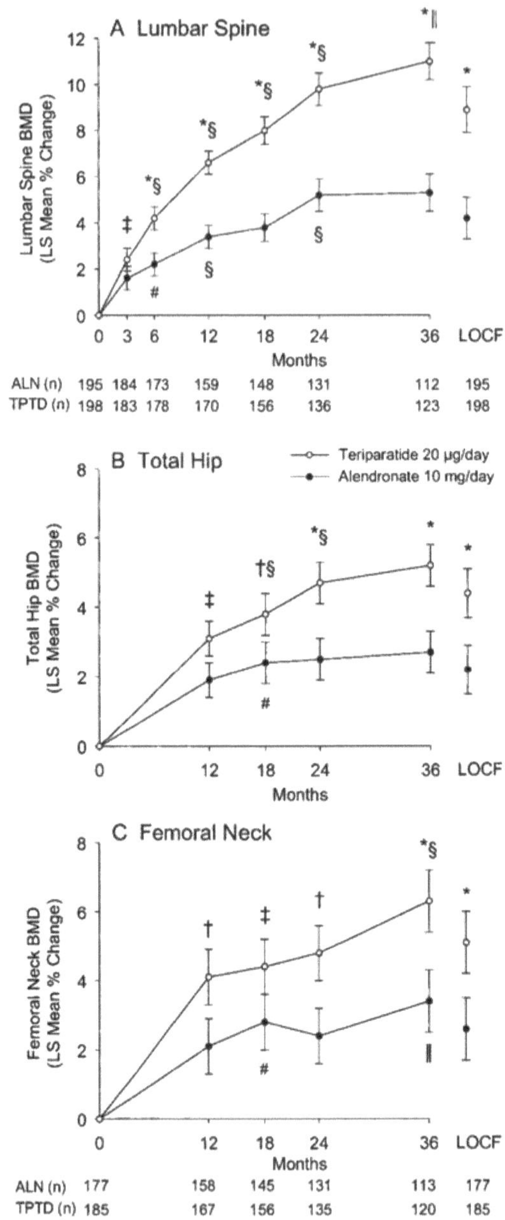

FIGURE 2.—Mean percent changes from baseline in lumbar spine (**A**), total hip (**B**), and femoral neck (**C**) bone mineral density (BMD) in the alendronate (ALN) group and teriparatide (TPTD) group. Numbers below the graph are the numbers of subjects assessed at each time point and for the last observation carried forward (LOCF) analysis and were identical for the total hip and femoral neck. Values are the least squares (LS) mean ± SEM. * = $P < 0.001$; † = $P < 0.01$; ‡ = $P < 0.05$ for the mean percent change from baseline in the teriparatide versus alendronate group. § = $P < 0.001$; † = $P < 0.01$, ‡ = $P < 0.05$ for the mean percent change from baseline within each treatment group for 6 versus 3 months, 12 versus 6 months, 18 versus 12 months, 24 versus 18 months, and 36 versus 24 months. (Courtesy of Saag KG, Zanchetta JR, Devogelaer J-P, et al. Effects of teriparatide versus alendronate for treating glucocorticoid-induced osteoporosis: thirty-six-month results of a randomized, double-blind, controlled trial. *Arthritis Rheum.* 2009;60:3346-3355.)

urinary calcium excretion may lead to physiological hyperparathyroidism in some cases, but not all.[3] Most studies correlate the magnitude of bone loss and fractures with the cumulative dose and duration of glucocorticoid therapy.[4]

Oral alendronate and risedronate have previously been shown to prevent bone loss in patients taking oral glucocorticoid therapy,[5-7] but these placebo-controlled studies were not powered to show fracture reduction. An initial report comparing teriparatide (human recombinant parathyroid hormone 1-34) with oral alendronate head-to-head showed that teriparatide increased lumbar spine and hip bone mineral density significantly more than alendronate in subjects with glucocorticoid-induced osteoporosis.[8] Teriparatide is a bone anabolic drug that increases cortical thickness and cancellous bone volume and connectivity, and improves cancellous bone plate-like structure. Teriparatide stimulates differentiation of bone lining cells and preosteoblasts along quiescent bone surfaces into osteoblasts, causes pre-existing osteoblasts to form new bone, and decreases osteoblast and osteocyte apoptosis.[9,10]

This 36-month, randomized, double-blind, controlled trial evaluated the effects of teriparatide 20 μg/d versus alendronate 10 mg/d in 428 subjects aged 22 to 89 years with osteoporosis. All subjects had received prednisone equivalent of ≥5 mg/d for ≥3 months prior to screening. The study showed significantly greater increases in lumbar spine (11.0% vs 5.3%), total hip (5.2% vs 2.7%), and femoral neck (6.3% vs 3.4%) BMD in subjects receiving teriparatide compared with alendronate. Teriparatide increased the markers of bone formation throughout the study, and a marker of bone resorption for the first 6 months, whereas alendronate decreased the markers of bone formation and resorption from 6 to 36 months. Teriparatide-treated subjects had significantly fewer radiographic vertebral fractures (3 in 173 subjects, 1.7%) than alendronate-treated subjects (13 in 169 subjects, 7.7%), with most fractures occurring in the first 18 months of treatment. There was no difference in nonvertebral fractures between the groups. Teriparatide-treated subjects had more pre-dose increased serum calcium levels (21% vs 7%). The study discontinuation rate at 36 months was 44%, but the rate was not different between the groups.

This study concluded that subjects with glucocorticoid-induced osteoporosis treated for 36 months with teriparatide had greater increases in BMD and fewer radiographic vertebral fractures than subjects treated with alendronate. While not powered to show prevention of fractures, this study showed a significant difference in a small number of radiographic vertebral fractures between the groups, despite an equally high study discontinuation rate in the two groups. The high discontinuation rate was attributed to the severity of underlying disease and multiple comorbid conditions. This is the first study to compare the effects of an anabolic agent and an anticatabolic agent head-to-head for the treatment of patients with glucocorticoid-induced osteoporosis.

B. L. Clarke, MD

References

1. Saag KG. Glucocorticoid-induced osteoporosis. *Endocrinol Metab Clin North Am.* 2003;32:135-157.

2. Canalis E, Mazzioti G, Giustina A, Bilezikian JP. Glucocorticoid-induced osteoporosis: pathophysiology and therapy. *Osteoporos Int.* 2007;18:1319-1328.
3. Rubin MR, Bilezikian JP. Clinical review 151 – the role of parathyroid hormone in the pathogenesis of glucocorticoid-induced osteoporosis: a re-examination of the evidence. *J Clin Endocrinol Metab.* 2002;87:4033-4041.
4. Kanis JA, Johansson H, Oden A, et al. A meta-analysis of prior corticosteroid use and fracture risk. *J Bone Miner Res.* 2004;19:893-899.
5. Cohen S, Levy RM, Keller M, et al. Risedronate therapy prevents corticosteroid-induced bone loss: a twelve-month, multicenter, randomized, double-blind, placebo-controlled, parallel-group study. *Arthritis Rheum.* 1999;42:2309-2318.
6. Reid DM, Hughes RA, Laan RF, et al. Efficacy and safety of daily risedronate in the treatment of corticosteroid-induced osteoporosis in men and women: a randomized trial. European Corticosteroid-Induced Osteoporosis Treatment Study. *J Bone Miner Res.* 2000;15:1006-1013.
7. Saag KG, Emkey R, Schnitzer TJ, et al. Alendronate for the prevention and treatment of glucocorticoid-induced osteoporosis. Glucocorticoid-Induced Osteoporosis Intervention Study Group. *N Engl J Med.* 1998;339:292-299.
8. Saag KG, Shane E, Boonen S, et al. Teriparatide or alendronate in glucocorticoid-induced osteoporosis. *N Engl J Med.* 2007;357:2028-2039.
9. Dobnig H, Turner RT. Evidence that intermittent treatment with parathyroid hormone increases bone formation in adult rats by activation of bone lining cells. *Endocrinology.* 1995;136:3632-3638.
10. Jilka RL, Weinstein RS, Bellido T, Roberson P, Parfitt AM, Manolagas SC. Increased bone formation by prevention of osteoblast apoptosis with parathyroid hormone. *J Clin Invest.* 1999;104:439-446.

Comparative Effects of Teriparatide and Strontium Ranelate on Bone Biopsies and Biochemical Markers of Bone Turnover in Postmenopausal Women With Osteoporosis

Recker RR, Marin F, Ish-Shalom S, et al (Creighton Univ, Omaha, NE; Lilly Res Centre, UK; Rambam Health Care Campus, Haifa, Israel; et al)
J Bone Miner Res 24:1358-1368, 2009

We assessed the effects on bone remodeling and histomorphometry after daily subcutaneous injections of teriparatide ($n = 39$, 20 μg/d) or oral strontium ranelate (SrR, $n = 40$, 2 g/d) in postmenopausal women with osteoporosis. Evaluable biopsies were obtained from 29 patients in the teriparatide group and 22 in the SrR group after 6 mo of treatment. The mean ± SD mineralization surfaces as a percent of bone surfaces (MS/BS, %) at the trabecular level were 7.73 + 1.48% for teriparatide and 5.25 ± 1.15% for SrR ($p = 0.219$) and at the endocortical level were 17.22 ± 3.06% and 9.70 ± 2.07%, respectively ($p = 0.052$). Cortical porosity was 5.40 ± 0.41% in the teriparatide and 4.14 ± 0.40% in the SrR group ($p = 0.037$). Teriparatide induced significant increases from baseline in bone formation and resorption markers, reaching statistical significance for amino-terminal propeptide of type I collagen (PINP) after 1 mo (+57%, $p \pm 0.001$). SrR induced small, but statistically significant, reductions from baseline in PINP at 3 (−14%, $p = 0.005$) and 6 mo (−19%, $p < 0.001$) and in serum β-C-terminal telopeptide of type I collagen (β-CTX) at 1 and 3 mo (−11%, for both,

$p < 0.05$). There were more patients with adverse events after SrR (70%) than teriparatide (41%) treatment ($p = 0.013$). In conclusion, the changes in biochemical markers of bone formation confirmed bone-forming activity of teriparatide but not of SrR treatment. The effects of SrR on bone remodeling and cell activity were modest, indicating that its effects on fracture reduction may be predominantly mediated through a different mechanism than that observed with anabolic or more potent antiresorptive agents.

▶ Most currently available therapies for osteoporosis, including bisphosphonates, raloxifene, calcitonin, and estrogen, inhibit bone resorption followed by a coupled decrease in bone formation. These changes significantly reduce fracture risk in treated patients, but they do not restore normal bone architecture.[1] Anabolic therapies, such as teriparatide (recombinant human parathyroid hormone 1-34) or parathyroid hormone (PTH) 1-84 directly stimulate bone formation and resorption on trabecular, periosteal, and endosteal surfaces when given in low-dose intermittent regimens.[2,3] These agents appear to increase the size and activity of the osteoblast lineage pool.[4] In vitro and animal studies have shown that strontium ranelate may dissociate the coupled bone resorption/formation process by stimulating bone formation and inhibiting bone resorption.[5-7] The large clinical trials with strontium ranelate showed slightly increased serum bone alkaline phosphatase, a marker of bone formation, and mildly decreased serum β-C-terminal telopeptide of type 1 collagen (β-CTX), a marker of bone resorption, but these changes were not significantly different from baseline.[8,9] Unfortunately, the clinical trials did not include paired iliac crest bone biopsy studies.

This study compared the effects of teriparatide 20 μg by subcutaneous injection each day and strontium ranelate 2 g orally each day for 6 months on bone remodeling and histomorphometry in a small group of postmenopausal women with osteoporosis. The teriparatide group contained 39 subjects and the strontium ranelate group contained 40 subjects, with evaluable biopsies obtained from 29 subjects in the teriparatide group and 22 in the strontium group. The bone marker data showed that teriparatide increased bone formation, but that strontium did not and that the bone remodeling and cell activity effects of strontium were modest. The study concluded that strontium may reduce fractures by mechanisms different from those seen with anabolic and more potent antiresorptive agents.

These findings make it clear that bone-active medications may have different mechanisms of action in rodent models and humans. Strontium ranelate does not appear to be a dual-acting agent that both decreases bone resorption and stimulates bone formation in humans, as initially proposed. Rat studies that showed a dual action of strontium ranelate used doses about 30 times the dose currently approved for use in humans. Future studies with controlled paired-biopsy studies over longer periods of time will be required to more accurately assess the effects of strontium ranelate on bone formation and remodeling.

B. L. Clarke, MD

References

1. Riggs BL, Parfitt AM. Perspective: drugs used to treat osteoporosis: the critical need for a uniform nomenclature based on their action on bone remodeling. *J Bone Miner Res.* 2005;20:177-184.
2. Canalis E, Giustina A, Bilezikian JP. Mechanisms of anabolic therapies for osteoporosis. *New Engl J Med.* 2007;357:905-916.
3. Lindsay R, Zhou H, Cosman F, Nieves J, Dempster DW, Hodsman AB. Effects on a one-month treatment with PTH (1-34) on bone formation on cancellous, endocortical, and periosteal surfaces of the human ilium. *J Bone Miner Res.* 2007;22: 495-502.
4. Goltzman D. Studies on the mechanisms of the skeletal anabolic action of endogenous and exogenous parathyroid hormone. *Arch Biochem Biophys.* 2008;473: 218-224.
5. Canalis E, Hott M, Deloffre P, Tsouderos Y, Marie PJ. The divalent strontium salt S12911 enhances bone cell replication and bone formation in vitro. *Bone.* 1996; 18:517-523.
6. Takahashi N, Sasaki T, Tsuoderos Y, Suda TS. 12911-2 inhibits osteoclastic bone resorption in vitro. *J Bone Miner Res.* 2003;18:1082-1087.
7. Marie PJ, Ammann P, Boivin G, Rey C. Mechanics of action and therapeutic potential of strontium in bone. *Calcif Tiss Int.* 2001;69:121-129.
8. Meunier PJ, Roux C, Seeman E, et al. The effects of strontium ranelate on the risk of vertebral fracture in women with postmenopausal osteoporosis. *New Engl J Med.* 2004;350:459-468.
9. Meunier PJ, Slosman D, Delmas P, et al. Strontium ranelate: dose-dependent effects in established postmenopausal osteoporosis: a 2-year randomized placebo-controlled trial. *J Clin Endocrinol Metab.* 2002;87:2060-2066.

A Randomized Trial of Vertebroplasty for Osteoporotic Spinal Fractures

Kallmes DF, Comstock BA, Heagerty PJ, et al (Mayo Clinic, Rochester, MN; the Univ of Washington, Seattle; et al)
N Engl J Med 361:569-579, 2009

Background.—Vertebroplasty is commonly used to treat painful, osteoporotic vertebral compression fractures.

Methods.—In this multicenter trial, we randomly assigned 131 patients who had one to three painful osteoporotic vertebral compression fractures to undergo either vertebroplasty or a simulated procedure without cement (control group). The primary outcomes were scores on the modified Roland–Morris Disability Questionnaire (RDQ) (on a scale of 0 to 23, with higher scores indicating greater disability) and patients' ratings of average pain intensity during the preceding 24 hours at 1 month (on a scale of 0 to 10, with higher scores indicating more severe pain). Patients were allowed to cross over to the other study group after 1 month.

Results.—All patients underwent the assigned intervention (68 vertebroplasties and 63 simulated procedures). The baseline characteristics were similar in the two groups. At 1 month, there was no significant difference between the vertebroplasty group and the control group in either the RDQ score (difference, 0.7; 95% confidence interval [CI], −1.3 to 2.8; $P = 0.49$) or the pain rating (difference, 0.7; 95% CI, −0.3 to 1.7; $P = 0.19$). Both groups had immediate improvement in disability and pain scores after the intervention. Although the two groups did not differ significantly on any secondary outcome measure at 1 month, there was a trend toward a higher rate of clinically meaningful improvement in pain (a 30% decrease from baseline) in the vertebroplasty group (64% vs. 48%, $P = 0.06$). At 3 months, there was a higher crossover rate in the control group than in the vertebroplasty group (43% vs. 12%, $P<0.001$). There was one serious adverse event in each group.

Conclusions.—Improvements in pain and pain-related disability associated with osteoporotic compression fractures in patients treated with vertebroplasty were similar to the improvements in a control group. (ClinicalTrials.gov number, NCT00068822.)

▶ Osteoporotic patients with vertebral fractures often experience significant pain, occasionally develop disability, and rarely experience death. Pain from vertebral fractures normally resolves gradually over several weeks to several months. Subjects with persistently painful fractures are often treated with percutaneous vertebroplasty in which polymethylmethacrylate (PMMA) is injected into the fractured vertebral body. This treatment has become accepted as an effective method of pain relief in recent years, and guidelines currently recommend vertebroplasty for vertebral fractures not responding to medical treatment.[1] The mechanism of pain relief with vertebroplasty has never been clearly demonstrated, although it is often assumed that stabilization of the fracture is the reason for pain relief. A number of case series and small, unblinded, nonrandomized, controlled studies have suggested that vertebroplasty is effective in relieving pain from vertebral fractures.[2-8]

This randomized controlled study compared the effectiveness of PMMA infusion during vertebroplasty with a simulated procedure without PMMA in 131 subjects with 1 to 3 painful osteoporotic vertebral fractures. Baseline characteristics of the 2 groups were not different, and the Roland-Morris Disability Questionnaire scores and subjects' pain ratings were not different 1 month after intervention, although there was a trend toward clinically meaningful pain improvement in the vertebroplasty group at 1 month. Both groups improved immediately after their intervention. At 3 months, there was a higher crossover rate in the control group than the vertebroplasty group. The authors concluded that improvements in back pain intensity, pain-related disability, and quality of life after vertebral fractures in subjects treated with vertebroplasty were similar to improvements in a control group.

These findings strongly suggest that factors other than PMMA infusion may have accounted for the observed clinical improvement after vertebroplasty. The authors point out that these factors may include effect of local anesthesia, expectations of pain relief, natural history of the fracture, and regression toward the mean. The effect of patient expectations of pain relief on the outcomes of the study are unclear, given that the magnitude of treatment effect in this study was larger than in other similar studies. The authors note that the trend toward clinically meaningful pain relief at 1 month, and the higher crossover rate in the control group at 3 months, could indicate that vertebroplasty was a more effective treatment for a subgroup of patients. This study did not address the effect of kyphoplasty on pain relief due to osteoporotic vertebral fractures.

B. L. Clarke, MD

References

1. McGraw JK, Cardella J, Barr JD, et al. Society of Interventional Radiology quality improvement guidelines for percutaneous vertebroplasty. *J Vasc Inter Radiol.* 2003;14:827-831.
2. Layton KF, Thielen KR, Koch CA, et al. Vertebroplasty, first 1000 levels of a single center: evaluation of the outcomes and complications. *AJNR Am J Neuroradiol.* 2007;28:683-689.
3. Voormolen MH, Mali WP, Lohle PN, et al. Percutaneous vertebroplasty compared with optimal pain medication treatment: short-term clinical outcome of patients with subacute or chronic painful osteoporotic vertebral compression fractures. *AJNR Am J Neuroradiol.* 2007;28:555-560.
4. Alvarez L, Alcaraz M, Perez-Higueras A, et al. Percutaneous vertebroplasty: functional improvement in patients with osteoporotic compression fractures. *Spine.* 2006;31:1113-1118.
5. Diamond TH, Bryant C, Browne L, Clark WA. Clinical outcomes after acute osteoporotic vertebral fractures: a 2-year non-randomised trial comparing percutaneous vertebroplasty with conservative therapy. *Med J Aust.* 2006;184:113-117.
6. Voormolen MH, Lohle PN, Lampmann LE, et al. Prospective clinical follow-up after percutaneous vertebroplasty in patients with painful osteoporotic vertebral compression fractures. *J Vasc Interv Radiol.* 2006;17:1313-1320.
7. Do HM, Kim BS, Marcellus ML, Curtis L, Marks MP. Prospective analysis of clinical outcomes after percutaneous vertebroplasty for painful osteoporotic vertebral body fractures. *AJNR Am J Neuroradiol.* 2005;26:1623-1628.
8. Kobayashi K, Shimoyama K, Nakamura K, Murata K. Percutaneous vertebroplasty immediately relieves pain of osteoporotic vertebral compression fractures and prevents prolonged immobilization of patients. *Eur Radiol.* 2005;15:360-367.

Denosumab in Men Receiving Androgen-Deprivation Therapy for Prostate Cancer

Smith MR, for the Denosumab HALT Prostate Cancer Study Group (Massachusetts General Hosp Cancer Ctr, Boston, MA; et al)

N Engl J Med 361:745-755, 2009

Background.—Androgen-deprivation therapy is well-established for treating prostate cancer but is associated with bone loss and an increased risk of fracture. We investigated the effects of denosumab, a fully human monoclonal antibody against receptor activator of nuclear factor-κB ligand, on bone mineral density and fractures in men receiving androgen-deprivation therapy for nonmetastatic prostate cancer.

Methods.—In this double-blind, multicenter study, we randomly assigned patients to receive denosumab at a dose of 60 mg subcutaneously every 6 months or placebo (734 patients in each group). The primary end point was percent change in bone mineral density at the lumbar spine at 24 months. Key secondary end points included percent change in bone mineral densities at the femoral neck and total hip at 24 months and at all three sites at 36 months, as well as incidence of new vertebral fractures.

Results.—At 24 months, bone mineral density of the lumbar spine had increased by 5.6% in the denosumab group as compared with a loss of 1.0% in the placebo group ($P < 0.001$); significant differences between the two groups were seen at as early as 1 month and sustained through 36 months. Denosumab therapy was also associated with significant increases in bone mineral density at the total hip, femoral neck, and distal third of the radius at all time points. Patients who received denosumab had a decreased incidence of new vertebral fractures at 36 months (1.5%, vs. 3.9% with placebo) (relative risk, 0.38; 95% confidence interval, 0.19 to 0.78; $P = 0.006$). Rates of adverse events were similar between the two groups.

Conclusions.—Denosumab was associated with increased bone mineral density at all sites and a reduction in the incidence of new vertebral fractures among men receiving androgendeprivation therapy for nonmetastatic prostate cancer. (ClinicalTrials.gov number, NCT00089674.)

▶ Denosumab is an emerging treatment for bone disease that is being investigated for treatment of nonmetastatic prostate cancer. This drug is a fully human monoclonal antibody to the receptor activator of nuclear factor-κB ligand (RANKL) that blocks recruitment, activation, and survival of osteoclasts.[1,2] Denosumab primarily prevents bone loss, so it might help prevent bone loss in patients with prostate cancer treated with androgen-deprivation therapy. Androgen-deprivation therapy for prostate cancer causes hypogonadotropic hypogonadism, which is associated with bone loss and fractures.[3-7] This clinical trial randomized 1468 men with nonmetastatic prostate cancer to receive either denosumab 60 mg by subcutaneous injection once every 6 months or placebo for 3 years. Subjects receiving denosumab experienced an increase in lumbar spine bone mineral density (BMD) of 5.6%, whereas subjects on placebo experienced a decrease of 1.0% over 2 years (Fig 2 in the original article). A difference in bone density between the 2 groups was seen as early as 1 month of treatment, and this difference persisted over 36 months. Denosumab was also associated with increased BMD at the total hip, femoral neck, and one-third distal radius across the duration of the study. Subjects receiving denosumab developed a cumulative incidence of new vertebral fractures of 1.5% over 3 years, whereas the placebo group experienced a cumulative incidence of 3.9%, for a reduction in new vertebral fractures of 62%. Adverse events were equally balanced between the denosumab and placebo groups.

This study demonstrates that denosumab is associated with increased BMD at the lumbar spine, hip, and wrist in men receiving androgen-deprivation therapy for prostate cancer. Denosumab also reduces new vertebral fractures in this population. These findings are important because androgen-deprivation therapy used in men with prostate cancer is associated with bone loss and fractures. Denosumab prevents bone loss and vertebral fractures in men with nonmetastatic prostate cancer receiving androgen-deprivation therapy.

B. L. Clarke, MD

References

1. Kearns AE, Khosla S, Kostenuik PJ. Receptor activator of nuclear factor kappaB ligand and osteoprotegerin regulation of bone remodeling in health and disease. *Endocr Rev.* 2008;29:155-192.
2. Hofbauer LC, Schoppet M. Clinical implications of the osteoprotegerin/RANK/RANKL system for bone and vascular diseases. *JAMA.* 2004;292:490-495.
3. Loblaw DA, Virgo KS, Nam R, et al. Initial hormonal management of androgen-sensitive metastatic, recurrent, or progressive prostate cancer: 2006 update of an American Society of Clinical Oncology practice guideline. *J Clin Oncol.* 2007;25:1596-1605.
4. Sharifi N, Gulley JL, Dahut WL. Androgen deprivation therapy for prostate cancer. *JAMA.* 2005;294:238-244.
5. Bolla M, Collette L, Blank L, et al. Long-term results with immediate androgen suppression and external irradiation in patients with locally advanced prostate cancer (an EORTC study): a phase III randomised trial. *Lancet.* 2002;360:103-108.
6. Messing EM, Manola J, Sarosdy M, Wilding G, Crawford ED, Trump D. Immediate hormonal therapy compared with observation after radical prostatectomy and pelvic lymphadenectomy in men with node-positive prostate cancer. *New Engl J Med.* 1999;341:1781-1788.
7. Michaelson MD, Marujo RM, Smith MR. Contribution of androgen deprivation therapy to elevated osteoclast activity in men with metastatic prostate cancer. *Clin Cancer Res..* 2004;10:2705-2708.

Novel Osteoporosis Therapies

Denosumab for Prevention of Fractures in Postmenopausal Women with Osteoporosis

Cummings SR, for the FREEDOM Trial (California Pacific Med Ctr Res Inst and Univ of California, San Francisco; et al)
N Engl J Med 361:756-765, 2009

Background.—Denosumab is a fully human monoclonal antibody to the receptor activator of nuclear factor-κB ligand (RANKL) that blocks its binding to RANK, inhibiting the development and activity of osteoclasts, decreasing bone resorption, and increasing bone density. Given its unique actions, denosumab may be useful in the treatment of osteoporosis.

Methods.—We enrolled 7868 women between the ages of 60 and 90 years who had a bone mineral density T score of less than −2.5 but not less than −4.0 at the lumbar spine or total hip. Subjects were randomly assigned to receive either 60 mg of denosumab or placebo subcutaneously every 6 months for 36 months. The primary end point was new vertebral fracture. Secondary end points included nonvertebral and hip fractures.

Results.—As compared with placebo, denosumab reduced the risk of new radiographic vertebral fracture, with a cumulative incidence of 2.3% in the denosumab group, versus 7.2% in the placebo group (risk ratio, 0.32; 95% confidence interval [CI], 0.26 to 0.41; $P<0.001$) — a relative decrease of 68%. Denosumab reduced the risk of hip fracture, with a cumulative incidence of 0.7% in the denosumab group, versus 1.2% in the placebo group (hazard ratio, 0.60; 95% CI, 0.37 to 0.97;

P = 0.04) — a relative decrease of 40%. Denosumab also reduced the risk of nonvertebral fracture, with a cumulative incidence of 6.5% in the denosumab group, versus 8.0% in the placebo group (hazard ratio, 0.80; 95% CI, 0.67 to 0.95; P = 0.01) — a relative decrease of 20%. There was no increase in the risk of cancer, infection, cardiovascular disease, delayed fracture healing, or hypocalcemia, and there were no cases of osteonecrosis of the jaw and no adverse reactions to the injection of denosumab.

Conclusions.—Denosumab given subcutaneously twice yearly for 36 months was associated with a reduction in the risk of vertebral, nonvertebral, and hip fractures in women with osteoporosis. (ClinicalTrials.gov number, NCT00089791.)

▶ Denosumab is an emerging treatment for postmenopausal osteoporosis. This fully human monoclonal antibody to the receptor activator of nuclear factor-κB ligand (RANKL) blocks recruitment, activation, and survival of osteoclasts.[1,2] The primary effect of denosumab is to prevent bone loss.[3-5] Based on its mechanism of action, this first in class medication may be useful for the treatment of bone diseases, including osteoporosis. Denosumab is currently being investigated for the treatment of postmenopausal osteoporosis, glucocorticoid-induced osteoporosis, and metastatic cancer in the skeleton.

This pivotal phase 3 fracture prevention trial randomized 7868 postmenopausal women with lumbar spine or total hip BMD T-scores between −2.5 and −4.0 to receive either denosumab 60 mg by subcutaneous injection once every 6 months or placebo for 3 years. Subjects receiving denosumab developed a cumulative incidence of new vertebral fractures over 3 years of 2.3%, whereas the placebo group experienced a cumulative incidence of 7.2% for a reduction in new vertebral fractures of 68% (Fig 1 in the original article). Denosumab reduced hip fractures by 40% and nonvertebral fractures by 20%. There was no reported increase in the risk of cancer, infection, cardiovascular disease, delayed fracture healing, or hypocalcemia in subjects receiving denosumab, and no cases of jaw osteonecrosis were seen. No injection reactions were seen with denosumab in this clinical trial.

Denosumab appears to be a very potent antiresorptive drug that effectively prevents vertebral, hip, and nonvertebral fractures in postmenopausal women with osteoporosis. The data available suggest that this drug is well tolerated and not associated with significant risk of adverse effects. The FDA reviewed denosumab for the treatment of postmenopausal osteoporosis in fall 2009, and requested further safety information. A final decision on approval is pending.

B. L. Clarke, MD

References

1. Kearns AE, Khosla S, Kostenuik PJ. Receptor activator of nuclear factor kappaB ligand and osteoprotegerin regulation of bone remodeling in health and disease. *Endocrine Rev.* 2008;29:155-192.
2. Hofbauer LC, Schoppet M. Clinical implications of the osteoprotegerin/RANK/RANKL system for bone and vascular diseases. *JAMA.* 2004;292:490-495.

3. Bone HG, Bolognese MA, Yuen CK, et al. Effects of denosumab on bone mineral density and bone turnover in postmenopausal women. *J Clin Endocrinol Metab*. 2008;93:2149-2157.
4. Brown JP, Prince RL, Deal C, et al. Comparison of the effect of denosumab and alendronate on BMD and biochemical markers of bone turnover in postmenopausal women with low bone mass: a randomized, blinded, phase 3 trial. *J Bone Mineral Res*. 2009;24:153-161.
5. Kendler DL, Roux C, Benhamou CL, et al. Effects of denosumab on bone mineral density and bone turnover in postmenopausal women transitioning from alendronate therapy. *J Bone Miner Res*. 2010;25:72-81.

Randomized Trial of Denosumab in Patients Receiving Adjuvant Aromatase Inhibitors for Nonmetastatic Breast Cancer

Ellis GK, Bone HG, Chlebowski R, et al (Seattle Cancer Care Alliance, WA; Michigan Bone and Mineral Clinic, Detroit; Univ of California at Los Angeles Med Ctr, Torrance; et al)
J Clin Oncol 26:4875-4882, 2008

Purpose.—Adjuvant aromatase inhibitor therapy is well established in postmenopausal women with hormone receptor–positive breast cancer, but such therapy is complicated by accelerated bone loss and increased fracture risk. We investigated the ability of denosumab, a fully human monoclonal antibody against receptor activator of nuclear factor-κB ligand, to protect against aromatase inhibitor–induced bone loss.

Patients and Methods.—Eligible women with hormone receptor–positive nonmetastatic breast cancer treated with adjuvant aromatase inhibitor therapy were stratified by duration of aromatase inhibitor therapy (≤ 6 *v* > 6 months), received supplemental calcium and vitamin D, and were randomly assigned to receive placebo ($n = 125$) or subcutaneous denosumab 60 mg ($n = 127$) every 6 months. At enrollment, all patients were required to have evidence of low bone mass, excluding osteoporosis. The primary end point was percentage change from baseline at month 12 in lumbar spine bone mineral density (BMD).

Results.—At 12 and 24 months, lumbar spine BMD increased by 5.5% and 7.6%, respectively, in the denosumab group versus placebo ($P < .0001$ at both time points). Increases were observed as early as 1 month and were not influenced by duration of aromatase inhibitor therapy. Increases in BMD were also observed at the total hip, total body, femoral neck, and the predominantly cortical one-third radius. Bone turnover markers decreased with denosumab treatment. Overall incidence of treatment-emergent adverse events (AEs) was similar between treatment groups.

Conclusion.—In women with nonmetastatic breast cancer and low bone mass who were receiving adjuvant aromatase inhibitor therapy, twice-yearly administration of denosumab led to significant increases in BMD over 24 months at trabecular and cortical bone, with overall AE rates similar to those of placebo.

▶ Denosumab is being investigated for the treatment of various bone diseases, including hormone receptor-positive nonmetastatic breast cancer in postmenopausal women being treated with adjuvant aromatase inhibitor therapy. Denosumab is a fully human monoclonal antibody to the receptor activator of nuclear factor-κB ligand (RANKL) that blocks recruitment, activation, and survival of osteoclasts.[1,2] Denosumab thereby blocks bone loss, so it might help prevent bone loss or fractures in patients with breast cancer treated with adjuvant aromatase inhibitor therapy. Aromatase inhibitor therapy for breast cancer causes marked suppression of serum estradiol that is associated with bone loss and fractures.[3-7]

This clinical trial randomized 252 women with hormone receptor-positive, nonmetastatic breast cancer being treated with adjuvant aromatase inhibitor therapy to receive either denosumab 60 mg by subcutaneous injection once every 6 months or placebo for 2 years. Subjects were stratified by the duration of aromatase inhibitor therapy (≤6 months vs >6 months). All subjects had low bone density, but not osteoporosis, and received calcium and vitamin D supplements. Subjects receiving denosumab experienced an increase in lumbar spine bone mass density (BMD) of 4.8%, whereas subjects on placebo experienced a decrease of 0.7%, over 12 months (Fig 2 in the original article). By 24 months, the difference between subjects receiving denosumab and placebo was 7.6%. A difference in bone density between the 2 groups was seen as early as 1 month of the treatment, independent of the duration of aromatase inhibitor therapy, and this difference persisted over 24 months. Denosumab was also associated with increased BMD at the total hip, femoral neck, one-third distal radius, and total body across the duration of the study. No vertebral fractures were seen in either group during the study. Nonvertebral and major nonvertebral fractures were not different between the groups. Adverse events were equally balanced between the denosumab and placebo groups.

This study demonstrates that denosumab over 2 years is associated with increased BMD at the lumbar spine, hip, wrist, and total body in women with low bone density who have hormone receptor-positive breast cancer and are receiving adjuvant aromatase inhibitor therapy. This study was not powered to show reduction in vertebral or other fractures in this population. These findings are significant because adjuvant aromatase inhibitor therapy used in women with nonmetastatic breast cancer is associated with bone loss and fractures. Denosumab prevents bone loss in women with nonmetastatic breast cancer receiving adjuvant aromatase inhibitor therapy.

B. L. Clarke, MD

References

1. Kearns AE, Khosla S, Kostenuik PJ. Receptor activator of nuclear factor kappaB ligand and osteoprotegerin regulation of bone remodeling in health and disease. *Endocr Rev.* 2008;29:155-192.
2. Hofbauer LC, Schoppet M. Clinical implications of the osteoprotegerin/RANK/RANKL system for bone and vascular diseases. *JAMA.* 2004;292:490-495.

3. Eastell R, Hannon R. Long-term effects of aromatase inhibitors on bone. *J Steroid Biochem Mol Biol.* 2005;95:151-154.
4. Baum M, Buzdar A, Cuzick J, et al. ATAC (Arimidex, Tamoxifen Alone or in Combination) Trialists' Group. Anastrozole alone or in combination with tamoxifen versus tamoxifen alone for adjuvant treatment of postmenopausal women with early-stage breast cancer: results of the ATAC (Arimidex, Tamoxifen, Alone or in Combination) trial efficacy and safety update analyses. *Cancer.* 2003;98:1802-1810.
5. Coombes RC, Hall E, Gibson LJ, et al. Intergroup Exemestane Study. A randomized trial of exemestane after two to three years of tamoxifen therapy in postmenopausal women with primary breast cancer. *New Engl J Med.* 2004;350: 1081-1092.
6. Goss PE, Ingle JN, Martino S, et al. A randomized trial of letrozole in postmenopausal women after five years of tamoxifen therapy for early-stage breast cancer. *New Engl J Med.* 2003;349:1793-1802.
7. Lonning PE, Geisler J, Krag LE, et al. Effects of exemestane administered for 2 years versus placebo on bone mineral density, bone biomarkers, and plasma lipids in patients with surgically resected early breast cancer. *J Clin Oncol.* 2005;23: 5126-5137.

Lasofoxifene in Postmenopausal Women with Osteoporosis

Cummings SR, Ensrud K, Delmas PD, et al (Univ of California, San Francisco; Univ of Minnesota and Veterans Affairs Med Ctr, Minneapolis; Université de Lyon and INSERM Res Unit 831, Lyon, France; et al)
N Engl J Med 362:686-696, 2010

Background.—The effects of lasofoxifene on the risk of fractures, breast cancer, and cardiovascular disease are uncertain.

Methods.—In this randomized trial, we assigned 8556 women who were between the ages of 59 and 80 years and had a bone mineral density T score of −2.5 or less at the femoral neck or spine to receive once-daily lasofoxifene (at a dose of either 0.25 mg or 0.5 mg) or placebo for 5 years. Primary end points were vertebral fractures, estrogen receptor (ER)–positive breast cancer, and nonvertebral fractures; secondary end points included major coronary heart disease events and stroke.

Results.—Lasofoxifene at a dose of 0.5 mg per day, as compared with placebo, was associated with reduced risks of vertebral fracture (13.1 cases vs. 22.4 cases per 1000 person-years; hazard ratio, 0.58; 95% confidence interval [CI], 0.47 to 0.70), nonvertebral fracture (18.7 vs. 24.5 cases per 1000 person-years; hazard ratio, 0.76; 95% CI, 0.64 to 0.91), ER-positive breast cancer (0.3 vs. 1.7 cases per 1000 person-years; hazard ratio, 0.19; 95% CI, 0.07 to 0.56), coronary heart disease events (5.1 vs. 7.5 cases per 1000 person-years; hazard ratio, 0.68; 95% CI, 0.50 to 0.93), and stroke (2.5 vs. 3.9 cases per 1000 person-years; hazard ratio, 0.64; 95% CI, 0.41 to 0.99). Lasofoxifene at a dose of 0.25 mg per day, as compared with placebo, was associated with reduced risks of vertebral fracture (16.0 vs. 22.4 cases per 1000 person-years; hazard ratio, 0.69; 95% CI, 0.57 to 0.83) and stroke (2.4 vs. 3.9 cases per 1000 person-years; hazard ratio, 0.61; 95% CI, 0.39 to 0.96) Both the lower and higher

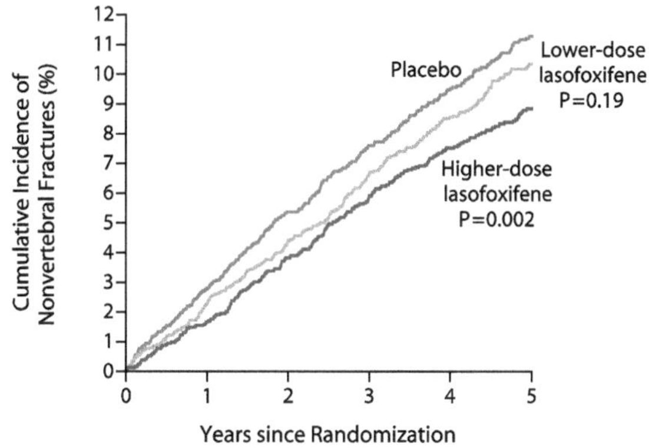

No. at Risk						
Lasofoxifene, 0.25 mg	2852	2745	2639	2520	2139	2002
Lasofoxifene, 0.5 mg	2852	2763	2647	2531	2150	2053
Placebo	2852	2731	2598	2479	2093	1979

FIGURE 1.—Cumulative incidence of nonvertebral fractures, according to study group. (Reprinted from Cummings SR, Ensrud K, Delmas PD, et al. Lasofoxifene in postmenopausal women with osteoporosis. *N Engl J Med.* 2010;362:686-696. Copyright 2010 Massachusetts Medical Society. All rights reserved.)

doses, as compared with placebo, were associated with an increase in venous thromboembolic events (3.8 and 2.9 cases vs. 1.4 cases per 1000 person-years; hazard ratios, 2.67 [95% CI, 1.55 to 4.58] and 2.06 [95% CI, 1.17 to 3.60], respectively). Endometrial cancer occurred in three women in the placebo group, two women in the lower-dose lasofoxifene group, and two women in the higher-dose lasofoxifene group. Rates of death per 1000 person-years were 5.1 in the placebo group, 7.0 in the lower-dose lasofoxifene group, and 5.7 in the higher-dose lasofoxifene group.

Conclusions.—In postmenopausal women with osteoporosis, lasofoxifene at a dose of 0.5 mg per day was associated with reduced risks of nonvertebral and vertebral fractures, ER-positive breast cancer, coronary heart disease, and stroke but an increased risk of venous thromboembolic events. (ClinicalTrials.gov number, NCT00141323.) (Fig 1).

▶ Early postmenopausal bone loss is primarily due to estrogen deficiency. Postmenopausal estrogen therapy helps prevent bone loss, lowers cholesterol, does not prevent cardiovascular disease, and increases risk of estrogen receptor (ER)-positive breast cancer, uterine cancer, stroke, and venous thromboembolic disease.[1] Selective ER modulators (SERMs) were developed to bind selectively to ER-α and ER-β, in an effort to produce tissue-selective effects that would increase the benefits, and reduce the risks, of native 17β-estradiol.[2]

Lasofoxifene is a nonsteroidal SERM that has been shown to decrease bone resorption, reduce bone loss, and lower low-density lipoprotein (LDL)-cholesterol in postmenopausal women.[3] The Postmenopausal Evaluation and Risk-Reduction with Lasofoxifene (PEARL) trial was conducted to determine if lasofoxifene would reduce fractures, ER-positive breast cancer, and cardiovascular disease in postmenopausal women with osteoporosis. This trial randomized 8556 women aged 59 to 80 years with bone mineral density (BMD) T-scores less than −2.5 at the femoral neck or lumbar spine to receive lasofoxifene 0.25 or 0.50 mg, or placebo, each day for 5 years. Higher-dose lasofoxifene reduced vertebral fractures by 42%, nonvertebral fractures by 24%, ER-positive breast cancer by 91%, coronary heart disease events by 32%, and stroke by 36% compared with placebo. Neither dose reduced risk of hip fracture. Lower-dose lasofoxifene reduced vertebral fractures by 31% and stroke by 39% compared with placebo. Lasofoxifene increased risk of venous thromboembolic events, similar to estrogen and other SERMs. Very few cases of endometrial cancer or hyperplasia were seen, and rates of death were not increased.

This study demonstrated that higher-dose lasofoxifene reduced risks of vertebral and nonvertebral fractures, ER-positive breast cancer, coronary heart disease, and stroke, but increased risk of venous thromboembolic events in postmenopausal women with osteoporosis. These findings illustrate that SERMs have multiple effects not limited to the skeleton, unlike other available antiresorptive agents. The decision to use a SERM or another antiresorptive agent should be based on the fracture reduction effects of the SERM, as well as consideration of the other benefits and risks of the SERM. The currently approved SERM raloxifene does not prevent nonvertebral fractures,[4] and neither raloxifene nor lasofoxifene prevent hip fractures. Future research may identify additional SERMs with more potent skeletal effects.

B. L. Clarke, MD

References

1. Rossouw JE, Anderson GL, Prentice RL, et al. Risks and benefits of estrogen plus progestin in healthy postmenopausal women: principal results from the Women's Health Initiative randomized controlled trial. *JAMA*. 2002;288:321-333.
2. Gennari L, Merlotti D, Valleggi F, Martini G, Nuti R. Selective estrogen receptor modulators for postmenopausal osteoporosis: current state of development. *Drugs Aging*. 2007;24:361-379.
3. McClung MR, Siris E, Cummings S, et al. Prevention of bone loss in postmenopausal women treated with lasofoxifene compared with raloxifene. *Menopause*. 2006;13:377-386.
4. Ettinger B, Black DM, Mitlak BH, et al. Reduction of vertebral fracture risk in postmenopausal women with osteoporosis treated with raloxifene: results from a 3-year randomized clinical trial. *JAMA*. 1999;282:637-645.

Osteoporosis in Other Settings

Bone Marrow Changes in Adolescent Girls With Anorexia Nervosa

Ecklund K, Vajapeyam S, Feldman HA, et al (Children's Hosp Boston, MA; et al)
J Bone Miner Res 25:298-304, 2009

Early osteoporosis is common among adolescent girls with anorexia nervosa (AN) and may result from premature conversion of red (RM) to yellow bone marrow. We performed right knee magnetic resonance imaging (MRI) on a 1.0 T extremity scanner in 20 patients and 20 healthy controls, aged 16.2 ± 1.6 years (mean ± SD). Coronal T_1-weighted (T_1W) images and T_1 maps were generated from T_1 relaxometry images. Blinded radiologists visually assessed RM in the distal femoral and proximal tibial metaphyses in T_1W images using a scale of signal intensity from 0 (homogeneous hyperintensity, no RM) to 4 (all dark, complete RM). Subjects with AN exhibited nearly twofold lower metaphyseal RM scores in both the femur (0.64 versus 1.22, $p = .03$) and tibia (0.54 versus 0.96, $p = .08$). In relaxometric measurements of four selected regions (femur and tibia amd epiphysis and metaphysis), subjects with AN showed higher mean epiphyseal but lower metaphyseal T_1. The net AN-control difference between epiphysis and metaphysis was 70 ms in the femur (+31 versus −35 ms, $p = .02$) and of smaller magnitude in the tibia. In relaxometry data from the full width of the femur adjacent to the growth plate, AN subjects showed mean T_1 consistently lower than in controls by 30 to 50 ms in virtually every part of the sampling region. These findings suggest that adolescents with AN exhibit premature conversion of hematopoietic to fat cells in the marrow of the peripheral skeleton potentially owing to adipocyte over osteoblast differentiation in the mesenchymal stem cell pool.

▶ Adolescent girls with anorexia nervosa have increased risk of low bone mineral density (BMD), early onset of osteoporosis, and increased fracture risk compared with healthy adolescent girls.[1-4] The pathophysiology of low BMD and fractures in anorexia nervosa is complex and involves alterations in serum estrogen, leptin, insulin-like growth factor-1 (IGF-1), growth hormone, and cortisol levels associated with low body weight. These hormonal changes are associated with abnormalities in osteoblast and osteoclast progenitors in the bone marrow.[5] Bone marrow mesenchymal stem cells appear to preferentially differentiate into adipocytes, rather than osteoblasts, leading to increased bone marrow fat and premature conversion to yellow marrow.

Previous studies of bone marrow in adolescents with anorexia nervosa have shown variable results. Increased bone marrow adipocytes have been associated with increased bone loss and severe weight loss.[6] MRI studies have shown a correlation between anemia and leukopenia and decreased total body fat mass.[7] MRI, CT, and bone marrow biopsy studies have shown red marrow cell hypoplasia, reduced cellularity, and increased yellow marrow in the lumbar vertebrae, pelvis, and femoral marrow spaces,[8] similar to what is seen in older adults with osteoporosis. Other studies have shown increased extracellular hyaluronic acid in marrow spaces, reduced red and yellow marrow, and increased free water content, possibly as a physiological response to reduced body weight.[9] Adolescent girls with anorexia nervosa may fail to develop their predicted peak bone mass because of alterations in their bone marrow composition and inhibition of osteoblast-mediated bone formation.

This study evaluated right knee MRI using a 1.0 T extremity scanner in 20 adolescent female subjects with anorexia nervosa and 20 healthy controls. Red marrow content in the distal femoral and proximal tibial metaphyses was assessed visually by radiologists blinded to subject disease status. The study showed that adolescents with anorexia nervosa have increased marrow fat in the peripheral skeleton, suggesting that mesenchymal stem cells preferentially differentiate into adipocytes rather than osteoblasts in this disorder.

These findings suggest a pathophysiological link between low bone density, osteoporosis, and increased fracture risk in adolescent girls with anorexia nervosa and bone marrow mesenchymal stem cell differentiation. Young women with anorexia nervosa appear to undergo premature conversion of red marrow to yellow marrow at an age when they should have a more heterogeneous marrow cellularity to support bone formation. These findings persisted even after adjustment for duration of amenorrhea and anorexia nervosa. This study suggests that premature accumulation of bone marrow fat may contribute to the skeletal pathophysiology seen in anorexia nervosa.

B. L. Clarke, MD

References

1. Misra M. Long-term skeletal effects of eating disorders with onset during adolescence. *Ann NY Acad Sci.* 2008;1135:212-218.
2. Bachrach LK, Guido D, Katzman D, Litt IF, Marcus R. Decreased bone density in adolescent girls with anorexia nervosa. *Pediatrics.* 1990;86:440-447.
3. Rigotti NA, Neer RM, Skates SJ, Herzog DB, Nussbaum SR. The clinical course of osteoporosis in anorexia nervosa. *JAMA.* 1991;265:1133-1138.
4. Gordon CM, Goodman E, Emans SJ, et al. Physiologic regulators of bone turnover in young women with anorexia nervosa. *J Pediatr.* 2002;141:64-70.
5. Di Iorgi N, Rosol M, Mittelman SD, Gilsanz V. Reciprocal relation between marrow adiposity and the amount of bone in the axial and appendicular skeleton of young adults. *J Clin Endocrinol Metab.* 2008;93:2281-2286.
6. Abella E, Feliu E, Granada I, et al. Bone marrow changes in anorexia nervosa are correlated with the amount of weight loss and not with other clinical findings. *Am J Clin Pathol.* 2002;118:582-588.
7. Geiser F, Murtz P, Lutterbey G, et al. Magnetic resonance spectroscopic and relaxometric determination of bone marrow changes in anorexia nervosa. *Psychosom Med.* 2001;63:631-637.
8. Vande Berg BC, Malghem J, Lecouvet FE, Lambert M, Maldague BE. Distribution of serous like bone marrow changes in the lower limbs of patients with anorexia nervosa: predominant involvement of the distal extremities. *Am J Radiol.* 1996; 166:621-625.
9. Vande Berg BC, Malghem J, Devuyst O, Maldague BE, Lambert MJ. Anorexia nervosa: correlation between MR appearance of bone marrow and severity of disease. *Radiology.* 1994;193:859-864.

Serum Dickkopf-1 is increased and correlates with reduced bone mineral density in patients with thalassemia-induced osteoporosis. Reduction post-zoledronic acid administration

Voskaridou E, Christoulas D, Xirakia C, et al (Laikon General Hosp, Athens; 251 General Air Force Hosp, Athens; et al)

Haematologica 94:725-728, 2009

Dickkopf-1 is an inhibitor of *Wnt* signaling, which is crucial for osteoblast differentiation. We evaluated serum levels of Dickkopf-1 in 66 patients with thalassemia-induced osteoporosis who received therapy with zoledronic acid in a placebo-controlled, randomized trial. At baseline, thalassemia patients had increased serum levels of Dickkopf-1 that correlated with reduced bone mineral density of the lumbar spine and the distal radius. High Dickkopf-1 also correlated with increased bone resorption and reduced bone formation markers. Zoledronic acid produced a reduction in serum Dickkopf-1, which was associated with bone mineral density increase after 12 months of therapy. On the contrary, placebo group showed a borderline increase of Dickkopf-1, which was higher in patients who showed deterioration in pain scores. These results suggest that Dickkopf-1 is implicated in the pathogenesis of osteoporosis in thalassemia and reveal Dickkopf-1 as a possible target for the development of novel agents for the management of thalassemia-induced osteoporosis.

▶ Dickkopf-1 (Dkk-1) is a soluble inhibitor of Wingless-type (Wnt)/canonical β-catenin signaling that stimulates osteoblast differentiation and function.[1] As a result of inhibition of Wnt/canonical β-catenin signaling, Dkk-1 inhibits new bone formation.[2] Dkk-1 overexpression in osteoblasts causes osteopenia and inhibits fracture repair.[3] Dkk-1 activation in osteoblasts is involved in development of glucocorticoid-induced osteoporosis and postmenopausal estrogen deficiency-related osteoporosis.[4] Dkk-1 has recently been associated with pathogenesis of cancer-related bone disease with Dkk-1 levels increased in patients with multiple myeloma[5] and breast cancer with bone metastasis.[6] Whether Dkk-1 might also be involved in the pathogenesis of osteoporosis associated with benign disorders is not clear.

Osteoporosis associated with thalassemia is attributed to bone marrow expansion, endocrine dysfunction, and iron overload.[7] In thalassemia, osteoclast activity and bone resorption are increased,[8] resulting in treatment with bisphosphonate therapy. However, osteoblast function is decreased in thalassemia, but the mechanism of decreased osteoblast function has not been established.

The authors evaluated serum levels of Dkk-1 in 66 patients (22 males and 44 females; median age 42 years) with thalassemia being treated as part of a randomized, placebo-controlled, phase II clinical trial with zoledronic acid for osteoporosis. Subjects were treated with zoledronic acid 4 mg intravenously over 15 minutes once every 3 or 6 months or placebo at the same intervals over 12 months. Baseline serum Dkk-1 levels in untreated subjects were increased compared with healthy controls (39.6 ± 16.6 vs 27.4 ± 9.7 pmol/L, $P < .0001$), and these levels correlated with lumbar spine and distal radius bone mineral density (BMD), increased bone resorption markers C-telopeptide of type-I collagen (CTX)-telopeptide and tartrate-resistant acid phosphatase isoform-5b (TRACP-5b), and decreased bone formation markers bone-specific alkaline phosphatase, osteocalcin, and C-terminal propeptide of type I collagen. Zoledronic acid treatment reduced serum Dkk-1 levels from 39.6 ± 16.6 pmol/L pretreatment to 28.9 ± 16.3 pmol/L after 12 months, $P = .004$, and this decrease was correlated with increased BMD. Dkk-1 levels were borderline-increased in placebo-treated subjects at 12 months, with higher levels in those with worsening pain scores. The authors concluded that Dkk-1 plays a role in the causation of osteoporosis associated with thalassemia.

These findings suggest that Dkk-1 and the Wnt signaling system play crucial roles in the pathophysiology of bone loss associated with disorders other than postmenopausal osteoporosis. The role of increased Dkk-1 levels in preservation of skeletal lytic lesions in multiple myeloma and metastatic breast cancer is well established. Lack of appropriate new bone formation due to increased Dkk-1 levels may be a common theme, even in disorders thought to be primarily due to increased bone resorption.

B. L. Clarke, MD

References

1. Glinka A, Wu W, Delius H, Monaghan AP, Blumenstock C, Niehrs C. Dickkopf-1 is a member of a new family of secreted proteins and functions in head induction. *Nature.* 1998;391:357-362.
2. MacDonald BT, Joiner DM, Oyserman SM, et al. Bone mass is inversely proportional to Dkk1 levels in mice. *Bone.* 2007;41:331-339.
3. Pinzone JJ, Hall BM, Thudi NK, et al. The role of Dickkopf-1 in bone development, homeostasis, and disease. *Blood.* 2009;113:517-525.
4. Wang FS, Ko JY, Lin CL, Wu HL, Ke HJ, Tai PJ. Knocking down dickkopf-1 alleviates estrogen deficiency induction of bone loss. A histomorphological study in ovariectomized rats. *Bone.* 2007;40:485-492.
5. Politou M, Heath DJ, Rahemtulla A, et al. Serum concentrations of Dickkopf-1 protein are increased in patients with multiple myeloma and reduced after autologous stem cell transplantation. *Int J Cancer.* 2006;119:1728-1731.
6. Voorzanger-Rousselot N, Goehrig D, Journe F, et al. Increased Dickkopf-1 expression in breast cancer bone metastases. *Br J Cancer.* 2007;97:964-970.
7. Voskaridou E, Terpos E. New insights into the pathophysiology and management of osteoporosis in patients with β thalassemia. *Br J Haematol.* 2004;127:127-139.
8. Voskaridou E, Kyrtsonis MC, Terpos E, et al. Bone resorption is increased in young adults with thalassemia major. *Br J Haematol.* 2001;112:36-41.

Mineral and Vitamin D Metabolism

Bone Mineralization Defects and Vitamin D Deficiency: Histomorphometric Analysis of Iliac Crest Bone Biopsies and Circulating 25-Hydroxyvitamin D in 675 Patients

Priemel M, von Domarus C, Klatte TO, et al (Univ Med Ctr Hamburg-Eppendorf, Germany)

J Bone Miner Res 25:305-312, 2010

Parathyroid hormone (PTH) is only one measurable index of skeletal health, and we reasoned that a histomorphometric analysis of iliac crest biopsies would be another and even more direct approach to assess bone health and address the required minimum 25-Hydroxyvitamin D [25(OH)D] level. A cohort from the northern European population with its known high prevalence of vitamin D deficiency therefore would be ideal to answer the latter question. We examined 675 iliac crest biopsies from male and female individuals, excluding all patients who showed any signs of secondary bone diseases at autopsy. Structural histomorphometric parameters, including osteoid indices, were quantified using the Osteomeasure System according to ASBMR standards, and serum 25(OH)D levels were measured for all patients. Statistical analysis was performed by Student's *t* test. The histologic results demonstrate an unexpected high prevalence of mineralization defects, that is, a pathologic increase in osteoid. Indeed, 36.15% of the analyzed patients presented with an osteoid surface per bone surface (OS/BS) of more than 20%. Based on the most conservative threshold that defines osteomalacia at the histomorphometric level with a pathologic increase in osteoid volume per bone volume (OV/BV) greater than 2% manifest mineralization defects were present in 25.63% of the patients. The latter were found independent of bone volume per trabecular volume (BV/TV) throughout all ages and affected both sexes equally. While we could not establish a minimum 25(OH)D level that was inevitably associated with mineralization defects, we did not find pathologic accumulation of osteoid in any patient with circulating 25(OH)D above 75 nmol/L. Our data demonstrate that pathologic mineralization defects of bone occur in patients with a serum 25(OH)D below 75 nmol/L and strongly argue that in conjunction with a sufficient calcium intake, the dose of vitamin D supplementation should ensure that circulating levels of 25(OH)D reach this minimum threshold (75 nmol/L or 30 ng/mL) to maintain skeletal health.

▶ Vitamin D and calcium are both important for maintenance of normal skeletal health. However, debate persists regarding the optimal amounts of vitamin D and calcium that older men and women require to protect their skeletal health.[1] It is widely agreed that vitamin D and calcium supplementation should be the first consideration in treatment regimens for osteoporosis.[2] Vitamin D and calcium supplementation helps offset low calcium intake or absorption that otherwise requires the skeleton to give up skeletal mineral to keep serum calcium levels in the normal range. Vitamin D and calcium together reduce increased skeletal bone turnover that results in increased bone fragility,[3] reduce fracture rates,[4] and improve neuromuscular function leading to decreased falls.[5]

It is generally agreed that serum 25-hydroxyvitamin D is the best measure of vitamin D status, but there is not yet a general consensus regarding the optimal vitamin D level for skeletal health. Recent studies have defined the optimal circulating serum 25-hydroxyvitamin D level to be the level required to maximally suppress parathyroid hormone secretion.[1] Multiple studies have shown that this threshold in adult humans is around a mean of 30 ng/mL, with a published range from 12 to 40 ng/mL.[6] Other indices of skeletal health could also be considered in helping to define the optimal serum 25-hydroxyvitamin D level, among them iliac crest bone histomorphometric mineralization.

The authors performed unlabeled iliac crest bone biopsies in 675 deceased male and female subjects at autopsy in one northern German city, excluding any subjects with obvious evidence of bone disease, and determined serum 25-hydroxyvitamin D levels in blood taken at the time of autopsy. Bone histomorphometry showed abnormally increased osteoid in 36.2% of subjects, with osteoid surface/bone surface greater than 20%. Osteoid volume/bone volume greater than 2% was found in 25.6% of subjects, regardless of age and sex. Pathological accumulation of osteoid or defective osteoid mineralization was not seen with serum 25-hydroxyvitamin D levels less than 30 ng/mL, although a lower threshold for serum 25-hydroxyvitamin D that was always associated with mineralization defects was not able to be determined.

This study concluded that serum 25-hydroxyvitamn levels above 30 ng/mL were not associated with mineralization abnormalities on iliac crest bone biopsies but did not determine a lower threshold at which vitamin D prevented osteomalacia in all subjects. These findings suggest that the optimal serum 25-hydroxyvitamin D level required to prevent mineralization defects may be somewhat variable but that all subjects did well with serum 25-hydroxyvitamin D levels above 30 ng/mL. Unfortunately, serum parathyroid hormone levels were not measured on the same blood samples to see whether they also correlated with the bone histomorphometric findings.

B. L. Clarke, MD

References

1. Dawson-Hughes B, Heaney RP, Holick MF, Lips P, Meunier PJ, Vieth R. Estimates of optimal vitamin D status. *Osteoporos Int.* 2005;16:713-716.
2. Rizzoli R, Boonen S, Brandi ML, Burlet N, Delmas P, Reginster JY. The role of calcium and vitamin D in the management of osteoporosis. *Bone.* 2008;42: 246-249.
3. Dawson-Hughes B, Harris SS, Krall EA, Dallal GE. Effect of calcium and vitamin D supplementation on bone density in men and women 65 years or age or older. *N Engl J Med.* 1997;337:670-676.
4. Trivedi DP, Doll R, Khaw KT. Effect of four monthly oral vitamin D3 (cholecalciferol) supplementation on fractures and mortality in men and women living in the community: randomized, double-blind, controlled trial. *BMJ.* 2003;326:469.
5. Bischoff-Ferrari HA, Dawson-Hughes B, Willett WC, et al. Effect of vitamin D on falls: a meta-analysis. *JAMA.* 2004;291:1999-2006.

6. Chapuy MC, Pamphile R, Paris E, et al. Combined calcium and vitamin D3 supplementation in elderly women: confirmation of reversal of secondary hyperparathyroidism and hip fracture risk: the Decalyos II study. *Osteoporos Int.* 2002;13:257-264.

Circulating Fibroblast Growth Factor 23 in Patients with End-Stage Renal Disease Treated by Peritoneal Dialysis is Intact and Biologically Active

Shimada T, Urakawa I, Isakova T, et al (Massachusetts General Hosp and Harvard Med School, Boston, MA; Kyowa Hakko Kirin Co., Ltd., Gunma, Japan; et al)

J Clin Endocrinol Metab 95:578-585, 2010

Context.—Fibroblast growth factor 23 (FGF23) regulates phosphorus homeostasis and vitamin D metabolism. Circulating FGF23 levels are elevated in inherited and acquired hypophosphatemic disorders that can cause rickets or osteomalacia. Particularly increased concentrations of FGF23 are observed in patients with chronic kidney disease (CKD), in which increased FGF23 is associated with more rapid disease progression, improved bone mineralization, the development of left ventricular hypertrophy, and increased mortality.

Objective.—Our objective was to determine whether the markedly elevated levels of immunoreactive FGF23 in CKD represent accumulation of intact, biologically active hormone, C-terminal cleavage fragments, or both.

Design.—Biologically active FGF23 in plasma from CKD patients treated by peritoneal dialysis was quantified using a cell-based Egr-1 reporter assay; bioactive FGF23 levels were compared with those measured with immunometric FGF23 assays detecting either intact hormone alone or intact hormone and C-terminal fragments.

Setting and Patients.—Adult and pediatric patients with end-stage renal disease treated with peritoneal dialysis participated in the study at a tertiary referral center.

Results.—Serially diluted patient samples revealed levels of bioactive FGF23 that ran in parallel to CHO cell-derived recombinant human FGF23. FGF23 bioactivity was inhibited by an anti-FGF23 antibody. Levels of bioactive and immunoreactive FGF23 were tightly correlated, and Western blot analysis of FGF23 immunoprecipitated with anti-FGF23 antibodies from plasma of dialysis patients revealed only a single prominent protein band, which was indistinguishable from recombinant intact FGF23, without clear evidence for FGF23 fragments.

Conclusions.—Our results provide strong evidence for the conclusion that virtually all circulating FGF23 in dialysis patients is intact and biologically active.

▶ Fibroblast growth factor-23 (FGF-23) is a hormone secreted by osteoblasts and osteocytes in bone. Serum FGF-23 regulates phosphorus metabolism by altering the expression of NPT2a and NPT2c, the sodium-dependent phosphate transporters in the proximal renal tubule. Increased serum FGF-23 levels increase the expression of these two transporters, thereby increasing urinary phosphorus excretion, which results in lower serum phosphorus levels. FGF-23 is also the most important negative regulator of renal 1α-hydroxylase expression, which prevents inappropriate increases in serum 1,25-dihydroxyvitamin D.[1]

Currently available immunoassays for serum FGF-23 detect this protein in serum or plasma. Increased levels of serum FGF-23, increased urinary phosphorus excretion, and inappropriately low serum,[1] 25-dihydroxyvitamin D levels are the hallmark of tumor-induced osteomalacia,[2] X-linked hypophosphatemia,[3] autosomal recessive hypophosphatemia,[4] and McCune-Albright syndrome.[5]

Increased serum FGF-23 is also characteristic of chronic kidney disease (CKD).[6] Serum FGF-23 levels increase in early-stage CKD, and progressively increase as renal function decreases further. Patients receiving renal replacement therapy with hemodialysis have serum FGF-23 levels that are 100 to 10 000 fold higher than the normal range for healthy subjects. It is unclear whether the currently available immunoassays detect whole-molecule FGF-23, C-terminal cleavage fragments of FGF-23, or both. This is important because several observational studies have shown correlation between increased serum FGF-23 and improved bone mineralization, more rapid progression of CKD, left ventricular hypertrophy, and mortality.

This study correlated biological activity of serum FGF-23 from adult and pediatric patients with CKD who were receiving peritoneal dialysis with serum immunoreactive FGF-23 levels. FGF-23 biological activity assessed by a cell-based early growth response-1 (Egr-1) reporter assay was tightly correlated with serum FGF-23 immunoreactivity, as measured by immunoassays measuring whole-molecule FGF-23 alone, or intact hormone and C-terminal fragments. Western blot analysis of FGF-23 immunoprecipitated by anti-FGF-23 antibodies from plasma showed only a single protein band. This protein band was not distinguishable from recombinant intact FGF-23, and was not clearly associated with FGF-23 fragments. These findings strongly suggest that CKD patients have increased serum FGF-23 that is predominantly in the intact form and biologically active.

This study suggests that C-terminal FGF-23 fragments do not accumulate in patients with CKD, unlike the situation with parathyroid hormone. The currently available FGF-23 assays only detect C-terminal fragments, so it is possible that N-terminal fragments may accumulate. However, the tight correlation between bioactivity and immunoreactivity in this study argues that this is unlikely. These findings are similar to studies of serum FGF-23 in patients with X-linked hypophosphatemia, autosomal recessive hypophosphatemia, and tumor-induced osteomalacia, in which FGF-23 predominantly circulates in the intact form. The only diseases currently known where FGF-23 circulates predominantly as fragments are rare genetic forms of tumoral calcinosis in which intact FGF-23 levels have been shown to be very low or undetectable.

B. L. Clarke, MD

References

1. Shimada T, Hasegawa H, Yamazaki Y, et al. FGF-23 in a potent regulator of vitamin D metabolism and phosphate homeostasis. *J Bone Miner Res.* 2004;19: 429-435.
2. Shimada T, Mizutani S, Muto T, et al. Cloning and characterization of FGF23 as a causative factor of tumor-induced osteomalacia. *Proc Natl Acad Sci USA.* 2001; 98:6500-6505.
3. Jonsson KB, Zahradnik R, Larsson T, et al. Fibroblast growth factor 23 in oncogenic osteomalacia and X-linked hypophosphatemia. *New Engl J Med.* 2003;348: 1656-1663.
4. Feng JQ, Ward LM, Liu S, et al. Loss of DMP1 causes rickets and osteomalacia and identifies a role for osteocytes in mineral metabolism. *Nat Genet.* 2006;38: 1310-1315.
5. Yamamoto T, Imanishi Y, Kinoshita E, et al. The role of fibroblast growth factor 23 for hypophosphatemia and abnormal regulation of vitamin D metabolism in patients with McCune-Albright syndrome. *J Bone Miner Res.* 2005;23:231-237.
6. Gutierrez O, Isakova T, Rhee E, et al. Fibroblast growth factor-23 mitigates hyperphosphatemia but accentuates calcitriol deficiency in chronic kidney disease. *J Am Soc Nephrol.* 2005;16:2205-2215.

Metabolic Bone Disease

Cinacalcet Treatment of Primary Hyperparathyroidism: Biochemical and Bone Densitometric Outcomes in a Five-Year Study

Peacock M, Bolognese MA, Borofsky M, et al (Indiana Univ School of Medicine, Indianapolis; Bethesda Health Res, MD; Clinical Res Ctr of Reading, West Reading, PA; et al)

J Clin Endocrinol Metab 94:4860-4867, 2009

Context.—Primary hyperparathyroidism (PHPT) is characterized by chronically elevated serum calcium and inappropriately normal or increased PTH.

Objective.—Our objective was to evaluate long-term tolerability, safety, and efficacy of cinacalcet in PHPT patients.

Design and Setting.—A 4.5-yr open-label extension study was conducted at 14 study centers in the United States.

Patients or Other Participants.—Forty-five subjects with PHPT from a double-blind, placebo-controlled, 1-yr trial were continued into this study.

Interventions.—After the parent study, all subjects were treated with 30 mg cinacalcet twice daily, increasing to 50 mg twice daily during the 12-wk titration if serum calcium levels were 10.3 mg/dl or higher and then maintained on cinacalcet for up to 4.5 yr.

Main Outcome Measures.—Assessments included serum calcium, PTH, phosphate and alkaline phosphatase, and areal bone mineral density (aBMD). Vital signs, safety chemistries and hematology, and adverse events were monitored throughout.

Results.—Compared with baseline, cinacalcet treatment improved biochemical measures of PHPT including reducing serum calcium and

PTH and increasing serum phosphate with slight increases in alkaline phosphatase. No changes in z-scores of a BMD at spine, hip, or wrist were seen with annual percent changes, consistent with reports for untreated postmenopausal women or PHPT patients. Safety biochemistries remained normal, and adverse events (most commonly arthralgia, myalgia, diarrhea, respiratory infection, and nausea) were mild to moderate in severity.

Conclusions.—Treatment of PHPT patients with cinacalcet for up to 5.5 yr maintained normocalcemia, reduced plasma PTH, increased serum phosphate and alkaline phosphatase with no significant effects on aBMD, and was well tolerated.

▶ Primary hyperparathyroidism is characterized by increased serum calcium and inappropriately normal or increased serum parathyroid hormone (PTH). This disorder may be associated with osteoporosis, fractures, decreased bone density, calcium-containing kidney stones, fatigue, neurocognitive dysfunction, or musculoskeletal symptoms, but most patients seen in the modern era do not have complications of the disorder, and are asymptomatic.[1] Parathyroidectomy is highly effective at curing this disorder, but medical treatment options are limited for subjects who fail surgery, have contraindications to surgery, refuse surgery, or do not meet current surgical guidelines.

The only medical therapy currently available to suppress PTH secretion is cinacalcet, but this agent is not approved to treat primary hyperparathyroidism in the United States. Cinacalcet is a calcimimetic agent that binds to calcium-sensing receptors on the parathyroid gland and increases their sensitivity to extracellular calcium, thereby rapidly and directly decreasing PTH secretion and serum calcium.[2-4] This agent is approved in the United States for the treatment of secondary hyperparathyroidism associated with chronic kidney disease in patients on dialysis treatment,[5-7] and parathyroid carcinoma.[8] In Europe, cinacalcet is approved for the treatment of hypercalcemia due to primary hyperparathyroidism in patients in whom parathyroidectomy is indicated based on serum calcium levels, but in whom parathyroidectomy is clinically inappropriate or contraindicated for other reasons.

This small study demonstrates that cinacalcet is effective and well tolerated by patients with mild to moderate primary hyperparathyroidism over 5.5 years of treatment. In this open-label extension of the previous 1-year randomized, placebo-controlled study,[9] 45 of the initial 78 patients were enrolled to continue cinacalcet starting at 30 mg twice daily, with dose titration up to 50 mg twice daily as needed during a 12-week titration phase. Compared with baseline, cinacalcet normalized serum calcium and decreased serum PTH over the duration of the study. Lumbar spine, hip, and wrist BMD remained stable throughout the course of the study. Safety biochemistries remained normal, and adverse events were limited to mild to moderate musculoskeletal pain, diarrhea, respiratory infection, and nausea.

These findings suggest that cinacalcet may be an effective option for the treatment of primary hyperparathyroidism in patients in whom parathyroidectomy is contraindicated or who have failed surgical correction. Treated subjects maintained normal serum calcium levels and stable BMD over 5.5 years, with no apparent significant adverse effects. Only 5 of 41 subjects required up-titration of their dose over 4.5 years during the open-label extension study, indicating that the abnormal parathyroid glands in these individuals did not expand their cell mass or secretory capacity sufficiently to require increasing doses of adequately controlled PTH secretion.

B. L. Clarke, MD

References

1. Bilezikian JP, Khan AA, Potts JT Jr. Third International Workshop on the Management of Asymptomatic Primary Hyperthyroidism. Guidelines for the management of asymptomatic primary hyperparathyroidism: summary statement from the third international workshop. *J Clin Endocrinol Metab.* 2009;94:335-339.
2. Nemeth EF, Fox J. Calcimimetic compounds: a direct approach to controlling plasma levels of parathyroid hormone in subjects with hyperparathyroidism. *Trends Endocrinol Metab.* 1999;10:66-71.
3. Shoback DM, Bilezikian JP, Turner SA, McCary LC, Guo MD, Peacock M. The calcimimetic cinacalcet normalizes serum calcium in subjects with primary hyperparathyroidism. *J Clin Endocrinol Metab.* 2003;88:5644-5649.
4. Marcocci C, Chanson P, Shoback D, et al. Cinacalcet reduces serum calcium concentrations in patients with intractable primary hyperparathyroidism. *J Clin Endocrinol Metab.* 2009;94:2766-2772.
5. Block GA, Martin KJ, de Francisco AL, et al. Cinacalcet for secondary hyperparathyroidism in patients receiving hemodialysis. *N Engl J Med.* 2004;350: 1516-1525.
6. Lindberg JS, Culleton B, Wong G, et al. Cinacalcet HCl, an oral calcimimetic agent for the treatment of secondary hyperparathyroidism in hemodialysis and peritoneal dialysis: a randomized, double-blind, multicenter study. *J Am Soc Nephrol.* 2005;16:800-807.
7. Messa P, Macario F, Yaqoob M, et al. The OPTIMA Study: assessing a new cinacalcet (Sensipar®/Mimpara®) treatment algorithm for secondary hyperparathyroidism. *Clin J Am Soc Nephrol.* 2008;3:36-45.
8. Silverberg SJ, Rubin MR, Faiman C, et al. Cinacalcet hydrochloride reduces the serum calcium concentration in inoperable parathyroid carcinoma. *J Clin Endocrinol Metab.* 2007;92:3803-3808.
9. Peacock M, Bilezikian JP, Klassen PS, Guo MD, Turner SA, Shoback D. Cinacalcet hydrochloride maintains long-term normocalcemia in patients with primary hyperparathyroidism. *J Clin Endocrinol Metab.* 2005;90:135-141.

Cinacalcet Reduces Serum Calcium Concentrations in Patients with Intractable Primary Hyperparathyroidism

Marcocci C, Chanson P, Shoback D, et al (Univ of Pisa, Italy; Hôpital de Bicêtre and Université Paris-Sud 11, Le Kremlin-Bicêtre, France; Univ of California, San Francisco; et al)

J Clin Endocrinol Metab 94:2766-2772, 2009

Context.—Patients with persistent primary hyperparathyroidism (PHPT) after parathyroidectomy or with contraindications to parathyroidectomy often require chronic treatment for hypercalcemia.

Objective.—The objective of the study was to assess the ability of the calcimimetic, cinacalcet, to reduce serum calcium in patients with intractable PHPT.

Design.—This was an open-label, single-arm study comprising a titration phase of variable duration (2–16 wk) and a maintenance phase of up to 136 wk.

Setting.—The study was conducted at 23 centers in Europe, the United States, and Canada.

Patients.—The study included 17 patients with intractable PHPT and serum calcium greater than 12.5 mg/dl (3.1 mmol/liter).

Intervention.—During the titration phase, cinacalcet dosages were titrated every 2 wk (30 mg twice daily to 90 mg four times daily) for 16 wk until serum calcium was 10 mg/dl or less (2.5 mmol/liter). If serum calcium increased during the maintenance phase, additional increases in the cinacalcet dose were permitted.

Main Outcome Measure.—The primary end point was the proportion of patients experiencing a reduction in serum calcium of 1 mg/dl or greater (0.25 mmol/liter) at the end of the titration phase.

Results.—Mean ± SD baseline serum calcium was 12.7 ± 0.8 mg/dl (3.2 ± 0.2 mmol/liter). At the end of titration, a 1 mg/dl or greater reduction in serum calcium was achieved in 15 patients (88%). Fifteen patients (88%) experienced treatment-related adverse events, none of which were serious. The most common adverse events were nausea, vomiting, and paresthesias.

Conclusions.—In patients with intractable PHPT, cinacalcet reduces serum calcium, is generally well tolerated, and has the potential to fulfill an unmet medical need.

▶ Some patients with primary hyperparathyroidism have persistent primary hyperparathyroidism after initial surgery or surgeries, or have contraindications to surgery and need treatment based on their degree of hypercalcemia. While most patients with primary hyperparathyroidism today are asymptomatic, some have complications or symptoms related to their hypercalcemia, including skeletal or kidney disease, gastrointestinal disturbances, or neuropsychiatric symptoms.[1] While parathyroidectomy by experienced surgeons cures 95% to 98% of patients with this condition, 5% to 12% may have persistent disease not cured at surgery or recurrent disease developing more than 6 months after surgery.[2-4] Patients with moderate to severe hypercalcemia, or those with symptoms, require treatment, but medical options are limited for those with persistent or recurrent disease or those with contraindications to surgery.

This small study demonstrates that cinacalcet is effective and well tolerated by patients with intractable primary hyperparathyroidism characterized by serum calcium greater than 12.5 mg/dL over up to 152 weeks of treatment. In this open-label single-arm study, 17 subjects were treated with cinacalcet starting at 30 mg twice daily, with dose titration up to 90 mg four times daily as needed, to obtain serum calcium ≤10 mg/dL during a 16-week titration phase. Further dose adjustment was allowed during the study if serum calcium increased during the maintenance phase of the study. Compared with baseline, cinacalcet decreased by ≥1.0 mg/dL in 88% of 15 subjects. Fifteen subjects developed treatment-related mild or moderate adverse events, most commonly nausea, vomiting, or paresthesias.

These findings provide evidence that cinacalcet may be a treatment option for patients with more severe intractable primary hyperparathyroidism. Cinacalcet was able to reduce serum calcium close to the normal range, and was also able to decrease parathyroid hormone (PTH) toward the normal range, with higher doses than used in a study of milder primary hyperparathyroidism.[5] This drug has the potential to improve metabolic parameters and fills an unmet need in patients with intractable primary hyperparathyroidism.

B. L. Clarke, MD

References

1. AACE/AAES Task Force on Primary Hyperparathyroidism. The American Association of Clinical Endocrinologists and the American Association of Endocrine Surgeons position statement on the diagnosis and management of primary hyperparathyroidism. *Endocr Pract.* 2005;11:49-54.
2. Boggs JE, Irvine GL 3rd, Carneiro DM, Molinari AS. The evolution of parathyroidectomy failures. *Surgery.* 1999;126:998-1002.
3. Hasse C, Sitter H, Brune M, Wollenteit I, Nies C, Rothmund M. Quality of life and patient satisfaction after reoperation for primary hyperparathyroidism: analysis of long-term results. *World J Surg.* 2002;26:1029-1036.
4. Hedback G, Oden A. Recurrence of hyperparathyroidism: a long-term follow-up after surgery for primary hyperparathyroidism. *Eur J Endocrinol.* 2003;148: 413-421.
5. Peacock M, Bolognese MA, Borofsky M, et al. Cinacalcet treatment of primary hyperparathyroidism: biochemical and bone densitometric outcomes in a five-year study. *J Clin Endocrinol Metab.* 2009;94:4860-4867.

Evaluation of MR spectroscopy and diffusion-weighted MRI in detecting bone marrow changes in postmenopausal women with osteoporosis

Tang GY, Lv ZW, Tang RB, et al (Affiliated Tenth People's Hosp of Tongji Univ, Shanghai, China)

Clin Radiol 65:377-381, 2010

Aim.—To prospectively investigate the role of MR spectroscopy (MRS) and diffusion-weighted magnetic resonance imaging (DWI) in assessing vertebral marrow changes in postmenopausal women with osteoporosis.

Materials and Methods.—Seventy-eight postmenopausal women (mean age 63.7 ± 3.5 years; range 55–81 years), who underwent dual-energy x-ray absorptiometry of the spine, were divided into three bone density groups (24 with normal, 25 with osteopaenic, and 29 with osteoporotic) based on T score. Both MRS and DWI of the L3 vertebral body were performed to calculate the marrow fat content and apparent diffusion coefficient (ADC). The results were compared between three groups and correlated with BMD.

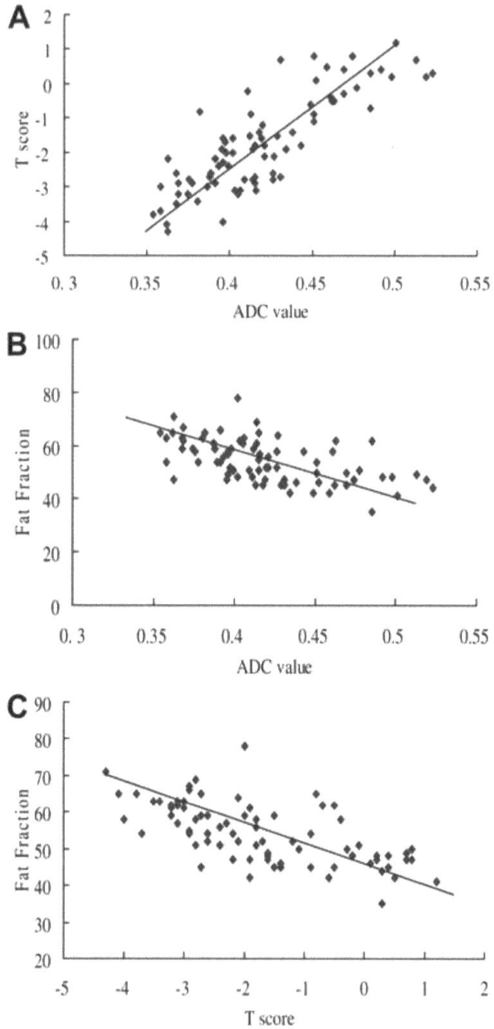

FIGURE 3.—(A) Scatterplot shows a positive correlation between ADC and DXA T-scores ($r = 0.835$, $P < 0.001$). (B) Scatterplot shows a negative correlation between ADC and Fat Fraction(FF) ($r = -0.554$, $P < 0.001$). (C) Scatterplot shows a negative correlation between DXA T-scores and Fat Fraction(FF) ($r = -0.639$, $P < 0.001$). (Reprinted from Tang GY, Lv ZW, Tang RB, et al. Evaluation of MR spectroscopy and diffusion-weighted MRI in detecting bone marrow changes in postmenopausal women with osteoporosis. *Clin Radiol.* 2010;65:377-381, with permission The Royal College of Radiologists.)

Results.—Vertebral marrow fat content was significantly increased in the osteoporotic group (59.97 ± 5.78%), when compared with that of the osteopaenic group (53.04 ± 7.66%, $p = 0.001$) and the normal bone density group (48.79 ± 7.1%, $p < 0.001$). ADC values in the osteoporotic, osteopaenic, and normal bone density groups were $0.39 \pm 0.02 \times 10^{-3}$ mm²/s, $0.41 \pm 0.02 \times 10^{-3}$ mm²/s, and $0.47 \pm 0.03 \times 10^{-3}$ mm²/s, respectively, with statistically significant difference ($P < 0.001$).

A statistically significant positive correlation between T scores and ADC existed ($r = 0.835$, $p < 0.001$). The vertebral marrow fat content was negatively correlated to the bone density ($r = -0.639$, $p < 0.001$) and to marrow ADC ($r = -0.554$, $p < 0.001$).

Conclusion.—The postmenopausal women with osteoporosis exhibited a corresponding increase in vertebral marrow fat content as the bone density decreased. Marrow fat content and ADC were related to the bone density. MRS and DWI are helpful in evaluating the bone marrow changes in postmenopausal women (Fig 3).

▶ Osteoporosis is common in aging humans and results in a reduction in bone mass, degeneration of microstructure of the bone, and increased risk of fractures. Dual-energy x-ray absorptiometry (DEXA) is commonly used to determine bone mineral density (BMD), but bone marrow quality also affects bone strength. In the study by Tang et al magnetic resonance spectroscopy and magnetic resonance imaging were also measured along with DEXA in postmenopausal women between the age of 55 and 81 years. As shown in Fig 3, they observed an inverse relationship between T score and bone fat fraction. The increase in bone marrow fat of the vertebral spine might reflect trabecular thinning. There are several limitations of the study. It was not determined that increased marrow fat correlated with fracture risk and if therapies for osteoporosis affected marrow fat. Further study is needed to determine the clinical usefulness of bone marrow fat analysis in the management of osteoporosis, which causes considerable morbidity and mortality in our aging population.

A. W. Meikle, MD

Pseudohypoparathyroidism and *GNAS* Epigenetic Defects: Clinical Evaluation of Albright Hereditary Osteodystrophy and Molecular Analysis in 40 Patients

Mantovani G, de Sanctis L, Barbieri AM, et al (Università degli Studi di Milano, Italy; Univ of Turin, Italy)

J Clin Endocrinol Metab 95:651-658, 2010

Context.—The two main subtypes of pseudohypoparathyroidism (PHP), PHP-Ia and -Ib, are caused by mutations in *GNAS* exons 1-13 and methylation defects in the imprinted *GNAS* cluster, respectively. PHP-Ia patients show Albright hereditary osteodystrophy (AHO) and resistance toward PTH and additional hormones, whereas PHP-Ib patients do not have AHO, and hormone resistance appears to be limited to PTH and TSH. Recently, methylation defects have been detected in few patients with PHP and mild AHO, indicating a molecular overlap between the two forms.

Objectives.—The aim of the study was to screen patients with clinically diagnosed PHP-Ia for methylation defects and to investigate the presence of correlations between the molecular findings and AHO severity.

Patients and Methods.—We investigated differential methylation of *GNAS* regions and STX16 microdeletions in genomic DNA from 40 patients with sporadic AHO and multihormone resistance, with no mutations in Gsα-coding *GNAS* exons.

Results.—Molecular analysis showed *GNAS* cluster imprinting defects in 24 of the 40 patients analyzed. No STX16 deletion was detected. The presence of imprinting defects was not associated with the severity of AHO or with specific AHO signs.

Conclusions.—We report the largest series of the literature of patients with clinical AHO and multihormone resistance and no mutation in the Gsα gene. Our findings of frequent *GNAS* imprinting defects further confirm the existence of an overlap between molecular and clinical features of PHP-Ia and PHP-Ib and highlight the necessity of a new clinical classification of the disease that takes into account the recent knowledge on the molecular basis underlying these defects.

▶ The 2 main types of genetic parathyroid hormone (PTH) resistance, known as pseudohypoparathyroidism types 1a and 1b, are associated with *GNAS* gene mutations in exons 1 to 13 in type 1a, and methylation defects in the imprinted *GNAS* cluster in type 1b.[1,2] Patients with pseudohypoparathyroidism type 1a are characterized by a skeletal phenotype known as Albright hereditary osteodystrophy as well as resistance to PTH and other hormones.[3] Those with pseudohypoparathyroidism type 1b do not have a recognized skeletal phenotype and appear to have more limited resistance to PTH and thyroid-stimulating hormone (TSH) only.[4] Recently, several patients with mild Albright hereditary osteodystrophy have been reported who had methylation defects usually associated with pseudohypoparathyroidism type 1b.[5-7] These findings suggest that both forms of pseudohypoparathyroidism type 1 may be characterized by methylation defects.

This study evaluated 40 patients clinically diagnosed with pseudohypoparathyroidism type 1a, with skeletal features of Albright hereditary osteodystrophy and resistance to multiple hormones, who did not have detectable *GNAS* mutations. Analysis of differential methylation of their *GNAS* regions and for genomic STX16 microdeletions showed that 24 patients had *GNAS* cluster imprinting defects without any detected STX16 microdeletions. These imprinting defects were not associated with the severity or specific skeletal features of Albright hereditary osteodystrophy.

These findings further confirm the molecular and skeletal phenotypic overlap between the current classification scheme for pseudohypoparathyroidism types 1a and 1b. This study contains the largest series of patients reported to date with clinical pseudohypoparathyroidism type 1a who did not have detectable *GNAS* coding exon mutations, and provides further evidence that a new clinical classification system for pseudohypoparathyroidism type 1 is necessary.

B. L. Clarke, MD

References

1. Weinstein LS, Yu S, Warner DR, Liu J. Endocrine manifestations of stimulatory G protein α-subunit mutations and the role of genomic imprinting. *Endocrine Rev.* 2001;22:675-705.
2. Aldred MA, Trembath RC. Activating and inactivating mutations in the human GNAS1 gene. *Hum Mutat.* 2000;16:183-189.
3. Bastepe M, Jüppner H. GNAS locus and pseudohypoparathyroidism. *Horm Res.* 2005;63:65-74.
4. Bastepe M, Fröhlich LF, Hendy GN, et al. Autosomal dominant pseudohypoparathyroidism type Ib is associated with a heterozygous microdeletion that likely disrupts a putative imprinting control element of GNAS. *J Clin Invest.* 2003; 112:1255-1263.
5. De Nanclares GP, Fernández-Rebollo E, Santin I, et al. Epigenetic defects of GNAS in patients with pseudohypoparathyroidism and mild features of Albright hereditary osteodystrophy. *J Clin Endocrinol Metab.* 2007;92:2370-2373.
6. Mariot V, Maupetit-Méhouas S, Sinding C, Kottler ML, Linglart A. A maternal epimutation of GNAS leads to Albright hereditary osteodystrophy and parathyroid hormone resistance. *J Clin Endocrinol Metab.* 2008;93:661-665.
7. Unluturk U, Harmanci A, Babaoglu M, et al. Molecular diagnosis and clinical characterization of pseudohypoparathyroidism type-Ib in a patient with mild Albright hereditary osteodystrophy-like features, epileptic seizures, and defective renal handling of uric acid. *Am J Med Sci.* 2008;336:84-90.

Randomized Trial of Intensive Bisphosphonate Treatment Versus Symptomatic Management in Paget's Disease of Bone

Langston AL, Campbell MK, Fraser WD, et al (Inst of Genetics and Molecular Medicine Univ of Edinburgh, UK; Univ of Aberdeen, UK; Univ of Liverpool, UK; et al)

J Bone Miner Res 25:20-31, 2010

Bisphosphonates are widely regarded as the treatment of choice for Paget's disease of bone (PDB) because of their potent inhibitory effects on bone turnover, but the effects of bisphosphonate therapy on symptoms and complications of PDB have been little studied. Here we report the results of a randomized trial that compared the effects of symptomatic treatment with intensive bisphosphonate therapy in a cohort of 1324 patients with PDB who were followed up for a median of 3 years (range 2 to 5 years). The symptomatic treatment group was treated only if they had pagetic bone pain, for which they were first given analgesics or anti-inflammatory drugs, followed by bisphosphonates if they did not respond. The intensive group received repeat courses of bisphosphonates irrespective of symptoms with the aim of reducing and maintaining serum alkaline phosphatase (ALP) levels within the normal range. The endpoints were fracture, orthopedic surgery, quality of life, bone pain, and hearing thresholds. Serum ALP levels were significantly lower in the intensive treatment group than in with the symptomatic treatment group within 4 months of commencing treatment and remained lower throughout the study ($p < .001$). There was no difference between the groups in quality of life (as assessed by the SF36 questionnaire), in overall bodily pain, or in pagetic bone pain. Hearing thresholds, as assessed by audiometry did not change significantly and did not differ between the treatment groups. Clinical fractures occurred in 46 of 661 patients (7.0%) in the intensive treatment group compared with 49 of 663 patients (7.4%) in the symptomatic treatment group, and orthopedic surgery was required in 50 of 661 patients (7.3%) in the intensive treatment group and in 55 of 663 patients (8.3%) in the symptomatic treatment group. These differences were not significant. Subgroup analyses of patients with elevated ALP levels at baseline and those who did or did not receive bisphosphonates during the study yielded similar results to those in the study group as a whole. We conclude that striving to maintain normal ALP levels with intensive bisphosphonate therapy confers no clinical advantage over symptom-driven management in patients with established PDB. Neither management strategy had a significant beneficial impact on pain or quality of life (Clinical trial registration number ISRCTN12989577).

▶ Symptomatic Paget disease of bone is currently most commonly treated with oral or intravenous bisphosphonates. These potent drugs effectively suppress osteoclast-induced bone turnover, which markedly reduces the inflammatory changes associated with Paget disease.[1,2] Up to 30% of patients with Paget disease develop complications such as bone deformity, fracture, deafness, or secondary osteoarthritis[3] that significantly impact the quality of life of affected patients.[4,5] In spite of the effective treatments available, no studies have addressed the effects of bisphosphonate therapy on symptoms and complications of Paget disease. It has been proposed that the goal of therapy for Paget disease should be to normalize bone turnover, because this might prevent disease progression and development of complications.[6]

This non-blinded, industry-funded study randomized 1324 subjects with Paget disease to receive symptomatic treatment or intensive bisphosphonate therapy for a median of 3 years. The symptomatic treatment group was treated only when they had pagetic bone pain, first with analgesics or antiinflammatory drugs, followed by bisphosphonates if they did not improve. The intensive treatment group received multiple courses of bisphosphonates without regard to symptoms, with the goal of suppressing and maintaining serum alkaline phosphatase in the normal range. Oral risedronate was chosen as the first-line treatment when treatment was recommended, with tiludronate, etidronate, and subcutaneous calcitonin permitted, and aminobisphosphonates were allowed only when response to the other agents was inadequate. Subjects receiving intensive treatment with bisphosphonates developed lower serum alkaline phosphatase levels by 4 months of commencing treatment and remained lower throughout the remainder of the study. There was no difference in overall pain, pagetic bone pain, bone fractures, requirement for orthopedic surgery, hearing loss, or quality of life between the groups, and hearing thresholds did not differ. Clinical fractures and orthopedic surgery occurred with equal frequency in the 2 groups. The authors concluded that keeping serum alkaline phosphatase in the normal range with intensive bisphosphonate therapy offered no greater clinical benefit than management based on symptoms, and that neither approach had significant beneficial effect on pain or quality of life.

This is the first Paget disease study to explore long-term clinical outcomes in patients randomized to receive intensive therapy or symptomatic treatment, rather than short-term changes in serum alkaline phosphatase. Previous studies have not correlated lower serum alkaline phosphatase levels with favorable clinical outcomes because most studies have been too short-term to allow correlation. This study showed that intensive therapy with oral risedronate and other bisphosphonates did not improve bone pain, hearing loss, or fracture over symptomatic treatment. The study permitted the use of oral non-aminobisphosphonates only, with intravenous pamidronate used in two different dosing regimens, depending on the study group. No subjects received intravenous zoledronic acid. Further studies are required to determine whether potent suppression of bone turnover caused by bisphosphonates is sufficient to reduce long-term complications of Paget disease of bone.

B. L. Clarke, MD

References

1. Reid IR, Miller P, Lyles K, et al. Comparison of a single infusion of zoledronic acid with risedronate for Paget's disease. *N Engl J Med.* 2005;353:898-908.
2. Siris ES, Weinstein RS, Altman R, et al. Comparative study of alendronate versus etidronate for the treatment of Paget's disease of bone. *J Clin Endocrinol Metab.* 1996;81:961-967.
3. Von Staa TP, Selby P, Leufkens HG, Lyles K, Sprafka JM, Cooper C. Incidence and natural history of Paget's disease of bone in England and Wales. *J Bone Miner Res.* 2002;17:465-471.
4. Langston AL, Campbell MK, Fraser WD, Maclennan G, Selby P, Ralston SH. Clinical determinants of quality of life in Paget's disease of bone. *Calcif Tiss Int.* 2007; 80:1-9.
5. Gold DT, Boisture J, Shipp KM, Pieper CF, Lyles KW. Paget's disease of bone and quality of life. *J Bone Miner Res.* 1996;11:1897-1904.
6. Lyles KW, Siris ES, Singer FR, Meunier PJ. A clinical approach to diagnosis and management of Paget's disease of bone. *J Bone Miner Res.* 2001;16:1379-1387.

6 Adrenal Cortex

Introduction

We have selected for the 2010 YEAR BOOK edition a series of articles to highlight the published focus on adrenal diseases during this period. Some of the articles emphasize recurrent themes, and others present novel investigative approaches. In the area of hyperaldosteronism, a group from Taipei, Taiwan, investigated causes of persistent hypertension after resection of an aldosterone-secreting adrenal adenoma and concluded that changes in kidney function play an important role. Using data from the ALOFT study, Freel et al examine the role of aldosterone in the insulin resistance of patients with heart failure in evaluating a cohort of 466 African American patients with hypertension. Kidambi et al indicate that aldosterone contributes to blood pressure variance in normal weight and overweight African American subjects. The aldosterone:renin ratio (ARR) is used routinely to screen patients for primary aldosteronism, but in a study 1172 individuals, Alvarez Madrazo et al find the ARR is influenced by genetic and environmental factors that need to be considered in interpreting results. Adrenal venous sampling is another key tool in the diagnosis of primary aldosteronism, and Auchus et al suggest ways in which the procedure can be improved. Patients with primary aldosteronism with bilateral adrenal cortical hyperplasia are usually treated medically with mineralocorticoid receptor antagonists. Based on the experience with 684 patients with this condition, Sukor et al provide good data in support of unilateral adrenalectomy in cases of asymmetrical hormone production.

Cushing's syndrome is another topic of interest—the syndrome is not always easy to diagnose, and the treatment can be challenging. Baid et al from the NIH report on their investigation of obese patients with some features of Cushing's and conclude that the yield among these patients is low, but the need to screen many of these individuals still remains. Kissane and Cendan report on their immediate postoperative experience with 80 patients undergoing laparoscopic adrenalectomy and emphasize that they require more intensive care and longer duration of hospitalization, especially among those requiring bilateral adrenalectomy. Pheochromocytomas and paragangliomas can be sporadic or part of familial genetic syndromes. In a study of 989 apparently nonsyndromic pheochromocytomas by a European-American study group, Erlic et al look at susceptibility genes and propose an algorithm for the genetic diagnosis of these patients. According to Fiebrich et al, localization of extra-adrenal pheochromocytomas or metastases in cases of malignant pheochromocytomas may be more effectively done using 6-[F-18]-fluorodihydroxyphenylalanine positron emission tomography.

We found several interesting articles on adrenal cortical tumors, and these were highlighted. Ballian et al revisit the issue of adrenal mass size as an indication of malignancy and need for adrenalectomy, and Piatidis et al challenge the definition of nonfunctioning incidentally discovered masses and potentially the indication for surgically removing these masses. Although there are several imaging criteria for determining the likelihood that a mass is benign, Groussin et al propose the use of positron emission tomography in the initial diagnosis of these masses. The future of targeted treatment of adrenal cancer lies in the discovery of specific molecular targets. We discuss 4 interesting studies that identify promising targets.

Three articles deal with testing and treatment of patients with adrenal insufficiency. A study by Paisley et al looks at the validity of peak cortisol response to stimulation as an indicator of cortisol production rate, and Perogamvros et al show good diagnostic sensitivity and specificity using salivary cortisol with liquid chromatography-tandem mass spectrometry. Debono et al have come up with a new hydrocortisone formulation to restore circadian rhythm in patients on glucocorticoid replacement therapy. Two articles focus on polycystic ovary (PCO) syndrome. Vassiliadi et al suggest increased cortisol production as an important pathogenic pathway, and Puurunen et al report increased androgen-secreting capacity in women with PCO remains high through menopause, at a time when women without PCO show a decline. Finally, we offer a pair of interesting research studies of adrenal cortical hyperplasia. Robinson-White et al investigated the possibility of treating Carney complex–associated tumors with 8-Cl-adenosine and its mechanism of action, and Tsiao et al characterized a large series of patients with ACTH-independent macronodular adrenal hyperplasia and found clinical and genetic heterogeneity in spite of phenotypic similarities.

We hope the reader will find our selections instructive and representative of some of the contributions to the adrenal literature over the past year.

David E. Schteingart, MD

Adrenal Function

^{18}F-Fluorodeoxyglucose Positron Emission Tomography for the Diagnosis of Adrenocortical Tumors: A Prospective Study in 77 Operated Patients

Groussin L, Bonardel G, Silvéra S, et al (Institut Cochin, Paris, France; Université Paris Descartes, France; Hôpital d'Instruction des Armées du Val de Grâce, Paris, France; et al)

J Clin Endocrinol Metab 94:1713-1722, 2009

Context.—Most adrenal incidentalomas are nonfunctioning adrenocortical adenomas (ACAs). Adrenocortical carcinomas (ACCs) are rare but should be recognized at an early stage.

Objective.—The objective of the study was to evaluate the usefulness of ^{18}Ffluorodeoxyglucose positron emission tomography (^{18}F-FDG PET) to predict malignancy in patients without a previous history of cancer.

Design.—This was a prospective, multicenter study from 2001 to 2006.

Setting.—The study was conducted at a network of seven university hospitals in Paris.

Patients.—Seventy-seven patients were included. All underwent surgery because of hypersecretory and/or growing benign lesions ($n = 18$), obvious ACCs ($n = 21$), or radiologically indeterminate lesions ($n = 38$).

Main Outcome Measure.—The degree of ^{18}F-FDG PET uptake [maximum standardized uptake value (maxSUV)] was related to the pathological findings serving as a reference, and its diagnostic value was compared with that of computerized tomography (CT) scan.

Results.—Pathology eventually diagnosed 43 ACAs, 22 ACCs, and 12 nonadrenocortical lesions. Using a cutoff value above 1.45 for adrenal to liver maxSUV ratio, the sensitivity and specificity to distinguish ACAs from ACCs were, respectively, 1.00 (95% confidence interval 0.85–1.00) and 0.88 (95% confidence interval 0.75–0.96). Among the 38 indeterminate lesions at CT scan, we could analyze a subgroup of 16 adrenocortical tumors with high unenhanced density (>10 HU) and an inappropriate washout: ^{18}F-FDG PET correctly predicted the benignity in 13 of 15 ACAs.

Conclusions.—In a multidisciplinary team approach, ^{18}F-FDG PET helps to manage suspicious CT scan lesions. An adrenal to liver maxSUV ratio less than 1.45 is highly predictive of a benign lesion.

► Distinguishing between benign and malignant nonfunctioning adrenal masses is critical in making a decision whether to surgically remove them. Several approaches based on size, lipid content, and washout of contrast have been used to make this distinction. We previously reported on the use of ^{18}F-fluorodeoxyglucose positron emission tomography ([^{18}F]-FDG PET)[1] in evaluating locally recurrent and metastatic adrenal cortical carcinoma and distinguishing these masses from benign concurrent lesions. Groussin et al studied 77 patients who were scheduled for surgery because of a functioning adrenal mass, indeterminate imaging, lipid poor on CT or MRI, or growing size with [^{18}F]-FDG PET. With a Maximal Standardized Uptake Value (Max SUV) adrenal lesion to liver < 1.45, they found high sensitivity (100%) and specificity (88%) in determining a lesion was benign. The conclusion is that in doubtful cases, this technique is very helpful in settling the question of whether the lesion is malignant.

D. E. Schteingart, MD

Reference

1. Mackie GC, Shulkin BL, Ribeiro RC, et al. Use of [18F]fluorodeoxyglucose positron emission tomography in evaluating locally recurrent and metastatic adrenocortical carcinoma. *J Clin Endocrinol Metab.* 2006;91:2665-2671.

Bone Morphogenetic Proteins 2 and 5 Are Down-regulated in Adrenocortical Carcinoma and Modulate Adrenal Cell Proliferation and Steroidogenesis

Johnsen IK, Kappler R, Auernhammer CJ, et al (Ludwig Maximilians Univ, Munich, Germany; Univ of Munich, Germany; et al)

Cancer Res 69:5784-5792, 2009

Bone morphogenetic proteins (BMP) have been shown to affect tumorigenesis in a variety of tumors. Quantitative PCR analysis revealed down-regulation of BMP2 and BMP5 in tissue samples from adrenocortical carcinoma and adrenocortical tumor cell lines compared with normal adrenal glands. Integrity of BMP-dependent pathways in these cell lines could be shown by activation of the Smad1/5/8 pathway with subsequent increase of ID protein expression upon incubation with BMP2 or BMP5. On a functional level, BMP treatment resulted in inhibition of cell proliferation and viability in a dose- and time-dependent manner. This growth inhibitory effect was associated with BMP-dependent reduction of AKT phosphorylation under baseline conditions and under insulin-like growth factor costimulation. Furthermore, steroidogenic function, including melanocortin-2 receptor and steroidogenic enzyme expressions, was profoundly reduced. *In vitro* demethylation treatment and overexpression of GATA6 resulted in reactivation of BMP-dependent pathways with concomitant modulation of steroidogenesis. Taken together, we show that loss of expression of members of the BMP family of ligands is a common finding in adrenocortical tumors and we provide evidence that BMP-dependent pathways are likely to be involved in the modulation of the malignant and functional phenotype of adrenocortical cancer cells.

▶ Of the various gene-regulated proteins in adrenal tumors, bone morphogenetic proteins (BMP) may play an important role in tumorigenesis. The availability of gene array technology has made it possible to compare benign adrenal cortical adenomas (ACA) and adrenal cortical carcinomas (ACC) and determine which genes are overexpressed or underexpressed and signal potential targets for therapy. Johnsen et al showed downregulation of BMP 2 and 5 in ACC but not in ACA. BMP appears to inhibit cell growth. When BMP was added to NCI-H295 and SW-13 cell cultures there was inhibition of cell proliferation and viability. BMPs are part of a cascade of transcription factors regulating cell growth, including SOX9, NF-κB and GATA. Expression of BMP may be regulated by a number of pharmacological agents, such as retinoic acid and protein kinase C activators. Activation of BMP expression by specific agents could be a strategy for antitumor therapy in ACC.

D. E. Schteingart, MD

High prevalence of autonomous cortisol and aldosterone secretion from adrenal adenomas

Piaditis GP, Kaltsas GA, Androulakis II, et al (General Hosp of Athens "G. Gennimatas", Greece; Univ of Athens, Greece)

Clin Endocrinol 71:772-778, 2009

Objectives.—Previous studies based on standard endocrine testing have shown a variable incidence of autonomous cortisol secretion (ACS) or autonomous aldosterone secretion (AAS) in patients with single adrenal adenomas (SAA). We tested whether the use of appropriate controls and modification of standard testing, aiming at eliminating interference from endogenous ACTH, reveals previously undetected subtle ACS and AAS by SAA.

Design.—Case control study.

Patients.—We investigated 151 patients with SAA and 72 matched controls with normal adrenal computerized tomography.

Measurements.—All participants had arterial blood pressure recorded, and serum cortisol and aldosterone measured before and after intravenous administration of 250 μg of ACTH, and following dexamethasone administration. Eighty-three patients and all the controls had serum aldosterone and renin measured before and after saline infusion, and after a second saline infusion following dexamethasone administration.

Results.—Using the mean + 2 SD values obtained from controls after dexamethasone administration and saline infusion following dexamethasone administration, normal cut-off values for cortisol (30·11 nm), aldosterone (67·59 pM), and aldosterone/renin ratio (9·74 pM/mU/l) were developed. Using these cut-off values, the estimated incidence of ACS and AAS in patients with SAA was 56·63% and 24·10%, respectively, whereas 12·05% had autonomous secretion of both cortisol and aldosterone. Systolic and diastolic arterial blood pressure correlated significantly with the aldosterone/renin ratio following ACTH stimulation ($P < 0{\cdot}0002$ and $P < 0{\cdot}001$, respectively), and after saline infusion following dexamethasone administration ($P < 0{\cdot}003$ and $P < 0{\cdot}002$, respectively).

Conclusions.—By applying new cut-offs, ACS and AAS in patients with a SAA is very common, and aldosterone secretion correlates with arterial blood pressure.

▶ This is a provocative article with potential consequence on the management of accidentally discovered adrenal adenomas. It reports higher than previously acknowledged cortisol and aldosterone secretion by apparently nonfunctioning adrenal tumors. The change comes from setting up new cutoff limits for the testing used to evaluate adrenal function. The study tested 151 patients with single adenomas and 72 matched control subjects with normal adrenals by tomography. Compared with controls, patients with single adenomas had relatively lower adrenocorticotropic hormone (ACTH) and renin, increased urinary-free cortisol, and greater cortisol response to ACTH stimulation. Using the new cutoff criteria, incidence of cortisol-secreting adenomas was 56.6%, aldosterone-secreting adenomas 24.1 %, and combined cortisol + aldosterone 12 %. That left 31% to 33 % of patients with adenoma with truly nonfunctioning tumors. The implication of these findings is significant. There are clinical consequences of chronic mild hypertension, glucose intolerance, insulin resistance, and metabolic syndrome, conditions that may occur even in patients with subclinical syndromes. The critical question is whether patients with low-grade hyperfunction should undergo adrenalectomy. Current recommendation is that patients with nonfunctioning adenomas should be followed without treatment, but if we follow the implications of this study to its natural conclusion, we will have to consider laparoscopic adrenalectomy and the cost:benefit ratio of such an approach, taking into account the surgical risk and cost involved. There is need to continue to accumulate longitudinal data regarding the metabolic consequence of treated versus nontreated disease.

D. E. Schteingart, MD

Inhibition of adrenocortical carcinoma cell proliferation by steroidogenic factor-1 inverse agonists

Doghman M, Cazareth J, Douguet D, et al (Université de Nice-Sophia Antipolis, Valbonne, France; et al)

J Clin Endocrinol Metab 94:2178-2183, 2009

Context.—Transcription factor steroidogenic factor-1 (SF-1) plays a pivotal role in the control of adrenocortical cell steroidogenesis and proliferation. *SF-1* amplification and overexpression are found in most cases of childhood adrenocortical tumors (ACTs).

Objective.—Our objective was to investigate the effect of SF-1 inverse agonists of the alkyloxyphenol and isoquinolinone classes on the proliferation of human adrenocortical cell lines expressing SF-1 (H295R), in conditions of basal and increased SF-1 expression, or negative for SF-1 expression (SW-13).

Main Outcome Measures.—Proliferation assays, immunoblots, flow cytometric analyses, steroid hormone assays, and reverse transcription quantitative PCR were used.

Results.—SF-1 inhibitors of the alkyloxyphenol class displayed a dosedependent inhibitory effect on both SF-1-positive and -negative ACT cells, whereas SF-1 inverse agonists of the isoquinolinone class selectively inhibited cell proliferation elicited by SF-1 overexpression. These drugs also inhibited stimulated steroid hormone secretion and CYP21 and CYP17 mRNA expression.

Conclusion.—SF-1 inhibitors may represent a useful tool in the chemotherapy of ACTs.

▶ Steroidogenic factor-1 (SF-1) is an orphan nuclear receptor that is expressed in the adrenal gland, gonads, spleen, ventromedial hypothalamus, and pituitary gonadotrope cells. It is essential in adrenal and gonadotrope development and deficiency of SF-1 in the adrenal and pituitary lead to adrenal insufficiency and hypogonadism. Targeted disruption of SF-1 in mice prevents gonadal and adrenal development and causes male-to-female sex reversal. Similar picture has been reported in children with SF-1 mutations. SF-1 regulates proliferation of human adrenal cortical cells and triggers adrenal tumor formation in mice. SF-1 may be an important factor in adrenal tumorigenesis. The ligand responsible for activation of SF-1 is unknown, but the receptor has high affinity for phosphatidylinositol bis- and triphosphate as well as C12-C16 fatty acids. In contrast, sphingosine acts as a negative regulator of SF-1 activity. Doghman et al report that transgenic H295R human adrenal cortical carcinoma cells overexpressing SF-1 were treated with SF-1 inverse agonists. Compounds of the isoQ class specifically inhibited cell proliferation. This effect appears to be SF-1 dependent because the same compound did not inhibit cell proliferation in another cell line (SW-13) that does not express SF-1. This is another example of potential molecular targets for inhibiting cell growth in adrenocortical carcinoma (ACC).

D. E. Schteingart, MD

Osteopontin stimulates invasion of NCI-h295 cells but is not associated with survival in adrenocorticol carcinoma

Weismann D, Briese J, Niemann J, et al (Univ Hosp of Würzburg, Germany)
J Pathol 218:232-240, 2009

Gene array studies indicated that osteopontin (OPN) mRNA is highly expressed in adrenocortical carcinomas (ACCs). OPN enhances invasiveness, proliferation, and metastasis formation, and is associated with poor survival in some malignant diseases. Integrin alphavbeta3 has been shown to mediate OPN effects on invasion. In this study, we demonstrated OPN and integrin alphavbeta3 expression in normal adrenal glands and benign adenomas, with staining seen exclusively in adrenocortical cells as well as even stronger staining in ACC. Western blot analysis confirmed overexpression of OPN in ACC ($p < 0.01$). With Matrigel invasion assays, we have shown that OPN greatly stimulates the invasiveness of NCI-h295 cells (>six-fold increase, $p < 0.001$). Transfection with integrin alphavbeta3 further increased invasiveness after OPN stimulation ($p < 0.001$). This increase was reversed by the addition of an anti-integrin beta3 antibody, indicating a functional relationship of OPN and integrin alphavbeta3 in ACC. With tissue arrays, we confirmed high OPN expression in 147 ACC samples. However, no association with survival was seen in Kaplan-Meier analysis including 111 patients with primary tumours graded for OPN staining and follow-up data available. In conclusion, our in vitro data indicate that OPN and integrin alphavbeta3 may act as a functional complex facilitating the invasiveness of adrenocortical tumours. This relationship remains of relevance to our understanding of carcinogenesis, but further studies are needed to address the physiological and pathological function of OPN in adrenal tissue.

▶ Osteopontin has been shown to increase cell proliferation and invasion in several malignant tumors, including lung and prostate cancer. Using Matrigel invasion assays, osteopontin was shown to increase proliferative and invasive characteristics in NCI-H295 cells. In microarray studies of adrenal tumors, Giordano et al showed that osteopontin is highly expressed in adrenocortical carcinoma (ACC).[1] Osteopontin is linked to metalloproteinase 9 pathways and binds to integrins $\alpha v\beta 3$. It is of interest that steroid hormones enhance osteopontin expression. If osteopontin plays a role in the progression of ACC, one wonders if it may explain the apparently worse course of patients with cortisol-secreting ACC.

D. E. Schteingart, MD

Reference

1. Giordano TJ, Thomas DG, Kuick R, et al. Distinct transcriptional profiles of adrenocortical tumors uncovered by DNA microarray analysis. *Am J Pathol.* 2003;162:521-531.

Revisiting Adrenal Mass Size as an Indication for Adrenalectomy

Ballian N, Adler JT, Sippel RS, et al (Univ of Wisconsin Hosp and Clinics, Madison)

J Surg Res 156:16-20, 2009

Background.—Diagnostic tests that can accurately differentiate between benign and malignant adrenal lesions are lacking. Mass size is currently utilized as an indication for adrenalectomy in patients with adrenal masses. However, the accuracy of this criterion and the ideal size threshold are unclear. The aim of the present study was to determine the frequency of using mass size as the only indication for adrenalectomy and the ideal size threshold for distinguishing malignant primary adrenal tumors from lesions that do not require surgical resection.

Patients and Methods.—The adrenalectomy database of the University of Wisconsin was retrospectively reviewed. Patients undergoing adrenalectomy for adrenal mass lesions were identified. Student's *t*-test and Fisher's exact test were used to compare continuous and noncontinuous variables respectively, with $P \leq 0.05$ representing significance.

Results.—Of 198 adrenalectomies performed between 1989 and 2007, 106 met inclusion criteria. There were no differences in age or gender distribution between patients with malignant and benign lesions. After complete clinical, imaging, and biochemical evaluation, mass size was the only indication for 16 adrenalectomies (15.1%). Adrenal mass size in these patients ranged from 3.3 to 14cm (mean 5.9 ± 0.6cm). Only three of these lesions (18.8%) proved malignant. In total, eight malignant tumors were identified in this series (7.5%, size range 4–14cm, mean 8.0 ± 1.3cm). Benign and non-neoplastic lesions accounted for the remaining masses (92.5%, size range 0.7–9.3cm, mean 3.6 ± 0.2cm) and were significantly smaller than malignant lesions ($P < 0.001$).

Conclusion.—Adrenal mass size is the only indication for adrenalectomy in a substantial number of patients. A size cut-off of 4cm would have led to resection of all primary malignant adrenal tumors in this series and reduced the number of adrenalectomies for benign disease.

▶ Accidentally found adrenal masses account for 3% to 5% of abdominal CT scans performed for abdominal complaints not directly attributed to adrenal disease. The main concerns in such discovery are whether the adrenal mass is functioning or nonfunctioning and benign or malignant. Function is usually determined by measuring plasma adrenocorticotropic hormone (ACTH) and serum cortisol, plasma renin and serum aldosterone, serum dehydroepiandrosterone (DHEA), and plasma-free normetanephrines. Most algorithms use tumor size as an indication of possible malignancy. Masses < 3 cm have high probability of being benign and > 6 cm of being malignant. Ballian et al, in a review of 198 adrenalectomies collected over an 18-year period, conclude that the critical size is 4 cm for capturing all adrenal malignancies. The problem with size alone as a criterion for adrenalectomy is that it misses early adrenal cortical carcinomas, the ones that have the best chance for surgical cure. Presently, we rely not only on size but also on radiographic appearance, such as regular contour and homogeneity, as well as lipid content and percent contrast washout. On CT or MRI, a lipid-rich mass is most likely benign and contrast washout of > 60% in 15 minutes is also consistent with a benign adrenal cortical adenoma.

D. E. Schteingart, MD

The glucocorticoid receptor is overexpressed in malignant adrenocortical tumors

Tacon LJ, Soon PS, Gill AJ, et al (Univ of Sydney, New South Wales, Australia; et al)

J Clin Endocrinol Metab 94:4591-4599, 2009

Context.—Adrenocortical carcinoma (ACC) is a rare tumor with a poor prognosis. The Weiss score is the most widely accepted method for distinguishing an ACC from an adrenocortical adenoma (ACA); however, in borderline cases, accurate diagnosis remains problematic. We recently discovered that the glucocorticoid receptor (GR) gene *NR3C1* is significantly up-regulated in ACCs compared with ACAs in global gene expression studies.

Objective.—Our objective was to study GR expression in adrenocortical tumors (ACTs) and to assess its utility as an adjunct to the Weiss score.

Design.—Microarray analysis, real-time quantitative RT-PCR (qPCR), immunohistochemistry, Western blot, and direct sequencing were performed.

Results.—Analysis of 28 ACTs by microarray and 49 ACTs by qPCR found *NR3C1* expression to be up-regulated in ACCs compared with ACAs ($P < 0.001$). Western blotting and RT-PCR confirmed the presence of the GRα isoform in ACCs, and no mutations were detected on direct sequencing. Immunohistochemistry for GR in an overlapping cohort of ACTs demonstrated strongly positive nuclear staining in 31 of 33 ACCs (94%), with negative staining in 40 of 41 ACAs (98%) ($P < 0.001$). This finding was validated in an external cohort of ACTs, such that 14 of 18 ACCs (78%) demonstrated positive nuclear staining whereas 32 of 33 ACAs (94%) were negative ($P < 0.001$).

Conclusions.—The immunohistochemical finding of nuclear GR staining identified ACCs with high diagnostic accuracy. We propose that GR immunohistochemistry may complement the Weiss score in the diagnosis of ACC in cases that display borderline histology. The possibility that GR is transcriptionally active in these tumors, and may therefore be a therapeutic target, requires further study.

▶ Another result of microarray analysis of adrenal cortical tumors is the finding that nuclear glucocorticoid receptor (GR) is overexpressed in malignant tumors. In a study by Tacon et al, the difference in GR expression between benign and malignant tumors was striking. Strongly positive nuclear staining for GR was seen in 94% of adrenocortical carcinoma (ACC) and negative staining in 98% of adrenocortical adenoma (ACA). This difference makes nuclear GR staining a good biomarker for malignancy and could be added to the histological criteria of the Weiss classification. The Weiss score has been used for years to diagnose ACC, but it is based mainly on histological features of the tumor. With the availability of molecular markers, such as nuclear GR and Ki67, the Weiss classification could be improved and made to more accurately determine prognosis.

Another molecular marker is the melanocortin 4 receptor (MC4R). It is found to have higher expression in functioning tumors but does not highlight cell proliferation or invasiveness. The relationship between nuclear GR and malignancy in patients with ACC raises the question whether GR antagonists may be useful in the treatment of these patients.

D. E. Schteingart, MD

Adrenal Hormone Secretion and Pathology

8-Cl-Adenosine Inhibits Proliferation and Causes Apoptosis in B-Lymphocytes via Protein Kinase A-Dependent and Independent Effects: Implications for Treatment of Carney Complex-Associated Tumors

Robinson-White AJ, Bossis I, Hsiao H-P, et al (Natl Insts of Health, Bethesda, MD; Univ of Maryland, College Park; et al)

J Clin Endocrinol Metab 94:4061-4069, 2009

Context.—Carney complex, a multiple neoplasia syndrome, characterized primarily by spotty skin pigmentation and a variety of endocrine and other tumors, is caused by mutations in *PRKAR1A*, the gene that codes for the RIα subunit of protein kinase A (PKA). PKA controls cell proliferation in many cell types. The cAMP analogue 8-Cl-adenosine (8-Cl-ADO) is thought to inhibit cancer cell proliferation.

Objective.—The objective of the study was to study the antiproliferative effects of 8-Cl-ADO on growth and proliferation in B-lymphocytes of Carney complex patients that have PKA defects and to determine whether 8-CL-ADO could be used as a therapeutic agent in the treatment of Carney complex-associated tumors.

Design.—We used a multiparametric approach (*i.e.* growth and proliferation assays, PKA, and PKA subunit assays, cAMP and ^{3}H-cAMP binding assays, and apoptosis assays) to understand the growth and proliferative effects of 8-Cl-ADO on human B-lymphocytes.

Results.—8-Cl-ADO inhibited proliferation, mainly through its intracellular transport and metabolism, which induced apoptosis. PKA activity, cAMP levels, and ^{3}H-cAMP binding were increased or decreased, respectively, by 8-Cl-ADO, whereas PKA subunit levels were differentially affected. 8-Cl-ADO also inhibited proliferation induced by G protein-coupled receptors for isoproterenol and adenosine, as well as proliferation induced by tyrosine kinase receptors.

Conclusions.—8-Cl-ADO in addition to unambiguously inhibiting proliferation and inducing apoptosis in a PKA-independent manner also has PKA-dependent effects that are unmasked by a mutant *PRKAR1A*. Thus, 8-Cl-ADO could serve as a therapeutic agent in patients with Carney complex-related tumors.

▶ Carney complex is characterized by primary pigmented micronodular adrenocortical hyperplasia (PPMAH) with Cushing's syndrome. The adrenal pathology is characterized by normal-weight glands, multiple functioning nodules <10 mm in size, internodular cortical atrophy, and brown intracellular pigment (lipofuscin). The Cushing's syndrome is adrenocorticotropic hormone (ACTH) independent with normal or high cortisol. Cortisol levels may increase paradoxically with dexamethasone in contrast to the suppression observed with pituitary ACTH-dependent disease or in people with normal hypothalamic-pituitary-adrenal (HPA) axis function. In addition to adrenal disease, patients may present with growth hormone-secreting pituitary adenomas, Sertoli cell calcifying testicular tumors, cardiac myxomas, pigmented cutaneous lesions (lentigo and blue nevi), cutaneous myxomas, and melanotic schwannomas. This familial disease has autosomal dominant transmission and is determined by inactivating germline mutation of protein kinase A-R1 alpha subunit (*PRKAR1A*) with genetic loci in 17q24 and 2p16 chromosomes. Protein kinase A (*PKA*) functions as a tumor suppressor gene and mutations lead to multiple neoplastic manifestations. The study by Robinson-White et al tests whether 8-Cl-adenosine can be used to inhibit proliferation and tumor formation in Carney tumors. Using transformed B lymphocytes from normal subjects and patients with Carney complex, they tested whether the compound inhibits lymphocyte proliferation and induces apoptosis in the Carney cells. 8-Cl-adenosine is an analogue of cAMP. It penetrates the cell membrane via facilitated diffusion through specialized membrane nucleoside carrier proteins termed equilibrate nucleoside transporters (ENTs) for subsequent metabolism via 3 main pathways, 2 of which lead to apoptosis as the main mechanism for inhibition of proliferation. Another mechanism involves alteration of the PKA pathway, 1 of the main defects in Carney tumors. This study nicely investigates the mechanism by which 8-Cl-adenosine induces inhibition of cell proliferation in vitro and provides proof of concept for potential testing in vivo and eventual targeted therapy for Carney tumors. The conclusions of the study need to be considered tentative, and the future of 8-Cl-adenosine as a therapeutic target for Carney complex is still to be determined, but it offers an interesting approach to therapy based on the molecular pathology uncovered in Carney tumors.

D. E. Schteingart, MD

Clinical and genetic heterogeneity, overlap with other tumor syndromes, and atypical glucocorticoid hormone secretion in adrenocorticotropin-independent macronodular adrenal hyperplasia compared with other adrenocortical tumors

Hsiao HP, Kirschner LS, Bourdeau I, et al (Natl Insts of Health, Bethesda, MD; Ohio State Univ, Columbus; Centre Hospitalier de l'Université de Montréal, Québec, Canada)

J Clin Endocrinol Metab 94:2930-2937, 2009

Objective.—ACTH-independent macronodular adrenal hyperplasia (AIMAH) is often associated with subclinical cortisol secretion or atypical Cushing's syndrome (CS). We characterized a large series of patients of AIMAH and compared them with patients with other adrenocortical tumors.

Design and Patients.—We recruited 82 subjects with: 1) AIMAH (n = 16); 2) adrenocortical cortisol-producing adenoma with CS (n = 15); 3) aldosterone-producing adenoma (n = 19); and 4) single adenomas with clinically nonsignificant cortisol secretion (n = 32).

Methods.—Urinary free cortisol (UFC) and 17-hydroxycorticosteroid (17OHS) were collected at baseline and during dexamethasone testing; aberrant receptor responses were also sought by clinical testing and confirmed molecularly. Peripheral and/or tumor DNA was sequenced for candidate genes.

Results.—AIMAH patients had the highest 17OHS excretion, even when UFCs were within or close to the normal range. Aberrant receptor expression was highly prevalent. Histology showed at least two subtypes of AIMAH. For three patients with AIMAH, there was family history of CS; germline mutations were identified in three other patients in the genes for menin (one), fumarate hydratase (one), and adenomatosis polyposis coli (*APC*) (one); a *PDE11A* gene variant was found in another. One patient had a *GNAS* mutation in adrenal nodules only. There were no mutations in any of the tested genes in the patients of the other groups.

Conclusions.—AIMAH is a clinically and genetically heterogeneous disorder that can be associated with various genetic defects and aberrant hormone receptors. It is frequently associated with atypical CS and increased 17OHS; UFCs and other measures of adrenocortical activity can be misleadingly normal.

▶ This is an interesting study of 82 patients admitted to the National Institutes of Health (NIH) between 2000 and 2008 for macronodular adrenal hyperplasia and adrenal cortical tumors. Some of the patients had adrenocorticotropic hormone (ACTH)-independent Cushing's syndrome and others had primary aldosteronism or nonfunctioning adenomas. The study attempted to compare ACTH-independent macronodular adrenal hyperplasia (AIMAH) with the other tumors using clinical, radiographic, biochemical, and genetic data, including determination of genetic mutations and identification of aberrant receptors. Several of the patients with AIMAH had germline mutations (multiple endocrine neoplasia I [*MEN-1*], fumarate hydratase, adenomatous polyposis [*APC*], and G-protein alpha-subunit [*GNAS*]). In contrast, there were no mutations detected in the other types of tumors. Aberrant receptors were prevalent among patients with AIMAH, the most common being vasopressin. Noteworthy in this series is the heterogeneity of the clinical, histological, and molecular presentations. The 2 histological subtypes include large nodules with internodular cortical atrophy and large nodules with internodular cortical hyperplasia. Biochemically, elevated urinary 17-hydroxycorticoid excretion was more the reliable expression of function than urinary-free cortisol, but the reason is unclear because 17-hydroxysteroids are less specific a measurement of cortisol secretion. The response to ovine CRH (oCRH) was not helpful in discriminating among various subtypes of pathology. Patients with higher cortisol production, as expected, had greater suppression of response. The importance of the study lies in the number of cases collected and some of the descriptive data but other than indicating heterogeneity, it does not shed new light on the pathogenesis of the syndrome of adrenal cortical nodular hyperplasia or adrenal tumorigenesis.

D. E. Schteingart, MD

Autoimmunity and Addison's Disease

A subnormal peak cortisol response to stimulation testing does not predict a subnormal cortisol production rate

Paisley AN, Rowles SV, Brandon D, et al (Christie Hosp, Manchester, UK)
J Clin Endocrinol Metab 94:1757-1760, 2009

Introduction.—The decision to commence lifelong glucocorticoid replacement therapy is often based on a cortisol stimulation test. We investigated the relationship between the peak cortisol response to insulin-induced hypoglycemia and daily cortisol production rate (CPR) to ascertain whether provocative tests are accurate in indicating the need to initiate lifelong glucocorticoid replacement.

Patients and Methods.—Ten patients (five male; mean age, 44 ± 13 yr) with pituitary disease and with demonstrably suboptimal peak cortisol response (350-500 nmol/liter) to insulin-induced hypoglycemia, underwent CPR measurement by isotope dilution using gas chromatography-mass spectrometry and 24-h urinary free cortisol (UFC).

Results.—The median baseline and peak cortisol attained with hypoglycemia were 284 (164-323) and 473.5 (366-494) nmol/liter, respectively. A strong positive correlation was seen between peak stimulated cortisol and CPR (adjusted for body surface area) ($r = 0.75$; $P = 0.02$), and in all patients CPR [4.6 (2.9-15.1) mg/d × m(2)] was within the reference range (2.1-12 mg/d × m(2)) or elevated (one patient). A wide range was found for 24-h UFC [116.5 (20.5-265.9) nmol/liter] in this group of patients, and this parameter lacked significant correlation with either serum cortisol concentration or CPR.

Conclusion.—This is the first study to demonstrate a significant correlation between CPR and peak cortisol values during hypoglycemic challenge. An inadequate cortisol response to hypoglycemia suggests the need for glucocorticoid cover at times of stress, but these data indicate that a suboptimal peak cortisol does not equate to a low CPR and should not be an automatic indication for lifelong glucocorticoid replacement therapy. UFC bears no relation to serum cortisol or CPR and is therefore unhelpful in assessment of such patients.

▶ We measure adrenal function taking into account several indices of cortisol secretion such as serum cortisol, urinary free cortisol, urinary excretion of cortisol metabolites, and the response of cortisol to stimulation with synthetic corticotropin and corticotropin-releasing hormone. The hypothalamic-pituitary-adrenal system is complex, and a single measurement does not tell the whole story but only 1 aspect of it. Measurement of cortisol production rates (CPR) has been possible for more than 50 years since they were first introduced by Cope and Black. Their procedure was based on a single-injection isotope dilution technique, with several caveats for proper interpretation. Normal range of production as calculated by this method was 12 to 22 mg/d. More recently, Paisley et al have used a method using a deuterated cortisol infusion over 24 hours that allows them to measure production rates over a 24-hour period. The calculated production rates thus obtained are lower than with previous methods—around 10 mg/d. These values correlate with peak cortisol values during hypoglycemia stimulation. The study concludes that patients with subnormal cortisol responses to hypoglycemia may not have a decreased CPR and should not automatically receive glucocorticoid replacement. They also dismiss the use of urinary-free cortisol to calculate the dose of cortisol during cortisol replacement. Experience teaches us otherwise. Measurement of urinary-free cortisol has been clinically useful to monitor the optimal dose of hydrocortisone to be administered in situations of primary or secondary adrenal insufficiency. Anecdotal reports relate patients who developed signs and symptoms of Cushing's disease during replacement with standard doses of cortisol and whose urinary-free cortisol was several fold above normal. Symptoms disappeared when the dose was adjusted in order to bring the urinary-free cortisol into the normal range. Measurement of CPR as proposed in this study is not clinically convenient and requires a specialized laboratory. Hypoglycemia is a good stress but uncomfortable to patients and dangerous to those with panhypopituitarism in whom glucose counterregulation is impaired. A safer method for testing these patients is a low-dose corticotropin stimulation test and measurement of urinary-free cortisol.

D. E. Schteingart, MD

Measurement of salivary cortisol with liquid chromatography-tandem mass spectrometry in patients undergoing dynamic endocrine testing

Perogamvros I, Owen LJ, Keevil BG, et al (Christie Hosp, Manchester, UK; Univ Hosp of South Manchester, UK)
Clin Endocrinol 72:17-21, 2010

Objective.—Liquid chromatography-tandem mass spectrometry (LC-MS/MS) eliminates cross-reactivity, which is a major limitation of immunoassays used for the measurement of salivary cortisol (SalC). We aimed to evaluate the potential of SalC measured by LC-MS/MS in patients undergoing assessment of the HPA axis.

Design and Patients.—Cross-sectional study of 78 patients admitted for routine testing in a specialized endocrine unit.

Measurements.—Matched serum and saliva samples were collected from 68 patients who had a short synacthen test (SST, 250 mcg im) and 10 patients who had an insulin tolerance test (ITT, insulin 0·15 U/kg iv). Serum cortisol (SerC) was measured with an automated immunoassay and SalC with LC-MS/MS. Adequate SerC responses were >500 nmol/l.

Results.—In all patients with adequate responses, the relative increase in SalC was significantly higher than that in SerC [6·4(0·3–26·1) *vs.* 1·0(0·3–4·9), $P < 0 \cdot 0001$)]. The SerC–SalC relationship was better explained by an exponential rather than a linear model ($R^2 = 0 \cdot 83$ *vs.* $R^2 = 0 \cdot 65$, both $P < 0 \cdot 0001$). Based on 59 patients with adequate SerC responses to an SST, an adequate SalC response was defined as 8·3 nmol/l. Seven patients following an SST and three patients following an ITT showed inadequate responses in both SerC and SalC, but two patients with CBG deficiency showed a low SerC with normal SalC.

Conclusions.—We have shown an excellent diagnostic sensitivity and specificity of LC-MS/MS SalC in the assessment of the HPA axis and superiority over SerC when CBG levels are altered. The exponential relationship between SerC and SalC supports the concept of CBG binding capacity saturation.

▶ Accurate measurement of cortisol is essential for proper interpretation of its concentration, especially when levels are minimally elevated or low. Another challenge is whether the measurement is in serum, saliva, or urine. Measurements in serum reflect total cortisol (protein bound 96% and free 4%) and can be affected by oral contraceptives, pregnancy, and familial decrease in corticosteroid-binding globulin (CBG), conditions that increase or decrease protein binding. In contrast, cortisol levels in urine and saliva reflect the level of free cortisol. The usefulness of measuring free cortisol is that as levels of total cortisol increase, there is a disproportionate increase in the free fraction as the CBG binding capacity is saturated. The relationship between total and free cortisol is exponential rather than linear. The study by Perogamvros et al confirms the sensitivity and specificity of salivary cortisol measured by liquid chromatography-tandem mass spectrometry (LC/MS), a procedure that eliminates cross reactivity with other steroids and can be used effectively under conditions of dynamic testing.

D. E. Schteingart, MD

Modified-release hydrocortisone to provide circadian cortisol profiles

Debono M, Ghobadi C, Rostami-Hodjegan A, et al (Univ of Sheffield, UK; et al)

J Clin Endocrinol Metab 94:1548-1554, 2009

Context.—Cortisol has a distinct circadian rhythm regulated by the brain's central pacemaker. Loss of this rhythm is associated with metabolic abnormalities, fatigue, and poor quality of life. Conventional glucocorticoid replacement cannot replicate this rhythm.

Objectives.—Our objectives were to define key variables of physiological cortisol rhythm, and by pharmacokinetic modeling test whether modified-release hydrocortisone (MR-HC) can provide circadian cortisol profiles.

Setting.—The study was performed at a Clinical Research Facility.

Design and Methods.—Using data from a cross-sectional study in healthy reference subjects (n = 33), we defined parameters for the cortisol rhythm. We then tested MR-HC against immediate-release hydrocortisone in healthy volunteers (n = 28) in an open-label, randomized, single-dose, cross-over study. We compared profiles with physiological cortisol levels, and modeled an optimal treatment regimen.

Results.—The key variables in the physiological cortisol profile included: peak 15.5 μg/dl (95% reference range 11.7–20.6), acrophase 0832 h (95% confidence interval 0759–0905), nadir less than 2 μg/dl (95% refence range 1.5–2.5), time of nadir 0018 h (95% confidence interval 2339–0058), and quiescent phase (below the mesor) 1943–0531 h. MR-HC 15 mg demonstrated delayed and sustained release with a mean (SEM) maximum observed concentration of 16.6 (1.4) μg/dl at 7.41 (0.57) h after drug. Bioavailability of MR-HC 5, 10, and 15 mg was 100, 79, and 86% that of immediate-release hydrocortisone. Modeling suggested that MR-HC 15–20 mg at 2300 h and 10 mg at 0700 h could reproduce physiological cortisol levels.

Conclusion.—By defining circadian rhythms and using modern formulation technology, it is possible to allow a more physiological circadian replacement of cortisol.

▶ Patients with adrenal insufficiency usually get replacement with hydrocortisone and fludrocortisone in standard doses. For hydrocortisone the dose is 20 to 25 mg in 3 unequally divided doses, and for fludrocortisone the dose is 0.05 to 0.2 mg/d. The smallest dose of hydrocortisone is administered in the evening to replicate a normal circadian rhythm. Every case requires customizing the dose according to the patient's response. Urinary-free cortisol and plasma renin are helpful in determining optimal replacement. The objective of normal replacement is to tailor the dose of hydrocortisone so that the urinary-free cortisol is in the middle of the normal range and to adjust the dose of fludrocortisone so that the renin concentration is normal. With standard replacement, patients occasionally complain of chronic fatigue, muscle aches, and tendency to hypoglycemia or symptoms of Cushing's syndrome. We prefer to use the shorter acting hydrocortisone rather than the longer acting prednisone or dexamethasone for greater flexibility of dosing. Hydrocortisone also allows for measurement of urinary-free cortisol. It is uncertain if the symptoms that patients complain of while on steroid replacement for adrenal insufficiency are due to an inability of these steroids to restore a normal circadian rhythm. Debono et al introduce a novel modified-release hydrocortisone preparation. Based on pharmacokinetic modeling, they recommend a twice-daily regimen with doses administered at 07:00 and 23:00 hours. Data will be needed to determine if patients treated with this preparation experience more normal metabolic parameters and better quality of life than those treated with the standard preparation.

D. E. Schteingart, MD

Cushing's Disease: Diagnosis and Treatment

Patients with Cushing's syndrome are care-intensive even in the era of laparoscopic adrenalectomy

Kissane NA, Cendan JC (Univ of Florida College of Medicine, Gainesville)
Am Surg 75:279-283, 2009

We report outcomes from laparoscopic adrenalectomy (LA) comparing patients with Cushing's syndrome with those with other adrenal pathology with respect to length of stay (LOS), overall complications, and financial implications. We conducted a retrospective review of 80 continuous patients (103 glands) undergoing LA. The clinical diagnoses were: hypercortisolism (Cushing' syndrome; n=33), hyperaldosteronism (Conn's syndrome; n=20), phaeochromocytoma (n=16), and neoplasm (others; n=11). Advanced care in the intermediate or intensive care unit was necessary in 27 patients, most frequently in our Cushing's population (16 of 33 [48%]). Six patients sustained major complications, including death in two patients; seven patients sustained minor complications. LOS was longer for patients with Cushing's syndrome (mean, 5.5 vs. 3.3 days; $P = 0.024$). Financially, patients with Cushing's syndrome had statistically higher total hospital ($P = 0.009$), advanced care ($P = 0.002$), and anesthetic costs ($P = 0.005$). LA in patients with Cushing's syndrome is associated with longer hospitalizations, more frequent major complications, and higher advanced care requirements, especially for patients undergoing bilateral adrenalectomy. Minor complications were infrequent and median LOS was brief regardless of diagnosis. Patients with Cushing's syndrome had higher costs for overall hospital charges, advanced care, and anesthesia.

▶ Laparoscopic adrenalectomy is the treatment of choice for patients with functioning adrenal cortical adenomas, Cushing's syndrome, or primary aldosteronism. Bilateral adrenalectomies can also be performed laparoscopically. In contrast, open adrenalectomy is recommended in all cases of suspected or confirmed adrenal cortical carcinoma. Laparoscopic adrenalectomy in such patients carries an increased risk of local recurrence or peritoneal spread. Kissane and Cendan report that the postoperative course of patients with Cushing's syndrome is fraught with more complications, longer length of stay, and higher cost. This is due to the greater morbidity associated with chronic cortisol excess and the susceptibility of these patients to acute problems. The complications may be systemic and metabolic as well as local because of infection, bleeding, and delayed wound healing. Whenever possible, these patients should be pretreated with adrenal suppressive drugs for a period of time to normalize cortisol levels and reverse some of the more serious metabolic components of Cushing's syndrome. This approach may improve glucose levels, blood pressure, and electrolytes and correct the patient's catabolic state. Patients with primary aldosteronism should be pretreated with mineralocorticoid receptor antagonists, such as spironolactone or eplerenone, which may render patients more stable in terms of potassium levels and hypertension.

D. E. Schteingart, MD

Persistent Adrenocorticotropin Response to Desmopressin in the Early Postoperative Period Predicts Recurrence of Cushing's Disease

Losa M, Bianchi R, Barzaghi R, et al (Università Vita-Salute, Milano, Italy)
J Clin Endocrinol Metab 94:3322-3328, 2009

Context.—Patients with Cushing's disease (CD) often show an ACTH and cortisol response to desmopressin (DDAVP).

Objective.—We tested whether persistence of a positive response to DDAVP after successful surgery identifies patients at risk of CD recurrence.

Design.—We prospectively included all CD patients who had a positive response to DDAVP before successful surgery from 1995 through 2007.

Setting.—The study was performed at a university hospital.

Patients.—One hundred seventy-four patients with CD, 148 women and 26 men, mean age 36.1 ± 0.8 yr, were studied. The median follow-up after surgery was 58 months (interquartile range 22–93 months).

Intervention.—DDAVP test was performed immediately before and after surgery.

Main Outcome Measure.—An ACTH and cortisol increment of at least 30 and 20% above baseline, respectively, were considered as a positive response to DDAVP. The risk of CD recurrence was analyzed according to the postoperative hormonal response to DDAVP.

Results.—Recurrence of CD occurred in 19 patients (10.9%). The recurrence-free survival at 5 yr was 89.8% [95% confidence interval (CI) 84.2–95.4]. Patients with a positive ACTH response had a 5-yr recurrence-free survival of 82.6% (95% CI 70.6–94.6%) as compared with 94.0% (95% CI 88.2–99.8%; $P < 0.01$) in patients without it. Multivariate analysis showed that persistence of a positive ACTH response to DDAVP was significantly associated with CD recurrence.

Conclusion.—Positive ACTH response to DDAVP after surgery is associated with an increased risk of CD recurrence. However, the specificity and predictive value of this finding are low.

► Success of transsphenoidal pituitary surgery (TSS) in patients with Cushing's disease can be determined by withdrawing steroids immediately after surgery and measuring adrenocorticotropic hormone (ACTH) and cortisol levels. Complete suppression of these levels has been an indication of successful surgery and long-term remission. In 10% to 20% of patients, active Cushing's disease persists after TSS and in another 10% Cushing's disease recurs after 6 to 36 months. Persistence of Cushing's disease is seen particularly in patients operated by inexperienced surgeons and in those with pituitary macroadenomas, in whom complete tumor resection is difficult. Recurrence has been observed even in patients who had demonstrated postoperatively suppressed ACTH and cortisol levels and restoration of suppressibility with dexamethasone. The recurrence is caused by regrowth of tumor in the same location as the original tumor, suggesting incomplete resection. As proposed by Losa et al, an alternative postoperative testing method consists of stimulation of ACTH secretion by desmopressin, a long-acting vasopressin analog active mainly in tumor cells but not in normal corticotropes. Response to desmopressin after TSS has helped to identify patients who will experience recurrence of Cushing's syndrome. In a study of 174 patients, those with persistence of response to desmopressin after TSS had a higher probability of recurrence. The limiting usefulness of this test was a relatively low sensitivity and specificity.

D. E. Schteingart, MD

Specificity of Screening Tests for Cushing's Syndrome in an Overweight and Obese Population

Baid SK, Rubino D, Sinaii N, et al (Natl Insts of Health, Bethesda, MD; The George Washington Univ Weight Management Program, DC)
J Clin Endocrinol Metab 94:3857-3864, 2009

Context.—Recent reports suggest a higher prevalence (1–5%) of Cushing's syndrome in certain patient populations with features of the disorder (*e.g.*, diabetes), but the prevalence in the over-weight and obese population is not known.

Objective.—The aim of the study was to evaluate the diagnostic performance of screening tests for Cushing's syndrome in overweight and obese subjects with at least two other features of the disorder.

Design and Setting.—We conducted a cross-sectional prospective study.

Subjects and Methods.—A total of 369 subjects (73% female) completed two or three tests: a 24-h urine cortisol, and/or late-night salivary cortisol, and/or 1 mg dexamethasone suppression test (DST). If any result was abnormal [based on laboratory reference range or cortisol after DST $\geq$1.8 μg/dl (50 nmol/liter)], tests were repeated and/or a dexamethasone-CRH test was performed. Subjects with abnormal DST results and a low dexamethasone level were asked to repeat the test with 2 mg of dexamethasone.

Results.—In addition to obesity, subjects had a mean of five to six features of Cushing's syndrome. None was found to have Cushing's syndrome. Test specificities to exclude Cushing's syndrome for subjects who completed three tests were: urine cortisol, 96% [95% confidence interval (CI), 93–98%]; DST, 90% (95% CI, 87–93%); salivary cortisol, 84% by RIA (95% CI, 79–89%) and 92% by liquid chromatography-tandem mass spectrometry (95% CI, 88–95%). The combined specificity (both tests normal) for all combinations of two tests was 84 to 90%, with overlapping CIs.

Conclusion.—These data do not support widespread screening of overweight and obese subjects for Cushing's syndrome; test results for such patients may be falsely abnormal.

▶ Patients who frequently appear to have Cushing's syndrome are frequently referred to specialized endocrine centers for evaluation. While the most severe cases can be easily diagnosed, borderline cases are much more challenging. The clinical manifestations of Cushing's syndrome involve nonspecific as well as specific symptoms and signs of hypercortisolism. Nonspecific findings include generalized obesity and hypertension, insulin-resistant diabetes mellitus, fatigue, irregular menses, hirsutism, irritability and depression, and all frequent comorbidities of obesity. The specific symptoms involve evidence of protein catabolism such as proximal muscle weakness, muscle atrophy, easy bruising, skin atrophy, atrophic striae, and osteopenia. Given the high prevalence of obesity and its comorbidities, the possibility of Cushing's syndrome should be considered and investigated by sensitive and specific diagnostic testing. This is what Baid et al have done in a series of 369 obese subjects attending a weight loss clinic who presented with at least 2 other features of Cushing's syndrome. In addition to obesity, these subjects had 5 to 6 features of Cushing's syndrome. Diagnostic studies included bedtime salivary cortisol, 24-hour urine cortisol, 1-mg dexamethasone suppression test, and Dex-CRH test. Some of these tests were repeated several times, and higher dose dexamethasone suppression was used in some cases. True Cushing's syndrome was rare. The conclusion of this elaborate study is that it did not support widespread screening of overweight and obese subjects for Cushing's syndrome. Results may be abnormal because of pseudo-Cushing's associated with obesity, a condition still not completely understood. The problem with the conclusion of this study is that patients with true Cushing's syndrome may not be diagnosed for at least 2 to 3 years and their symptoms were attributed to changes in eating habits, aging, hypothyroidism, depression, etc. I prefer to have a low threshold of suspicion and screen patients with at least a 2-hour urinary free cortisol and 1-mg dexamethasone suppression test. Patients can be quite miserable while they wait for a correct diagnosis and appropriate treatment.

D. E. Schteingart, MD

Use of morning serum cortisol level after transsphenoidal resection of pituitary adenoma to predict the need for long-term glucocorticoid supplementation

Marko NF, Gonugunta VA, Hamrahian AH, et al (Cleveland Clinic, OH)
J Neurosurg 111:540-544, 2009

Object.—Accurate assessment of the hypothalamic-pituitary-adrenal (HPA) axis is critical for appropriate management of the disease in patients with pituitary adenoma after transsphenoidal resection. The authors examine the role of the morning total serum cortisol level in the early post-operative period as a predictor of long-term HPA function.

Methods.—Morning total serum cortisol was measured in 83 patients on postoperative Day 1 (or Day 2 if the patient received glucocorticoids during surgery) after transsphenoidal surgery for pituitary adenoma. These results were compared with those of definitive assays of HPA function performed at 1–3 months postoperatively, including cortrosyn/synacthen stimulation test (CST), insulin tolerance test (ITT), and metyrapone test (MTT). The ability of the early-postoperative morning cortisol level to predict HPA function was determined using standard confusion matrix calculations and receiver-operator control curve analysis.

Results.—The authors found that an early postoperative morning total cortisol level ≥ 15 μg/dl is a sensitive and accurate predictor of normal HPA function in the postoperative period (sensitivity 80.5%, specificity 66.7%, positive predictive value 96.9%).

Conclusions.—A morning total cortisol level ≥ 15 μg/dl in the early postoperative period after transsphenoidal surgery for pituitary adenomas is a good predictor of normal HPA function. This test has good sensitivity and accuracy and correlates well with the results of additional, definitive assays of HPA function (CST, ITT, and MTT) performed at 1–3 months postoperatively. Accordingly, it is the authors' practice to avoid exogenous perioperative glucocorticoid supplementation in patients with normal preoperative HPA function and postoperative morning total cortisol levels ≥ 15 μg/dl 1–2 days after transsphenoidal pituitary adenomectomy.

▶ Patients who undergo pituitary surgery for a pituitary adenoma run the risk of hypopituitarism. Of the various pituitary hormone deficiencies, secondary adrenal insufficiency is the immediately serious condition. Patients are usually covered with glucocorticoid replacement until such time they can be properly tested. However, prolonged replacement may by itself induce secondary adrenal insufficiency. The question is when and how to test these patients. Marko et al propose testing patients undergoing transsphenoidal surgery for non-Cushing's pituitary adenomas immediately after surgery. They do not cover patients with glucocorticoids and test their adrenal function immediately after surgery. A postoperative cortisol level > 15 μg/dL predicts normal function several months later. Risk of hypopituitarism is greater in patients with pituitary macroadenomas. Other pituitary hormones also need to be tested and replaced if necessary. A combined pituitary function test could be a useful means of assessing the postoperative integrity of pituitary function.

D. E. Schteingart, MD

Pheochromocytomas: Diagnosis and Treatment

6-[F-18]Fluoro-L-Dihydroxyphenylalanine Positron Emission Tomography Is Superior to Conventional Imaging with ^{123}I-Metaiodobenzylguanidine Scintigraphy, Computer Tomography, and Magnetic Resonance Imaging in Localizing Tumors Causing Catecholamine Excess

Fiebrich H-B, Brouwers AH, Kerstens MN, et al (Univ Med Ctr Groningen, The Netherlands; et al)

J Clin Endocrinol Metab 94:3922-3930, 2009

Context.—Catecholamine excess is rare, but symptoms may be life threatening.

Objective.—The objective of the study was to investigate the sensitivity of 6-[F-18]fluoro-L-dihydroxyphenylalanine positron emission tomography (^{18}F-DOPAPET), compared with ^{123}I-metaiodobenzylguanidine (^{123}I-MIBG) scintigraphy and computer tomography (CT)/magnetic resonance imaging (MRI) for tumor localization in patients with catecholamine excess.

Design and Setting.—All consecutive patients with catecholamine excess visiting the University Medical Center Groningen, Groningen, The Netherlands, between March 2003 and January 2008 were eligible.

Patients.—Forty-eight patients were included. The final diagnosis was pheochromocytoma in 40, adrenal hyperplasia in two, paraganglioma in two, ganglioneuroma in one, and unknown in three.

Main Outcome Measures.—Sensitivities and discordancy between ^{18}F-DOPA PET, ^{123}I-MIBG, and CT or MRI were analyzed for individual patients and lesions. Metanephrines and 3-methoxytyramine in plasma and urine and uptake of ^{18}F-DOPAwith PET were measured to determine the whole-body metabolic burden and correlated with biochemical tumor activity. The gold standard was a composite reference standard.

Results.—^{18}F-DOPA PET showed lesions in 43 patients, ^{123}I-MIBG in 31, and CT/MRI in 32. Patient-based sensitivity for ^{18}F-DOPA PET, ^{123}I-MIBG, and CT/MRI was 90, 65, and 67% ($P < 0.01$ for ^{18}F-DOPA PET *vs.* both ^{123}I-MIBG and CT/MRI, $P = 1.0$ ^{123}I-MIBG *vs.* CT/MRI). Lesion-based sensitivities were 73, 48, and 44% ($P = 0.001$ for ^{18}F-DOPA PET *vs.* both ^{123}I-MIBG and CT/MRI, $P = 0.51$ ^{123}I-MIBG *vs.* CT/MRI). The combination of ^{18}F-DOPA PET with CT/MRI was superior to ^{123}I-MIBG with CT/MRI (93 *vs.* 76%, $P < 0.001$). Whole-body metabolic burden measured with ^{18}F-DOPA PET correlated with plasma normetanephrine ($r = 0.82$), urinary normetanephrine ($r = 0.84$), and metanephrine ($r = 0.57$).

Conclusion.—To localize tumors causing catecholamine excess, ^{18}F-DOPA PET is superior to ^{123}I-MIBG scintigraphy and CT/MRI.

▶ The diagnosis of pheochromocytoma should be established first by the accurate assessment of catecholamine excess, using plasma-free and urinary normetanephrine measurements. It is important to understand the pitfalls and confounding factors in the measurement of catecholamines, including diet, renal function, etc. Localization of the lesion usually involves imaging with CT/MRI and in questionable cases, ^{123}I-MIBG. The study by Fiebrich et al proposes a new imaging technique with [18F] DOPA PET that shows greater sensitivity than MIBG (90% vs 65%). The combination of [18F] DOPA PET and CT/MRI was superior to MIBG/CT/MRI (93% vs 76%).

The majority of pheochromocytomas are intra-adrenal and easily detected using CT/MRI. MIBG scanning is useful only in questionable cases where it is uncertain whether the adrenal lesion is cortical or medullary. MIBG and [18F] DOPA PET are of maximal use in the detection of extra-adrenal pheos and paragangliomas in familial cases and in patients with metastatic malignant pheochromocytomas.

D. E. Schteingart, MD

Clinical Predictors and Algorithm for the Genetic Diagnosis of Pheochromocytoma Patients

Erlic Z, for the European-American Pheochromocytoma Study Group (Albert-Ludwigs-Univ, Freiburg, Germany; et al)

Clin Cancer Res 15:6378-6385, 2009

Purpose.—Six pheochromocytoma susceptibility genes causing distinct syndromes have been identified; approximately one of three of all pheochromocytoma patients carry a predisposing germline mutation. When four major genes (*VHL*, *RET*, *SDHB*, *SDHD*) are analyzed in a clinical laboratory, costs are ~$3,400 per patient. The aim of the study is to systematically obtain a robust algorithm to identify who should be genetically tested, and to determine the order in which genes should be tested.

Experimental Design.—DNA from 989 apparently nonsyndromic patients were scanned for germline mutations in the genes *VHL*, *RET*, *SDHB*, *SDHC*, and *SDHD*. Clinical parameters were analyzed as potential predictors for finding mutations by multiple logistic regression, validated by bootstrapping. Cost reduction was calculated between prioritized gene testing compared with that for all genes.

Results.—Of 989 apparently nonsyndromic pheochromocytoma cases, 187 (19%) harbored germline mutations. Predictors for presence of mutation are age <45 years, multiple pheochromocytoma, extra-adrenal location, and previous head and neck paraganglioma. If we used the presence of any one predictor as indicative of proceeding with gene testing, then 342 (34.6%) patients would be excluded, and only 8 carriers (4.3%) would be missed. We were also able to statistically model the priority of genes to be tested given certain clinical features. E.g., for patients with prior head and neck paraganglioma, the priority would be *SDHD*>*SDHB*>*RET*>*VHL*. Using the clinical predictor algorithm to prioritize gene testing and order, a 44.7% cost reduction in diagnostic process can be achieved.

Conclusions.—Clinical parameters can predict for mutation carriers and help prioritize gene testing to reduce costs in nonsyndromic pheochromocytoma presentations.

▶ Most pheochromocytomas are sporadic benign adrenal medullary tumors but 10% are malignant, 10% extra-adrenal, and 10% familial. Some of these cases are part of a syndrome and accompanied by syndromic clinical manifestations, such as in neurofibromatosis 1, von Hippel-Landau disease, multiple endocrine neoplasia (MEN 2 a and b), and the paraganglioma/pheochromocytoma syndrome. These genetic conditions have a well-characterized germline mutation leading to the syndrome, and genetic testing is important to detect family members not yet affected. Among the apparently sporadic cases, germline mutations may also be present in 19% of the cases. Although endocrine genetic evaluation and testing is recommended in cases of extra-adrenal pheochromocytoma, multiple pheochromocytomas, and a history of head and neck paraganglioma, carrying out this testing in every case can be costly. The study by Erlic et al for the European-American Pheochromocytoma Study Group focuses on 989 nonsyndromic cases and attempts to prioritize which genes should be tested to reduce the cost of the diagnostic process. These data are important to create a more cost-effective diagnostic evaluation of such patients.

D. E. Schteingart, MD

Primary Aldosteronism

Aldosterone Contributes to Blood Pressure Variance and to Likelihood of Hypertension in Normal-Weight and Overweight African Americans

Kidambi S, Kotchen JM, Krishnaswami S, et al (Med College of Wisconsin, Milwaukee)

Am J Hypertens 22:1303-1308, 2009

Background.—Hypertension and obesity are highly prevalent among African Americans (AAs). We have previously reported that both plasma aldosterone (PA) and body mass index (BMI) are higher in hypertensive than in normotensive AAs. This study evaluates the relative contributions of adiposity and PA to hypertension in AAs.

Methods.—A total of 466 AAs (50% hypertensive, 51% women) were evaluated in a Clinical Research Center by stratifying them into three subgroups based on BMI (normal weight, overweight, and obese). Anthropometric measurements, ambulatory blood pressure (BP), fasting glucose, insulin, 24-h urine sodium and potassium, creatinine clearance, standing PA and plasma renin activity (PRA) were measured. Insulin resistance was estimated by the homeostasis model assessment.

Results.—Compared to normotensives, hypertensives had higher BMI, waist circumference (WC), and were more insulin resistant ($P \leq 0.01$). When stratified by BMI, hypertensives in each BMI strata had higher PA ($P \leq 0.05$) and lower PRA ($P \leq 0.01$) compared to normotensives. Compared to normotensives, WC was greater in overweight and obese hypertensives, but not in normal-weight hypertensives. In the overall sample, age, WC, PA, and PRA were the major contributors to BP variance and to hypertension. Among normal-weight subjects, PA and PRA significantly predicted BP and the odds ratio for hypertension, whereas WC had no predictive value.

Conclusions.—PA, but not WC, is associated with BP and likelihood of hypertension in normal-weight AAs, whereas both WC and PA are predictive of hypertension in overweight and obese individuals. This suggests that aldosterone antagonists may be useful for the treatment of hypertension among AAs, regardless of BMI.

▶ Continuing with the role of aldosterone in the hypertension of normal-weight and overweight African Americans (AA), the study by Kidambi et al in 466 AA shows a link between aldosterone levels and risk of hypertension in both normal-weight and overweight individuals. Waist circumference, a measure of visceral obesity, was a concurrent factor in obese AA individuals. Together with other reports in the literature, there is evidence that because aldosterone is associated with a risk for hypertension even in the absence of primary aldosteronism, treatment with aldosterone receptor antagonists (spironolactone and eplerenone) should be considered in these patients.

D. E. Schteingart, MD

Aldosterone status associated with insulin resistance in patients with heart failure—data from the ALOFT study

Freel EM, Tsorlalis IK, Lewsey JD, et al (Univ of Glasgow, UK; et al)

Heart 95:1920-1924, 2009

Background.—Aldosterone has a key role in the pathophysiology of heart failure. In around 50% of such patients, aldosterone "escapes" from inhibition by drugs that interrupt the renin-angiotensin axis; such patients have a worse clinical outcome. Insulin resistance is a risk factor in heart failure and cardiovascular disease. The relation between aldosterone status and insulin sensitivity was investigated in a cohort of heart failure patients.

Methods.—302 patients with New York Heart Association (NYHA) class II-IV heart failure on conventional therapy were randomised in the ALiskiren Observation of heart Failure Treatment study (ALOFT), designed to test the safety of a directly acting renin inhibitor. Plasma aldosterone and 24-hour urinary aldosterone excretion, as well as fasting insulin and homeostasis model assessment of insulin resistance (HOMA-IR) were measured. Subjects with aldosterone escape and high urinary aldosterone were identified according to previously accepted definitions.

Results.—20% of subjects demonstrated aldosterone escape and 34% had high urinary aldosterone levels. At baseline, there was a positive correlation between fasting insulin and plasma ($r = 0.22$ $p < 0.01$) and urinary aldosterone($r = 0.19$ $p < 0.03$). Aldosterone escape and high urinary aldosterone subjects both demonstrated higher levels of fasting insulin ($p < 0.008$, $p < 0.03$), HOMA-IR ($p < 0.06$, $p < 0.03$) and insulin-glucose ratios ($p < 0.006$, $p < 0.06$) when compared to low aldosterone counterparts. All associations remained significant when adjusted for potential confounders.

Conclusions.—This study demonstrates a novel direct relation between aldosterone status and insulin resistance in heart failure. This observation merits further study and may identify an additional mechanism that contributes to the adverse clinical outcome associated with aldosterone escape.

▶ Several articles over the past 10 years have emphasized the role of aldosterone in the pathogenesis of hypertension and cardiovascular and renal disease. The effect is not through the effect of aldosterone as a mineralocorticoid receptor agonist but a direct effect on myocardial and renal structure and function. Aldosterone antagonists, such as spironolactone and eplerenone have been suggested for the treatment of acute systolic and diastolic heart failure, refractory hypertension to antihypertensive drugs, hypertension in patients with abdominal/visceral obesity, prevention of cardiovascular events in patients with vascular disease and treatment, and prevention of cerebrovascular infarction. Significant increases in plasma aldosterone associated with decreases in plasma renin activity have been described in African-Americans with hypertension and metabolic syndrome.[1] The study by Freel et al shows an association between aldosterone and insulin resistance. In a study of 302 patients with heart failure on conventional therapy randomized into the Aliskirin Observation of Heart Failure Treatment (ALOFT) trial, there was a direct correlation between aldosterone levels and insulin resistance as measured by homeostasis model assessment (HOMA). A relationship between aldosterone and glucose tolerance was first described by Jerome Conn in patients with primary aldosteronism. It was suggested then that hypokalemia impaired insulin secretion and caused a delay in insulin release following ingestion of glucose in a pattern similar to patients with type 2 diabetes mellitus. This glucose intolerance was observed in 50% of patients with primary aldosteronism and was reversible with potassium repletion. More recently, it was shown that these patients have diminished insulin sensitivity and that aldosterone decreases expression of insulin substrate[1] and induces insulin resistance at the vascular level via oxidative stress.[2,3] Another study showed higher prevalence of metabolic syndrome in primary aldosteronism than essential hypertension.[4]

D. E. Schteingart, MD

References

1. Kidambi S, Kotchen JM, Grim CE, et al. Association of adrenal steroids with hypertension and the metabolic syndrome in blacks. *Hypertension.* 2007;49:704.
2. Mosso LM, Carvajal CA, Maiz A, et al. A possible association between primary aldosteronism and a lower beta-cell function. *J Hypertens.* 2007;25:2125-2130.

3. Hitomi H, Kiyomoto H, Nishiyama A, et al. Aldosterone suppresses insulin signaling via the downregulation of insulin receptor substrate-1 in vascular smooth muscle cells. *Hypertension*. 2007;50:750.
4. Fallo F, Veglio F, Bertello C, et al. Prevalence and characteristics of the metabolic syndrome in primary aldosteronism. *J Clin Endocrinol Metab*. 2006;91:454.

Association of Kidney Function With Residual Hypertension After Treatment of Aldosterone-Producing Adenoma

Wu V-C, on behalf of the TAIPAI Study Group (Natl Taiwan Univ Hosp, Taipei; et al)
Am J Kidney Dis 54:665-673, 2009

Background.—Autonomous secretion of aldosterone in patients with primary aldosteronism increases glomerular filtration rate and causes kidney damage. The influence of a mild decrease in kidney function on residual hypertension after adrenalectomy is unexplored.

Study Design.—Nonconcurrent prospective study.

Setting & Participants.—The study was based on the Taiwan Primary Aldosteronism Investigation (TAIPAI) database. 150 patients (61 men; overall mean age, 47.2 ± 11.6 years) with a diagnosis of aldosterone-producing adenoma had undergone unilateral adrenalectomy at National Taiwan University Hospital from July 1999 to January 2007.

Predictor.—Presurgery estimated glomerular filtration rate (eGFR).

Outcomes & Measurements.—Residual hypertension after adrenalectomy, defined either as less than 75% of recorded blood pressure measurements with systolic blood pressure less than 140 mm Hg and diastolic blood pressure less than 90 mm Hg or requiring antihypertensive medications during the first year after surgery.

Results.—Before surgery, 27 (18%), 72 (48%), and 51 (34%) patients had moderately to severely decreased (<60 mL/min/1.73 m^2), mildly decreased ($60 \leq$ eGFR < 90 mL/min/1.73 m^2), or nondecreased eGFR (≥ 90 mL/min/1.73 m^2), respectively. After surgery, 16 (59.3%), 29 (40.3%), and 10 (19.3%) patients in each category had postsurgery residual hypertension. Compared with patients without decreased eGFR before surgery, adjusted odds ratios for postsurgery residual hypertension were 2.7 (95% confidence interval, 1.03 to 7.0; $P = 0.04$) and 2.8 (95% confidence interval, 1.05 to 9.3) for mildly and moderately to severely decreased eGFR, respectively.

Limitations.—Arbitrary definition for residual hypertension.

Conclusions.—Two-thirds of patients with aldosterone-producing adenoma were cured of hypertension by means of unilateral adrenalectomy. Kidney function impairment, even mild, appears to be associated with a high incidence of postsurgery residual hypertension.

▶ Improvement of hypertension and normalization of serum potassium are observed in 100% of patients with primary aldosteronism, but cure of hypertension is found in only 50%. Possible factors proposed for the persistence of hypertension were duration of sustained hypertension and renal disease. Excess aldosterone causes cardiovascular fibrosis through increased expression of plasminogen activator inhibitor 1 (PAI-1), transforming growth factor (TGF) β1, and reactive oxygen species. The study by Wu et al from the Taiwan Primary Aldosteronism Investigation (TAIPAI) Study Group in a group of 150 patients with aldosterone-producing adenomas shows a correlation between renal damage as indicated by the decrease in glomerular filtration rate (GFR) and persistence of hypertension.

D. E. Schteingart, MD

Familial and Phenotypic Associations of the Aldosterone Renin Ratio

Alvarez-Madrazo S, Padmanabhan S, Mayosi BM, et al (Univ of Glasgow, UK; Univ of Oxford, UK; et al)

J Clin Endocrinol Metab 94:4324-4333, 2009

Context.—The aldosterone to renin ratio (ARR) is a marker of aldosterone excess, widely used to screen for primary aldosteronism (PA). The significance of a raised ARR in normotensive and hypertensive subjects and the phenotypic and familial factors affecting it are unclear.

Objective.—We estimated the distribution and heritability of the ARR and tested for associations between ARR and blood pressure (BP) with 11 polymorphisms at the *CYP11B1/CYP11B2* locus.

Design and Setting.—A total of 1172 individuals from 248 Caucasian families ascertained via a hypertensive proband were evaluated.

Main Outcome Measure.—Plasma aldosterone was measured by RIA, and plasma renin concentration was measured by the LIAISON Direct Renin chemiluminescent immunoassay.

Results.—Unadjusted and adjusted ARR were continuously distributed in normotensives and hypertensives, with no evidence of a cutoff that would identify a separate population with PA. Median ARR was 4.19 ng/liter per mIU/liter (range, 0.04–253.16). ARR levels were higher in females and associated with age, body mass index, and potassium. Antihypertensive agents had significant predictable effects on the ARR. Renin was negatively associated, and ARR was positively associated with ambulatory BP readings ($P < 0.001$) in subjects not taking antihypertensives. The heritability of the ARR was 38.1% ($P < 10^{-8}$). Plasma aldosterone, but not ARR, was influenced by the intron 2 conversion variation in the *CYP11B2* gene ($\beta = -0.07$; $P = 0.04$).

Conclusions.—The ARR is continuously distributed, is influenced by genetic and environmental factors, and is not a marker of a distinct pathological abnormality but possibly reflects the long-term influence of aldosterone on cardiovascular homeostasis.

▶ The diagnosis of primary aldosteronism (PA) is suspected in patients with hypertension and unprovoked hypokalemia and in people with drug-resistant hypertension. Over the past few decades, the prevalence of this condition has gradually increased with better detection criteria. Key in establishing the diagnosis is the combination of high aldosterone and suppressed renin with an aldosterone:renin ratio (ARR) of 20:40 and a serum aldosterone >15 ng/dL. Additional testing includes demonstration of lack of suppression of aldosterone with a saline infusion or with captopril. CT or MRI of the adrenal glands look for a single adenoma or bilateral adrenal enlargement. The possibility of subclinical aldosteronism has been entertained in patients with hypertension but normal serum electrolytes who have a relatively high ARR. The reliability of the ARR in the diagnosis of PA has been investigated in several reports. In a recent study by Rossi et al, ARR showed a highly significant within-patient correlation ($r = 0.69$; $P < .0001$) and reproducibility.[1] Only 7% of the value fell outside of the 95% confidence interval (CI) for the between-test difference and accuracy of ARR for pinpointing PA patients was 80%. The reproducibility of the ARR supports its use for screening patients with PA, but many factors may affect the result as shown by Alvarez Madrazo et al in 1172 individuals evaluated via a hypertensive proband. According to this study, the ARR is influenced by familial and phenotypic factors, which include gender, body mass index (BMI), sampling conditions, antihypertensive drugs, and estrogen status. The ARR was positively correlated with female gender, age, daytime systolic pressure, potassium, diuretics, and β-blockers and negatively correlated with BMI and angiotensin-converting enzyme (ACE) inhibitor use. ARR appears to be a strongly heritable phenomenon, but the specific genetic locus is not clearly determined. The study also finds that the adjusted ARR is a continuously distributed variable within normal and hypertensive populations, which makes it difficult to establish a cutoff point for the diagnosis of PA. Most subjects studied, regardless of blood pressure status, had an ARR of 10 and with increase in this value the proportion of hypertensive subjects also increased. It may be necessary to use other tests, such as saline infusion or captopril, to better define patients with PA.

D. E. Schteingart, MD

Reference

1. Rossi GP, Seccia TM, Palumbo G, et al. Within-patient reproducibility of the aldosterone: renin ratio in primary aldosteronism. *Hypertension*. 2010;55:83.

Rapid cortisol assays improve the success rate of adrenal vein sampling for primary aldosteronism

Auchus RJ, Michaelis C, Wians FH Jr, et al (UT Southwestern Med Ctr, Dallas, TX)

Ann Surg 249:318-321, 2009

Objective.—We hypothesized that an adrenal vein sampling (AVS) algorithm incorporating rapid cortisol assays, which enables resampling of the adrenal veins, would improve the success rate by a team of radiologists.

Summary Background Data.—AVS is the most accurate means to localize aldosterone production in primary aldosteronism (PA). However, cannulation of the right adrenal vein (RAV) is difficult, and success is assumed from venography without the support of steroid assays. Furthermore, few institutions can assign all studies to 1 dedicated and experienced AVS interventional radiologist.

Methods.—Retrospective chart review of patients with PA at our university hospitals who underwent AVS. We compared results for 30 AVS studies incorporating rapid cortisol assays with 30 conventional AVS studies.

Results.—The success rate for the control period was 73% (22/30 studies). For the first 30 studies after incorporating rapid cortisol assay, the success rate increased to 97% (29/30 studies). Resampling the RAV was required for 2 studies, and prolonged sheath insertion did not cause any complications.

Conclusions.—High AVS success rates may be achieved by a team of interventional radiologists at 1 center using defined AVS protocols. Rapid cortisol assay allows for resampling of the RAV and improves AVS success rates.

▶ Adrenal vein sampling (AVS) has become the gold standard in primary aldosteronism (PA) for the differential diagnosis of a single unilateral adrenal adenoma and bilateral adrenal cortical hyperplasia. The distinction is important because adrenalectomy is the treatment of choice for a unilateral adenoma and medical treatment with aldosterone receptor antagonists for bilateral hyperplasia. The major problem in conducting accurate and reliable AVS is proper adrenal vein catheterization, given that the right adrenal vein is short and juxtaposed to the hepatic vein with accessory veins that dilute the concentration of the hormone being measured.[1] Failure to catheterize the adrenal vein, even if the tip of the catheter is in its proximity, will result in dilution of the aldosterone concentration and misinterpretation of results with erroneous lateralization of aldosterone production. To confirm the correct position of the catheters, angiographers use a normal co-secreted hormone like cortisol for guidance. When properly placed, cortisol levels are equally high in both adrenal veins and have a gradient between central and peripheral vein values. A discrepancy in cortisol concentration between the left and the right adrenal veins would indicate catheter misplacement. Auchus et al propose the measurement of cortisol during the procedure to confirm catheter placement. This measurement may take up to 2 hours during which patients continue with their sheaths in place and if the cortisol level is found to be low, the catheterization is repeated. The delay in obtaining a result is related to the logistics of getting samples to the laboratory and getting them analyzed. With cortisol monitoring, the success rate of AVS rises from 73% to 97%. While the idea of measuring cortisol during the sampling procedure is attractive (we do this with parathyroid hormone [PTH] measurement during parathyroid surgery), the time it takes to measure cortisol will have to be abbreviated. With automated techniques, the actual cortisol measurement can be completed in just a few minutes. The logistics need to be simplified for this strategy to be practical.

D. E. Schteingart, MD

Reference

1. Miotto D, De Toni R, Pitter G, et al. Impact of accessory hepatic veins on adrenal vein sampling for identification of surgically curable primary aldosteronism. *Hypertension.* 2009;54:885-889.

Role of unilateral adrenalectomy in bilateral primary aldosteronism: A 22-Year single center experience

Sukor N, Gordon RD, Ku YK, et al (Univ of Queensland School of Medicine, Australia; et al)

J Clin Endocrinol Metab 94:2437-2445, 2009

Objective.—The aim of the study was to examine blood pressure and biochemical responses to unilateral adrenalectomy in patients with bilateral primary aldosteronism (PA) and identify predictive parameters.

Context.—PA considered due to bilateral autonomous production of aldosterone is usually treated medically. Unilateral adrenalectomy has been considered ineffective. Because quality outcome data are lacking and medical treatment may cause adverse effects or fail to control hypertension, defining the role for unilateral adrenalectomy in bilateral PA is an important clinical issue.

Design and Setting.—Between 1984 and 2004, 51 of 684 patients diagnosed with bilateral PA underwent unilateral adrenalectomy. This report is based on the records of the 40 considered suitable for inclusion, who were followed for at least 12 (median, 56.4) months.

Results.—Hypertension was cured in 15% of patients and improved in 20%, usually within 1 yr of unilateral adrenalectomy. The proportion with controlled hypertension was significantly ($P < 0.001$) higher after adrenalectomy (65%) than before (25%). Mean systolic ($P < 0.001$) and diastolic ($P < 0.001$) blood pressure, left ventricular mass index ($P < 0.05$), plasma upright aldosterone ($P < 0.05$), and aldosterone/renin ratio ($P < 0.001$) fell. Serum creatinine independently predicted hypertension cure.

Conclusion.—Although this retrospective analysis of patients from a single center does not permit prediction of response rates among patients diagnosed elsewhere, it suggests that unilateral adrenalectomy can be beneficial in some patients with apparent bilateral PA and should not be dismissed as a treatment option.

▶ Treatment of primary aldosteronism (PA) secondary to bilateral hyperplasia has been medical with the use of mineralocorticoid receptor antagonists, such as spironolactone or eplerenone. In the case of suboptimal response, or patient's reluctance to take chronic pharmacological treatment, several groups have performed unilateral laparoscopic adrenalectomy. This is particularly an option when patients have hyperplasia with a distinct nodule in 1 gland and asymmetric secretion of aldosterone established during adrenal venous sampling. The adrenalectomy would be directed to the most active side. Sukor et al report on their experience over a decade in which unilateral adrenalectomy was performed in 51 of 684 patients diagnosed with bilateral PA. Hypertension was cured in 15% and improved in 20%. The proportion of patients in whom the hypertension was better controlled after the unilateral adrenalectomy (65%) was higher than before (25%). The subject is still controversial, but in selected cases, the improvement in control of hypertension and the reduction in drug use and cost associated with unilateral adrenalectomy recommends consideration of this procedure in the treatment of PA with bilateral disease.

D. E. Schteingart, MD

7 Reproductive Endocrinology

Introduction

This year's selections include many articles related to menopause, aging, hypogonadism in men, and hormonal influences on bone metabolism.

Puurunen and associates observe that all adrenal androgen production capacity remained high in women with polycystic ovary syndrome even to menopause.

Several markers of ovarian failure have been studied. The observations of Knauff and associates observed that anti-müllerian hormone was a more consistent determinate of the clinical degree of follicle pool depletion in young women with elevated FSH levels than other markers studied.

Estrogen is known to influence the development of fat cells; in the study by Goulart and associates, they reported that estrogen receptor 1 gene polymorphisms were associated with a decreased risk of obesity in women.

La Marca et al made the interesting observation that women with primary ovarian insufficiency due to autoimmunity of steroidogenic cells still had preservation of a pool of functioning follicles with the potential for fertility.

In postmenopausal women with diabetes, adiposity and insulin resistance accounted for most of the association of bioavailable testosterone, but not all of the association with estradiol and sex hormone binding globulin (Kalyani et al).

Sensitive and specific markers for polycystic ovary syndrome were sought by Stener-Victorin et al. They observed that the combination of elevated estrone and free testosterone appeared to give the best discrimination for high sensitivity and specificity for women with polycystic ovary syndrome (PCOS) compared with those without PCOS.

Cussons et al observed that young non-obese women with no biochemical evidence of insulin resistance with polycystic ovary syndrome, had abnormal vascular function, but normal arterial stiffness when compared with age-matched controls. They speculate as to whether or not this abnormality leads to a greater risk of cardiovascular disease.

The studies of Valkenburg et al observed genetic polymorphisms of gonadotropin-releasing hormone and gonadotrophic hormone receptors in patients with PCOS, and this altered the phenotype.

Non-alcoholic fatty liver disease is common in patients with polycystic ovary syndrome. Vassilatou and Associates observed that women with PCOS increased androgen bioavailability was associated with non-alcoholic fatty liver disease.

Sir-Petermann et al investigated girls before puberty and noted that metabolic and reproductive abnormalities were observed during puberty in daughters of women with PCOS.

Vitamin D deficiency has been extensively studied in various disorders particularly over the past 3-4 years. The study by Kotsa determined that vitamin D therapy reduced insulin resistance in women with PCOS.

The influence of sex steroids on femur strength was investigated by Travison et al, and they observed that the best correlate was the association with circulating estradiol, which was partially mediated by body composition.

Hammoud et al investigated the effect of a Roux-en-Y gastric bypass surgery on sex steroids and quality of life in obese men. They observed a marked improvement in hormonal profiles in men after substantial weight loss with Roux-en-Y gastric bypass, but not in the control group.

Bhasin and associates investigated the effect of human growth hormone and testosterone on propeptide type 3 procollagen and reported that procollagen may be an early biomarker of the anabolic effects of growth hormone and testosterone in men.

Aromatase inhibitors are known to increase testosterone levels in men. Burnett-Bowie et al evaluated the influence of aromatase inhibitor on sex hormone levels and on bone mineral density. They concluded that aromatase inhibition does not improve bone health in aging men with low or low-normal testosterone levels.

The combination of testosterone and growth hormone was shown to improve body composition and muscle performance in older men as investigated by Sattler and associates.

Recently, heightened interest in the influence of testosterone on frailty in older men has been observed. Cawthon and associates reported that low levels of biotestosterone were independently associated with the worse baseline fragility status.

Koutsari investigated the effect of dehydroepiandrosterone and testosterone replacement in hormonally deficient men and women on the effects of fatty acid metabolism. They found that dehydroepiandrosterone did not influence fat partitioning, and postabsorptive lipolysis and testosterone only partially corrected these effects.

In recent years, there has been increased interest in the influence of anabolic steroids on mortality. Guder et al observed that low levels of androgens had an adverse influence on outcome in patients with heart failure.

A search has been conducted for many years for an anabolic agent that would not influence prostate. Min and associates reported on a novel synthetic androgen receptor ligand that selectively modulates the androgen receptor and produces androgenic metabolic effects with little impact on prostate growth or prostate specific antigen.

Park et al made the interesting observation that 17 beta estradiol at low concentration acts through a distinct pathway in normal versus benign prostatic hyperplasia derived prostate stromal cells.

Jones and associates investigated a noncompetitive androgen receptor inhibitor in an attempt to apply the inhibitor to treatment of androgen-dependent disorders or diseases.

A. Wayne Meikle, MD

Female Reproductive Function and Menopause

Adrenal Androgen Production Capacity Remains High up to Menopause in Women with Polycystic Ovary Syndrome

Puurunen J, Piltonen T, Jaakkola P, et al (Oulu Univ Hosp, Finland)
J Clin Endocrinol Metab 94:1973-1978, 2009

Introduction.—Hyperandrogenism is one of the main features of polycystic ovary syndrome (PCOS). Of circulating androgens, 50% of androstenedione and testosterone are of ovarian and adrenal origin, whereas dehydroepiandrosterone (DHEA) and DHEA sulfate are almost uniquely of adrenal origin. Our previous studies have indicated that ovarian androgen production capacity is enhanced in women with PCOS, and it remains high until late reproductive age. To study whether this also applies to adrenal androgen production, ACTH tests were performed in healthy women and in women with PCOS.

Materials.—Sixty-nine healthy women (aged 19–62 yr; body mass index 19.2–35.0 kg/m^2) and 58 women with previously diagnosed PCOS (aged 18–59 yr; body mass index 19.0–42.9 kg/m^2) participated in the study.

Methods.—The subjects underwent ACTH stimulation tests, and serum cortisol, 17-hydroxyprogesterone, androstenedione, testosterone, DHEA, and DHEA sulfate levels were analyzed at 0, 30, and 60 min.

Results.—Basal and ACTH-stimulated levels of most adrenal androgens decreased in healthy women with age, whereas in women with PCOS, only the concentrations of basal serum 17-hydroxyprogesterone decreased, and all areas under the curve (AUCs) remained unchanged and significantly higher (except for DHEA) than those in control women. Likewise, at the menopausal transition, pre- and postmenopausal women with PCOS exhibited mainly unchanged and higher basal androgen and AUC levels.

Conclusions.—Similarly to ovarian endocrine function, serum adrenal steroid levels and adrenal steroid production capacity remain enhanced at least up to menopause in women with PCOS (Fig 2).

▶ Androgens in women are derived from ovarian and adrenal sex steroid secretion. The ovary is under control of luteinizing hormone (LH) and follicle-stimulating hormone (FSH) and the adrenal androgens are largely regulated

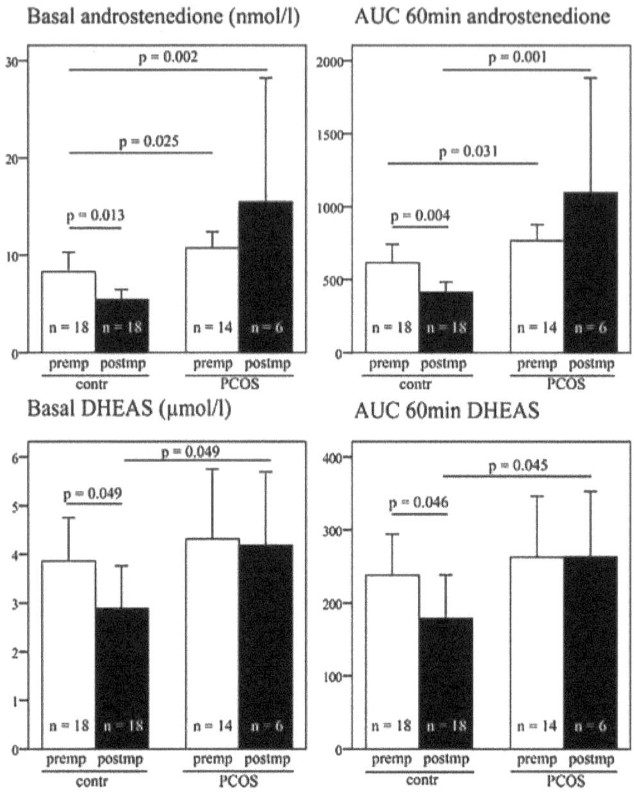

FIGURE 2.—Basal and ACTH-stimulated (AUC, 60 min) A and DHEAS levels in premenopausal (premp) and postmenopausal (postmp) control women and women with PCOS. contr, Control. (Reprinted from Puurunen J, Piltonen T, Jaakkola P, et al. Adrenal androgen production capacity remains high up to menopause in women with polycystic ovary syndrome. *J Clin Endocrinol Metab.* 2009;94:1973-1978, with permission from The Endocrine Society.)

by adrenocorticotropin hormone (ACTH). In women with polycystic ovary syndrome (PCOS) the adrenal is the main source of dehydroepiandrosterone (DHEA) and DHEA sulfate (DHEAS), and the ovary secretes about 60% of androstenedione and 60% of testosterone. Peripheral tissues convert androstenedione and DHEA into testosterone and estradiol. PCOS affects 4% to 11% of women and excess ovarian androgen occurs in approximately 20% to 60% of women, while adrenal androgen excess, mainly from DHEAS, occurs in about 15% to 60% of women. Puurunen et al investigated the adrenal androgen production capacity in aging women with PCOS compared with normal women. They observed that basal and ACTH-stimulated adrenal androgen decreased with age in normal healthy women. In contrast, women with PCOS had sustained adrenal steroid production, with the exception of a decrease in basal 17-hydroxyprogesterone. Thus, up to menopause women with PCOS have enhanced adrenal androgen production compared with normal women.

A. W. Meikle, MD

Anti-Müllerian Hormone, Inhibin B, and Antral Follicle Count in Young Women with Ovarian Failure

Knauff EAH, Eijkemans MJC, Lambalk CB, et al (Univ Med Ctr, Utrecht, The Netherlands; Vrije Universiteit Med Ctr, Amsterdam, The Netherlands; et al)
J Clin Endocrinol Metab 94:786-792, 2009

Context.—Ovarian dysfunction is classically categorized on the basis of cycle history, FSH, and estradiol levels. Novel ovarian markers may provide a more direct insight into follicular quantity in hypergonadotropic women.

Objective.—The objective of the study was to investigate the distribution of novel ovarian markers in young hypergonadotropic women as compared with normogonadotropic regularly menstruating women.

Design.—This was a nationwide prospective cohort study.

Setting.—The study was conducted at 10 hospitals in The Netherlands.

Patients.—Women below age 40 yr with regular menses and normal FSH (controls; n = 83), regular menstrual cycles and elevated FSH [incipient ovarian failure (IOF); n = 68]; oligomenorrhea and elevated FSH [referred to as transitional ovarian failure (TOF); n = 79]; or at least 4 months amenorrhea together with FSH levels exceeding 40 IU/liter [premature ovarian failure (POF); n = 112].

Main Outcome Measures.—Serum levels of anti-Müllerian hormone (AMH), inhibin B, and antral follicle count (AFC) was measured.

Results.—All POF patients showed AMH levels below the fifth percentile (p_5) of normoovulatory women. Normal AMH levels (>p_5) could be identified in 75% of IOF, 33% of TOF patients, and 98% of controls. AFC and AMH levels changed with increasing age ($P < 0.0001$), whereas inhibin B did not ($P = 0.26$). AMH levels were significantly different

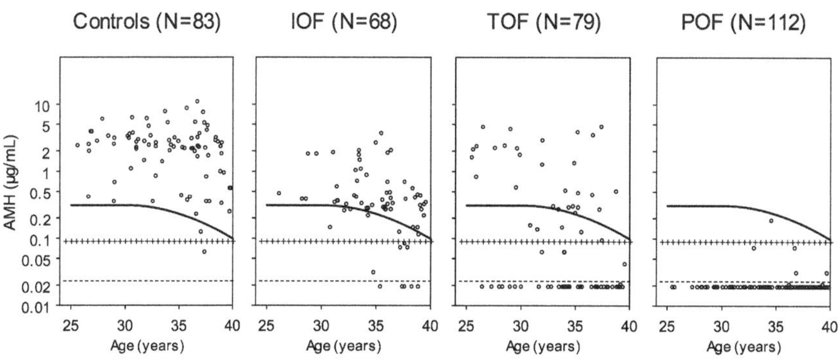

FIGURE 2.—Individual AMH levels (log scale) in relation to age in regularly menstruating controls and three subgroups of patients with elevated FSH levels. The *black lines* indicate the P_5 value for age. The +++++ lines indicate the menopausal threshold value for AMH (0.086 µg/ml); the *dashed* lines indicate the lower level of detection of the AMH assay (0.023 µg/ml) (24). (Reprinted from Knauff EAH, Eijkemans MJC, Lambalk CB, et al. Anti-Müllerian hormone, inhibin b, and antral follicle count in young women with ovarian failure. *J Clin Endocrinol Metab.* 2009;94:786-792, with permission from The Endocrine Society.)

between TOF and IOF over the entire age range, whereas AFC became similar for TOF and IOF at higher ages.

Conclusions.—Compared with inhibin B and AFC, AMH was more consistently correlated with the clinical degree of follicle pool depletion in young women presenting with elevated FSH levels. AMH may provide a more accurate assessment of the follicle pool in young hypergonadotropic patients, especially in the clinically challenging subgroups of patients with elevated FSH and regular menses (*i.e.* IOF) and in hypergonadotropic women with cycle disturbances not fulfilling the POF diagnostic criteria (*i.e.* TOF) (Fig 2).

▶ The World Health Organization has 3 classifications for abnormal ovarian function. These classifications are mainly based on serum concentrations of FSH and estradiol. Serum FSH is regulated by feedback responses from estradiol and inhibin. Idiopathic premature ovarian failure (POF), transitional ovarian failure (TOF), and incipient ovarian failure (IOF) were investigated. Because women are delaying their pregnancies, many of them have elevated FSH concentrations, suggesting pending ovarian failure. But, FSH has not been a reliable predictor of fertility potential in these women. In this study, they investigated the distribution of ovarian markers in young hypergonadotropic women compared with normogonadotrophic regularly menstruating women. Anti-Müllerian hormone (AMH) correlated better with the clinical degree of the ovarian follicle pool than inhibin and antral follicle count. A limitation of the current study is that it is a cross-sectional investigation. Long-term study is needed to establish that AMH can predict the clinical outcome in young women with hypergonadotropism.

A. W. Meikle, MD

Estrogen receptor 1 gene polymorphisms and decreased risk of obesity in women

Goulart AC, Zee RYL, Rexrode KM (Brigham and Women's Hosp and Harvard Med School, Boston, MA)
Metabolism 58:759-764, 2009

Estrogen receptor α gene (*ESR1*) polymorphisms have been associated with several diseases, but whether they are associated with obesity is uncertain. To elucidate the role of genetic variation in the ESR1 gene with body mass index (BMI), 543 white women (median age, 63 years) from the Women's Health Study were examined. Most were postmenopausal (99.3%). The relationships between rs2234693 and rs9340799 genotypes and their associated haplotypes with obesity (BMI $\geq$30 kg/m^2) and overweight (BMI $\geq$25 kg/m^2) were evaluated. Among women with the rs2234693 TT genotype, 18.3% were obese, whereas only 8.2% of those with the CC genotype were obese ($P = .04$). In a logistic regression model assuming additive inheritance, rs2234693 was associated with decreased

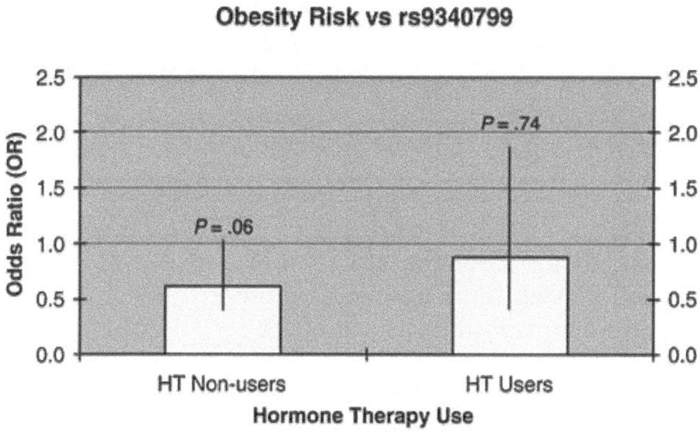

FIGURE 2.—Obese women (≥30.0 kg/m^2) were compared with women with BMI less than 30.0 kg/m^2, according to HT use. P values were obtained from multivariate logistic regression (adjusted for age at randomization, age at menopause, exercise, educational level, alcohol consumption, smoking status, total fat adjusted for energy intake). (Reprinted from Goulart AC, Zee RYL, Rexrode KM Estrogen receptor 1 gene polymorphisms and decreased risk of obesity in women. *Metabolism*. 2009;58:759-764, with permission from Elsevier Inc.)

odds of obesity (BMI ≥30 kg/m^2) (crude odds ratio = 0.63, 95% confidence interval = 0.44-0.90, P =.01). For rs9340799, only an inverse trend was observed for BMI (P =.08). Haplotypes that included the variant C allele were associated with a reduced risk of obesity (crude odds ratio = 0.65, 95% confidence interval = 0.44-0.94, P =.02 for C-G). The rs2234693 C allele of *ESR1* and its associated genotypes and haplotypes were inversely and consistently associated with obesity. One or more copies of the C allele were associated with decreased risk of obesity in white postmenopausal women (Fig 2).

▶ Obesity is a complex disease that is influenced by genetic and environmental factors. The Human Obesity Gene Map listed the receptor gene, estrogen receptor α gene (*ESRI*), as one of many candidate genes associated with obesity. Expression of *ESRI* has been related to menopausal status and obesity in women, and polymorphisms have been associated with variations in body mass index (BMI) and waist circumference. The study of Goulart et al investigated the relationship of 2 polymorphisms in *ESRI* (rs2234693) and (rs9340799) with risk of overweight or obesity in white postmenopausal women. They observed that one or more copies of the C allele were associated with decreased risk of obesity in postmenopausal women. A strength of the study is that it was a large study in postmenopausal women. A weakness is that the women were white so that the results cannot be extrapolated to other racial or ethnic groups. There is no direct evidence for a causal relationship of the polymorphisms and obesity.

A. W. Meikle, MD

Primary Ovarian Insufficiency due to Steroidogenic Cell Autoimmunity Is Associated with a Preserved Pool of Functioning Follicles

La Marca A, on behalf of the Italian Addison Network (Univ of Modena and Reggio Emilia, Italy; et al)

J Clin Endocrinol Metab 94:3816-3823, 2009

Context.—Primary ovarian insufficiency (POI) is defined as hypergonadotropic amenorrhea before the age of 40 yr. In 4–5% of patients with POI, an ovarian autoimmune process is present.

Design.—Serum concentrations of antimüllerian hormone (AMH) have been determined in 26 women with POI due to steroidogenic cell autoimmunity (SCA-POI), 66 with nonautoimmune idiopathic POI (iPOI), 40 postmenopausal women (PMW), and 44 healthy fertile women (HW). SCA-POI was diagnosed according to presence of steroidogenic enzyme autoantibodies (17α-hydroxylase, side chain cleavage, and 21-hydroxylase autoantibodies).

Results.—AMH concentrations were significantly higher in women with SCA-POI than women with iPOI ($P = 0.018$) or PMW ($P = 0.03$) but significantly lower than HW ($P < 0.0001$). AMH was detected in 11 of 26 women with SCA-POI (42%) and seven of 66 with iPOI (11%) ($P = 0.002$). Serum concentrations above the fifth percentile of the normal range (0.6 ng/ml) were detected in nine of 26 women with SCA-POI (35%) and four of 66 with iPOI (6%) ($P = 0.001$). Eight of 12 women with SCA-POI with less than 5 yr (67%) and one of 14 with longer disease duration (7%) had AMH concentrations within the normal range ($P = 0.003$). AMH concentrations correlated inversely with disease duration in women with SCA-POI (rho = −0.563, $P = 0.003$) but not women with iPOI. AMH correlated inversely with FSH serum concentrations in HW (rho = −0.584, $P < 0.001$) but not PMW or women with POI.

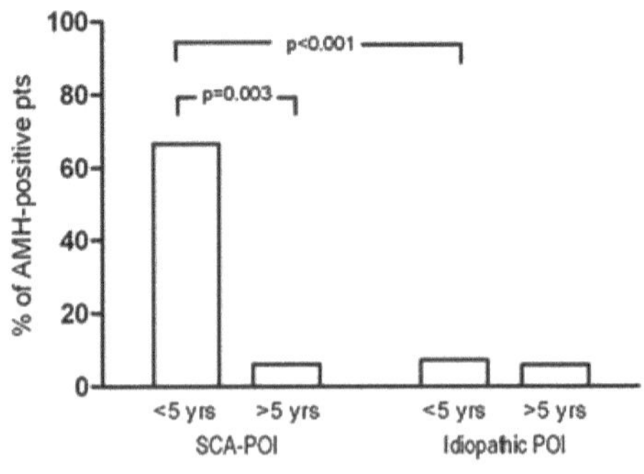

FIGURE 2.—Frequency of women with either SCA-POI or idiopathic POI, with AMH serum concentrations above the fifth percentile of normal values, according to time of blood sampling after clinical diagnosis of ovarian insufficiency. (Reprinted from La Marca A, on behalf of the Italian Addison Network. Primary ovarian insufficiency due to steroidogenic cell autoimmunity is associated with a preserved pool of functioning follicles. *J Clin Endocrinol Metab.* 2009;94:3816-3823, with permission from The Endocrine Society.)

Conclusions.—Two thirds of women with recent-onset SCA-POI had normal AMH concentrations. Women with SCA-POI, differently from those with iPOI, present a preserved ovarian follicle pool for several years after diagnosis of ovarian insufficiency (Fig 2).

▶ Primary ovarian insufficiency (POI) is characterized by hypergonadotropic hypogonadism, estrogen deficiency and infertility before 40 years of age, and it affects about 1% of women. A portion of these women have circulating autoantibodies against steroidogenic enzymes that characterize their POI and are classified as steroidogenic cell autoimmunity (SCA-POI). These patients have increased serum concentrations of inhibin B and total inhibin with a follicle-stimulating hormone (FSH) to luteinizing hormone (LH) ratio often less than 1. Thus, they have antibodies toward the theca cells but not the granulosa cells. Antimüllerian hormone (AMH) is the best marker for estimation of the ovarian follicle pool. The women with SCA-POI have preservation of the ovarian follicle pool for several years after the onset of ovarian insufficiency. An AMH concentration in women with various forms of ovarian insufficiency shows modest overlap in values in women with natural menopause and idiopathic POI and healthy women. Further refinement is needed to clearly differentiate patients with various forms of ovarian failure, but this is a good start.

A. W. Meikle, MD

The Association of Endogenous Sex Hormones, Adiposity, and Insulin Resistance with Incident Diabetes in Postmenopausal Women

Kalyani RR, Franco M, Dobs AS, et al (Johns Hopkins Univ, Baltimore, MD; Centro Nacional Investigación Cardiovascular, Madrid, Spain; et al)

J Clin Endocrinol Metab 94:4127-4135, 2009

Context.—In postmenopausal women, endogenous bioavailable testosterone (T) and estradiol (E2) have been positively associated, and SHBG has been negatively associated, with incident type 2 diabetes (T2DM). Previous studies have not explored possible factors explaining these relationships.

Objective.—Our objective was to examine the association of endogenous sex hormones with incident T2DM in postmenopausal women and possible explanatory factors.

Design, Setting, and Participants.—The Multi-Ethnic Study of Atherosclerosis (MESA) is a prospective study that included 1612 postmenopausal women aged 45–84 yr, followed between the years 2000–2006, who were not taking hormone replacement therapy, had no prevalent cardiovascular disease or diabetes, and had complete ascertainment of sex hormones.

Main Outcome Measures.—T2DM was defined based on fasting glucose and/or treatment for diabetes.

Results.—There were 116 incident cases of diabetes during follow-up. Across higher quartiles of bioavailable T and E2 and lower quartiles of SHBG, we found significantly greater hazards of developing incident T2DM (all *P* for trend ≤ 0.001). After adjustment for body mass index and insulin resistance estimated by homeostasis model assessment of insulin resistance, bioavailable T was no longer associated with incident T2DM. The associations of E2 and SHBG with incident T2DM were partially explained by body mass index and insulin resistance but persisted in fully adjusted models (both *P* for trend <0.02). Dehydroepiandrosterone had no relationship with incident T2DM.

Conclusions.—Adiposity and insulin resistance explained most of the association of bioavailable T but only partially explained the associations of E2 and SHBG with incident T2DM among postmenopausal women.

▶ Studies have shown that higher bioavialable testosterone (BT) and estradiol and lower sex hormone-binding globulin (SHBG) are associated with glucose intolerance and type II diabetes in postmenopausal women. This study by Kalyani et al extended previous investigations by controlling for factors that might contribute to these associations. The measurement of hormonal relationships with risk of diabetes and glucose intolerance might aid in identifying high-risk postmenopausal women. However, the cutoff concentrations for the risk need better definition than provided in this study. In this study, adiposity and insulin resistance explained most of the relationship between BT and incident diabetes type II but only partially accounted for the association of estradiol and SHBG with incident type II diabetes. The adrenal androgen dehydroepiandrosterone (DHEA) showed no association with risk of diabetes. The influence of sex steroids on insulin responsiveness, secretion, and action are poorly understood. Further investigation is needed to establish the mechanism by which sex hormones might affect the risk of diabetes type II and their influences on glucose transport and metabolism.

A. W. Meikle, MD

PCOS

Are There Any Sensitive and Specific Sex Steroid Markers for Polycystic Ovary Syndrome?

Stener-Victorin E, Holm G, Labrie F, et al (Univ of Gothenburg, Sweden; CHUL Res Ctr, Quebec, Canada)

J Clin Endocrinol Metab 95:810-819, 2010

Context.—Despite the high prevalence of hyperandrogenemia, the principal biochemical abnormality in women with polycystic ovary syndrome (PCOS), a definitive endocrine marker for PCOS has so far not been identified.

Objective.—To identify a tentative diagnostic marker for PCOS, we compared serum levels of sex steroids, their precursors, and main metabolites in women with PCOS and controls.

Design and Methods.—In this cross-sectional study of 74 women with PCOS and 31 controls, we used gas and liquid chromatography/mass spectrometry to analyze serum sex steroid precursors, estrogens, androgens, and glucuronidated androgen metabolites; performed immunoassays of SHBG, LH, and FSH; and calculated the LH/FSH ratio.

Results.—Androgens and estrogens, sex steroid precursors, and glucuronidated androgen metabolites were higher in women with PCOS than in controls. In multivariate logistic regression analyses, estrone and free testosterone were independently associated with PCOS. The odds ratios per SD increase were 24.2 for estrone [95% confidence interval (CI), 4.0–144.7] and 12.8 for free testosterone (95% CI, 3.1–53.4). In receiver operating characteristic analyses, the area under curve was 0.93 for estrone (95% CI, 0.88–0.98) and 0.91 for free testosterone (95% CI, 0.86–0.97), indicating high sensitivity and specificity.

Conclusion.—Women with PCOS have elevated levels of sex steroid precursors, estrogens, androgens, and glucuronidated androgen metabolites as measured with a specific and sensitive mass spectrometry-based technique. The combination of elevated estrone (>50 pg/ml) and free testosterone (>3.3 pg/ml) appeared to discriminate with high sensitivity and specificity between women with and without PCOS.

▶ Polycystic ovary syndrome (PCOS) is a common disorder in reproductive women and is characterized by polycystic ovaries, infertility with oligomenorrhea, and hyperandrogenism. The sex steroid abnormalities include both ovarian and adrenal hormones. Excess testosterone is secreted by the ovaries and androstenedione by both the adrenal glands and ovary and dehydroepiandrosterone (DHEA) and DHEA sulfate (DHEAS) from the adrenal glands. Because sex hormone-binding globulin (SHBG) usually tends to be reduced, free testosterone has been a better marker of hyperandrogenism than total testosterone. Radiometric assays have limitations in sensitivity and reproducibility in measurement of testosterone in women. Stener-Victorin et al, as reported in their study, overcame methodological issues by using liquid chromatographic/tandem mass spectrometry (LC/MS/MS) for measurement of sex steroids and their glucuronide metabolites. While most of the steroids measured and the ratio of LH/FSH were statistically significantly different between controls and patients with PCOS, estrone had 95% receiver operator area under the curve of 0.93 (confidence limits [CLs] of 0.88-0.98) and 0.91 for free testosterone (95% CL, 0.86-0.97). When both estrone and free testosterone were used, the limits were even higher. With the combination of estrone (> 50 pg/mL) and free testosterone (> 3.3 pg/mL), the discrimination for PCOS produced high sensitivity and sensitivity with a CL of 0.90 to 0.98.

A. W. Meikle, MD

Dissociation of endothelial function and arterial stiffness in nonobese women with polycystic ovary syndrome (PCOS)

Cussons AJ, Watts GF, Stuckey BGA (Keogh Inst for Med Res, Nedlands, Western Australia; Univ of Western Australia)
Clin Endocrinol 71:808-814, 2009

Objective.—Polycystic ovary syndrome (PCOS) is associated with cardiovascular risk but it is not clear if this is independent of obesity and insulin resistance. This study therefore investigates endothelial function and arterial stiffness in nonobese, noninsulin resistant women with PCOS.

Design.—This is cross-sectional case–control study.

Patients.—A total of 19 young women with PCOS, with body mass index (BMI) <30 kg/m^2, and 19 healthy controls matched for age and BMI were included in the study.

Measurements.—Endothelial function was assessed with flow mediated dilatation (FMD) of the brachial artery, while arterial stiffness was assessed with pulse wave velocity (PWV) and augmentation index (AI).

Results.—There were no significant differences between PCOS and control subjects when assessing the following clinical and biochemical variables: blood pressure, homeostasis model assessment insulin-resistance index, lipids and oestradiol. Women with PCOS had higher free androgen index scores (5·14 ± 3·47 *vs.* 3·25 ± 1·42, $P = 0{\cdot}036$). The PCOS subjects had significantly lower FMD of the brachial artery compared with the controls (6·5 ± 2·9% *vs.* 10·5 ± 4·0%, $P < 0{\cdot}01$). There were no significant differences in markers of arterial stiffness (PWV 5·8 ± 1·1 *vs.* 6·0 ± 1·0, $P = 0{\cdot}58$, AI 16·5 ± 10·2 *vs.* 20·3 ± 10·2, $P = 0{\cdot}25$).

Conclusions.—Women with polycystic ovary syndrome who are young, nonobese, and have no biochemical evidence of insulin resistance, have

TABLE 2.—Blood Pressure, Heart Rate, Flow Mediated Dilatation of the Brachial Artery (FMD), Glyceryl Trinitrate Mediated Dilatation of the Brachial Artery (GTN-MD) and Arterial Stiffness Indices for PCOS and Control Subjects

	PCOS ($n = 19$)	Control ($n = 19$)	P-value
Systolic blood pressure (mmHg)	108 ± 9	106 ± 12	0·70
Diastolic blood pressure (mmHg)	64 ± 7	62 ± 10	0·70
Heart rate (bpm)	62 ± 12	67 ± 7	0·20
Pulse pressure (mmHg)	46 ± 10	45 ± 8	0·77
FMD (%)	6·49 ± 2·89	10·46 ± 4·04	<0·01
FMD increase (%)	3·41 ± 2·94	7·83 ± 4·13	<0·01
GTN-MD (%)	19·88 ± 7·88	27·84 ± 7·30	<0·01
GTN-MD increase (%)	16·83 ± 7·94	25·22 ± 7·38	<0·01
Pulse wave velocity (m/s)	5·81 ± 1·12	6·00 ± 0·98	0·5
Augmentation index (%)	16·47 ± 10·19	20·31 ± 10·21	0·25

Mean (SD) shown.

abnormal vascular function, but normal arterial stiffness, when compared with age and weight matched control subjects. Whether this leads to a greater risk of cardiovascular disease requires further investigation (Table 2).

▶ Polycystic ovary syndrome (PCOS) is a common disorder of reproductive age women, and is characterized by oligomenorrhea and hyperandrogenism. Other clinical findings that are associated with PCOS include cardiovascular risk, insulin resistance, obesity, type II diabetes, dyslipidemia, and sleep apnea. Endothelial dysfunction and arterial stiffness are implicated in the pathogenesis of atherosclerosis and risk factors for cardiovascular events. Flow-mediated dilatation of the brachial artery is a measure of conduit endothelial function and glyceryl trinitrate-mediated dilatation is reflection of vasodilatation capacity and function of vascular smooth muscle. Nonobese women with or without PCOS were studied, and the authors observed that women with PCOS exhibited abnormal vascular function but normal arterial stiffness. The women with PCOS did not have evidence of insulin resistance. The authors speculate that low estrogen at mid cycle and lack of an ovulatory surge might account for the abnormal vascular function in women with PCOS. Study of these factors long-term is needed to test this hypothesis.

A. W. Meikle, MD

Genetic polymorphisms of GnRH and gonadotrophic hormone receptors affect the phenotype of polycystic ovary syndrome

Valkenburg O, Uitterlinden AG, Piersma D, et al (Univ Med Ctr, Rotterdam, The Netherlands; et al)

Hum Reprod 24:2014-2022, 2009

Background.—Polycystic ovary syndrome (PCOS) is a complex genetic disorder. Multiple functional polymorphisms have been identified in genes that regulate the hypothalamic–pituitary–gonadal (HPG) axis that regulates ovarian function. The present study aims to examine the influence of genetic variants of the HPG-axis on the severity of clinical features of PCOS and disease susceptibility.

Methods.—We included 518 Caucasian PCOS women and 2996 unselected controls from the general population (the Rotterdam study). Genotype distributions were compared between patients and controls. Subsequently, associations with clinical features of PCOS were studied. Single nucleotide polymorphisms were selected in GnRH (Trp16Ser [rs6185]), the FSH-receptor (FSHR, Ala307Thr [rs6165] and Asn680Ser [rs6166]) and the LH-receptor (18insLQ, Asn291Ser [rs12470652] and Ser312Asn [rs2293275]).

Results.—FSHR Ser^{680} was associated with higher levels of gonadotrophic hormones (FSH: $P < 0.01$, LH: $P = 0.01$), and testosterone ($P = 0.05$) and a higher frequency of hyperandrogenism ($P = 0.04$). No differences in risk for PCOS in association with the FSH-receptor variants were observed.

Conclusion.—Genetic variants of the HPG-axis were associated with a modest but significant effect on the phenotype of PCOS. FSHR variants were strongly associated with the severity of clinical features of PCOS, such as levels of gonadotrophic hormones and the presence of hyperandrogenism, but not disease risk.

▶ Polycystic ovary syndrome (PCOS) occurs in 5% to 8% of reproductive age women and is characterized with anovulation, androgen excess, and polycystic ovaries. These women also have alterations of function of the hypothalamic-pituitary axis associated with increased frequency and amplitude of the gonadotropin-releasing hormone (GnRH) pulses. These alterations in gonadotropin secretion tend to result in elevated luteinizing hormone (LH) relative to follicle-stimulating hormone (FSH). Valkenburg and associates investigated genetic polymorphisms of GnRH and gonadotropic hormone receptors in women with PCOS compared with a control group. They observed that FSHR Ser^{680} associated with higher concentrations of FSH, LH, and testosterone, but FSH-receptor (FSHR) variants were not an apparent risk for PCOS. However, the FSHR variants were strongly associated with the hormone alterations in PCOS. They propose that a decrease in FSHR sensitivity might disturb normal follicle formation resulting in a decreased production of estradiol and inhibin B that exert inhibitory feedback on the pituitary gland. The increased concentrations of the gonadotropins could then result in elevated androgen concentrations from persistent stimulation of theca cells of the ovaries by LH. In support of this they observed a significant association of LH and testosterone but not adrenal androgens.

A. W. Meikle, MD

Increased androgen bioavailability is associated with non-alcoholic fatty liver disease in women with polycystic ovary syndrome

Vassilatou E, Lafoyianni S, Vryonidou A, et al ('Amalia Fleming' General Hosp, Melissia, Athens, Greece; 'Red Cross Hosp', Athens, Greece; et al)

Hum Reprod 25:212-220, 2010

Background.—Increased prevalence of abnormal aminotransferase levels and/or ultrasonographic evidence of hepatic steatosis (HS) have been found in women with polycystic ovary syndrome (PCOS). However, factors associated with non-alcoholic fatty liver disease (NAFLD) in PCOS are still under investigation. The aim of this case–control study was to investigate the presence of NAFLD and to assess factors associated with this condition in PCOS patients.

Methods.—A prospective study of 57 premenopausal PCOS patients and 60 age-and weight-matched control women, with a history of no or minimal alcohol consumption was conducted. Anthropometric variables,

TABLE 5.—Multivariate Logistic Regression Results for Hepatic Steatosis as a Dependent Variable ($n = 117$)

Independent Variable	Multivariate Analysis OR	(95%CI)	*P*-value
HOMA-IR	1.67	(1.09–2.56)	0.017
HDL-cholesterol	0.90	(0.86–0.97)	0.003
SHBG	0.90	(0.85–0.94)	<0.001
FAI	1.31	(1.10–1.57)	0.002
PCOS	3.55	(1.03–12.25)	0.044

Adjusted for age, BMI and WC. Significant *P*-values <0.05 are bold.
FAI: free androgen index; HOMA-IR: homeostasis model assessment of insulin resistance; SHBG: sex hormone binding globulin.

biochemical and hormonal parameters were determined and NAFLD was evaluated by abdominal ultrasonography and biochemical testing, after excluding causes of secondary liver disease. Insulin resistance was assessed by homeostasis model assessment of insulin resistance (HOMA-IR) and free androgen index (FAI) was calculated.

Results.—PCOS patients had an increased prevalence of HS [21/57 patients (36.8%) versus 12/60 controls (20.0%), $P < 0.05$] and abnormal (≥40 IU/l) serum aminotransferase levels [13/57 patients (22.8%) versus 2/60 controls (3.3%), $P < 0.01$] than controls. All patients and controls with metabolic syndrome had HS. Factors associated with HS were PCOS diagnosis, older age, increased BMI, waist circumference (WC), HOMA-IR and FAI values and decreased high-density lipid cholesterol and sex hormone binding globulin levels. PCOS patients had an OR of 3.55 (95% CI: 1.02–5.35) for HS versus controls, after adjustment for age, BMI and WC.

Conclusion.—SNAFLD is common in PCOS patients and increased androgen bioavailability may be implicated, in combination with metabolic abnormalities. Liver evaluation is proposed in PCOS patients, especially in those with metabolic syndrome (Table 5).

▶ Non-alcoholic fatty liver disease (NAFLD) is a common disorder causing fatty liver, liver dysfunction, and fibrosis. It is markedly increased in obesity, type II diabetes, dyslipidemia, insulin resistance, the metabolic syndrome, and polycystic ovary syndrome (PCOS). Simple steatosis is considered a benign condition, but progresses to non-alcoholic steatohepatitis (NASH). PCOS affects 5% to 8% of premenopausal women and is characterized by hyperandrogenism and ovulatory dysfunction, and a higher percentage have the metabolic syndrome. This study concluded that increased bioavailable androgens (BA) might be implicated in the pathogenesis of NAFLD. While increased BA was an expected finding from decreased sex hormone binding globulin (SHBG) both in controls and PCOS patients with hepatic steatosis, the finding was only significant in women with increased total androgen concentrations. The influence of hyperandrogenism in the pathogenesis of NAFLD requires further investigation. Abdominal adiposity and more severe dyslipidemia are also implicated in the NAFLD in women with PCOS. It is important to evaluate patients with PCOS for NASH in an attempt to reverse it to minimize its effects on liver dysfunction and development of cirrhosis.

A. W. Meikle, MD

Metabolic and Reproductive Features before and during Puberty in Daughters of Women with Polycystic Ovary Syndrome

Sir-Petermann T, Codner E, Pérez V, et al (Univ of Chile, Santiago; et al)

J Clin Endocrinol Metab 94:1923-1930, 2009

Context.—A significant proportion of the first-degree female relatives of women with polycystic ovary syndrome (PCOS) may be at risk for developing PCOS. However, it is not known at which stage of pubertal development the hormonal and metabolic abnormalities ensue in PCOS.

Objective.—The aim of the study was to assess the reproductive and metabolic profiles of daughters of women with PCOS (PCOSd) during the peripubertal period, a stage during which the gonadal axis is activated and PCOS may become clinically manifest.

Design.—Ninety-nine PCOSd [30 prepubertal and 69 pubertal (Tanner II-V)] and 84 daughters of control women (Cd) (20 prepubertal and 64 pubertal) were studied. An oral glucose tolerance test, a GnRH agonist test (leuprolide acetate, 10 μg/kg sc), and a transabdominal ultrasound

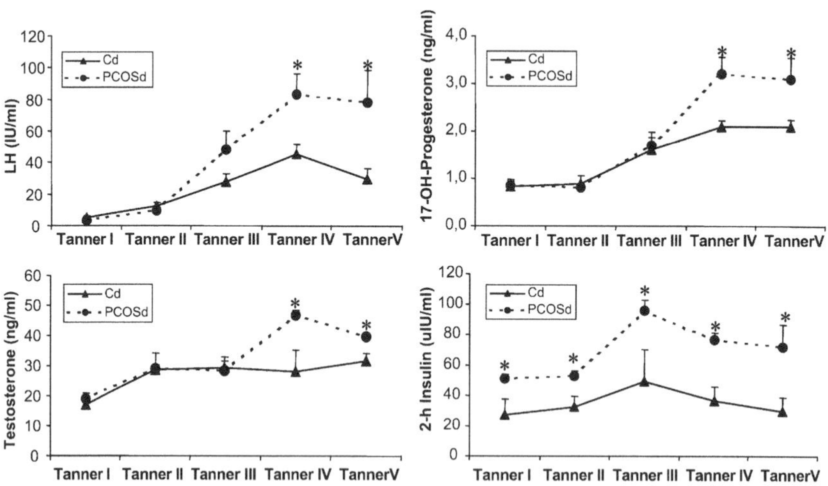

FIGURE 2.—LH, 17-OHP, and testosterone (LC-MS/MS) levels after stimulation with leuprolide acetate and the insulin levels after the glucose load (2-h) in PCOSd and Cd. Values are expressed as mean ± SEM. *, $P < 0.05$. (Reprinted from Sir-Petermann T, Codner E, Pérez V, et al. Metabolic and reproductive features before and during puberty in daughters of women with polycystic ovary syndrome. *J Clin Endocrinol Metab.* 2009;94:1923-1930, with permission from The Endocrine Society.)

were performed. Gonadotropins, sex steroids, SHBG, glucose, insulin, and lipids were determined.

Results.—Both groups had similar chronological ages and body mass index SD scores according to Tanner stage distribution. Ovarian volume and 2-h insulin were significantly higher in PCOSd compared to Cd at all Tanner stages. In Tanner stages IV and V, basal testosterone and post-stimulated LH, testosterone, and 17-hydroxyprogesterone concentrations were significantly higher in PCOSd compared to Cd.

Conclusions.—Hyperinsulinemia and an increased ovarian volume are present in PCOSd before the onset of puberty and persist during pubertal development. The biochemical abnormalities of PCOS appear during late puberty. Considering the early onset and the nature of the alterations, PCOSd constitute a high-risk group for metabolic and reproductive derangements (Fig 2).

▶ Polycystic ovary syndrome (PCOS) affects 5% to 10% of adult women, and is characterized by chronic anovulation and hyperandrogenism. Most of them have insulin resistance and are at high risk for type II diabetes mellitus and the metabolic syndrome. In most girls the clinical features begin after adolescence, but in some, clinical features can be recognized during the peripubertally. PCOS has a strong hereditary component. In the study by Sir-Petermann et al, daughters of women with PCOS were evaluated for their metabolic and hormonal abnormalities. High serum insulin concentrations and increased ovarian volume were observed before the onset of puberty and hormonal abnormalities characteristic of PCOS, such as increased luteinizing hormone (LH), testosterone, and 17 hydroxyprogesterone serum concentrations, were observed in late puberty. The clinical features of hyperandrogenism may not become apparent during early puberty because the effects of androgen excess may be delayed. They propose that the hyperinsulinemia may increase follicle-stimulating hormone (FSH) response to increase the number of ovarian follicles and increase the LH response on thecal cells of the ovary to increase testosterone production. Sensitive and specific measurements of sex steroids were critical for making the observations in these adolescents.

A. W. Meikle, MD

Adrenal androgen production capacity remains high up to menopause in women with polycystic ovary syndrome

Puurunen J, Piltonen T, Jaakkola P, et al (Oulu Univ Hosp, Finland)
J Clin Endocrinol Metab 94:1973-1978, 2009

Introduction.—Hyperandrogenism is one of the main features of polycystic ovary syndrome (PCOS). Of circulating androgens, 50% of androstenedione and testosterone are of ovarian and adrenal origin, whereas dehydroepiandrosterone (DHEA) and DHEA sulfate are almost uniquely of adrenal origin. Our previous studies have indicated that ovarian androgen production capacity is enhanced in women with PCOS, and it remains high until late reproductive age. To study whether this also applies to adrenal androgen production, ACTH tests were performed in healthy women and in women with PCOS.

Materials.—Sixty-nine healthy women (aged 19-62 yr; body mass index 19.2-35.0 kg/m2) and 58 women with previously diagnosed PCOS (aged 18-59 yr; body mass index 19.0-42.9 kg/m2) participated in the study.

Methods.—The subjects underwent ACTH stimulation tests, and serum cortisol, 17-hydroxyprogesterone, androstenedione, testosterone, DHEA, and DHEA sulfate levels were analyzed at 0, 30, and 60 min.

Results.—Basal and ACTH-stimulated levels of most adrenal androgens decreased in healthy women with age, whereas in women with PCOS, only the concentrations of basal serum 17-hydroxyprogesterone decreased, and all areas under the curve (AUCs) remained unchanged and significantly higher (except for DHEA) than those in control women. Likewise, at the menopausal transition, pre- and postmenopausal women with PCOS exhibited mainly unchanged and higher basal androgen and AUC levels.

Conclusions.—Similarly to ovarian endocrine function, serum adrenal steroid levels and adrenal steroid production capacity remain enhanced at least up to menopause in women with PCOS.

▶ Postpubertal hirsutism and irregular menses can be the manifestations of late-onset congenital adrenal hyperplasia (CAH) or polycystic ovary (PCO) syndrome. The diagnosis is made by measuring androgen levels (testosterone, androstenedione, and dehydroepiandrosterone) and the 17-hydroxyprogesterone or 17-hydroxypregnenolone response to corticotrophin. These patients used to be treated with low doses of corticosteroids for several years, with normalization of menses and decrease in body hair growth. In subsequent decades, emphasis was placed on oral contraceptives as a way to suppress ovarian androgen production and spironolactone to inhibit 5α-reductase and block conversion of testosterone to DHT. Corticosteroid suppression was limited to patients with late onset CAH. Treatment was usually interrupted when women obtained fertility and satisfactory control of hirsutism. Recent studies again emphasize the adrenal contribution to the hormonal abnormalities observed in PCO. Puurunen et al measured androgen and cortisol levels before and after corticotrophin stimulation to determine whether the levels changed as women got older and reached menopause. They studied 58 PCO women of different ages and compared them with 69 healthy women. For data analysis, subjects were separated into 3 age clusters: <30, 31 to 40, and 41 to menopause. They found that androgen and cortisol levels were higher in PCO women than control, and the difference persisted until menopause. Whereas normal women showed a decline in basal and stimulated androgen levels with age, PCO women did not decline. The study supports the view that adrenocortical steroids are involved in PCO and that this is not just an ovarian condition. It rehabilitates the rationale for using glucocorticoid suppression as a treatment for PCO.

D. E. Schteingart, MD

Increased 5 alpha-reductase activity and adrenocortical drive in women with polycystic ovary syndrome

Vassiliadi DA, Barber TM, Hughes BA, et al (Univ of Birmingham, UK)

J Clin Endocrinol Metab 94:3558-3566, 2009

Context.—Polycystic ovary syndrome (PCOS) is characterized by hyperandrogenism, anovulation, and susceptibility to the metabolic syndrome. Altered peripheral cortisol metabolism has been reported in PCOS, but also in simple obesity.

Objective.—The aim of the study was to describe cortisol metabolism and metabolic characteristics of a large PCOS cohort and to delineate the effect of obesity by comparison to body mass index (BMI)-matched controls.

Design and Setting.—We conducted an observational, cross-sectional study at outpatient clinics of two secondary/tertiary care centers.

Patients or Other Participants.—A total of 178 PCOS patients fulfilling Rotterdam criteria and 100 BMI-matched controls participated in the study.

Intervention.—The study included 24-h urine collection for steroid metabolite excretion and fasting blood samples, followed by an oral glucose tolerance test.

Main Outcome Measures.—We measured urinary steroid metabolites including glucocorticoids and androgens and the ratios reflecting enzymatic activities involved in peripheral cortisol and androgen metabolism, 5 alpha-reductase, and 11 beta-hydroxysteroid dehydrogenase types 1 and 2. We also measured circulating levels of glucose, insulin, dehydroepiandrosterone, dehydroepiandrosterone sulfate, and testosterone and calculated homeostasis model assessment.

Results.—Total androgen metabolites were higher in PCOS patients compared to BMI-matched controls (4,105 ± 2,047 vs. 2,532 ± 1,610 microg/24 h for the nonobese; 5,547 ± 2,911 vs. 2,468 ± 1,794 microg/24 h for the obese; both $P < 0.001$). Total glucocorticoid metabolites were higher in obese PCOS vs. controls (10,786 ± 3,852 vs. 8,834 ± 4,487 microg/24 h; $P = 0.001$). 5 alpha-Reductase activity correlated with BMI, insulin levels, and homeostasis model assessment. Both obese and nonobese PCOS patients had higher 5 alpha-reductase activity than controls (all $P < 0.05$). 11 beta- Hydroxysteroid dehydrogenase activities did not differ between PCOS and controls.

Conclusions.—PCOS is associated with enhanced androgen and cortisol metabolite excretion and increased 5 alphareductase activity that cannot be explained by obesity alone. Increased adrenal corticosteroid production represents an important pathogenic pathway in PCOS.

▶ Polycystic ovary (PCO) syndrome is one of the most common gynecological problems experienced by women in the reproductive age. The pathogenesis of this condition is probably multifactorial. For example, disruption of pituitary gonadotropin secretion leads to anovulation, increased intraovarian androgen synthesis leads to virilization of various degrees, insulin resistance leads to hyperinsulinemia that also stimulates ovarian androgen synthesis, and defects in adrenal steroidogenesis lead to increased androgen synthesis. Obesity is common among patients with PCO, and its role, along with the associated insulin resistance, is not totally clear. There are nonobese women with PCO and they may also be insulin resistant. Vassiliadi et al studied 178 women with PCO and compared them with 100 weight-matched controls. They measured androgen and cortisol metabolites to assess the enzymatic activity involved in peripheral cortisol and androgen metabolism, levels of adrenal (dehydroepiandrosterone) and ovarian androgens (testosterone), and insulin sensitivity. They found that women with PCO had higher total androgen and cortisol metabolites as well as 5α-reductase activity (conversion of testosterone to the more active dihydrotestosterone), but no difference in the activity of 11β-hydroxysteroid dehydrogenase (converting cortisol to cortisone or vice versa). The increase in 5α-reductase activity may be linked to insulin resistance or to increases in cortisol secretion, but the cause is still unknown. This report emphasizes an increase in cortisol metabolite excretion as playing a role in PCO. Abnormalities in cortisol secretion, turnover, and clearance have been described in obesity for almost 5 decades, but this study speculates that this abnormality plays a pathogenic role in PCO. It is likely that like in any syndrome, there are various pathogenic mechanisms involved causing a single phenotypic picture.

D. E. Schteingart, MD

Role of vitamin D treatment in glucose metabolism in polycystic ovary syndrome

Kotsa K, Yavropoulou MP, Anastasiou O, et al (Aristotle Univ of Thessaloniki, Greece)

Fertil Steril 92:1053-1058, 2009

Objective.—To determine the effect of treatment with vitamin D_3 analogue in the parameters of glucose metabolism in obese women with polycystic ovary syndrome (PCOS).

Design.—Observational study.

Setting.—Obese women with PCOS in an academic research environment.

Patient(s).—Fifteen obese women (mean age 28 ± 1.3 years, mean body mass index 32.55 ± 0.43) with documented chronic anovulation and hyperandrogenism were recruited into the study.

Intervention(s).—Alphacalcidol (1-α-hydroxyvitamin D_3) was administered orally 1 μg/day for 3 months. All subjects underwent a frequently sampled IV glucose tolerance test after a 10- to 12-hour overnight fast during a spontaneous bleeding episode before and after treatment with alphacalcidol.

Main Outcome Measure(s).—Peripheral insulin resistance and insulin effectiveness were estimated with minimal model.

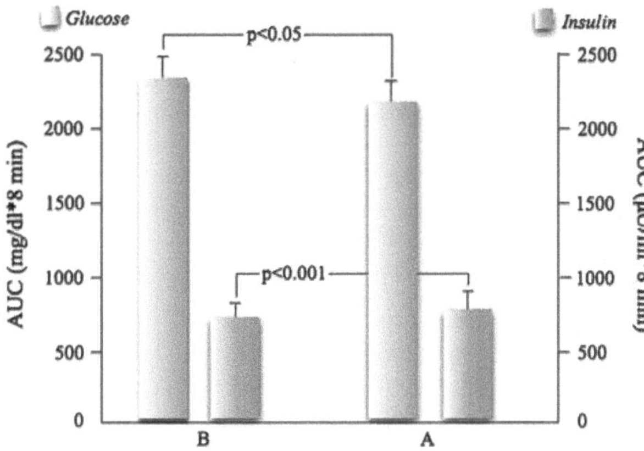

FIGURE 1.—Changes in glucose and insulin concentration during the first phase of insulin secretion (AUC_{1-8}) before and after treatment with alphacalcidol. Values are mean + SE. B = before treatment; A = after treatment. (Reprinted from Kotsa K, Yavropoulou MP, Anastasiou O, et al. Role of vitamin D treatment in glucose metabolism in polycystic ovary syndrome. *Fertil Steril.* 2009;92:1053-1058, with permission from the American Society for Reproductive Medicine.)

Result(s).—The first phase of insulin secretion was significantly increased after treatment with alphacalcidol. A favorable statistically significant change also was observed in the lipid profile.

Conclusion(s).—Treatment with the vitamin D_3 analogue (alphacalcidol) could be of value in the management of PCOS (Fig 1).

▶ Vitamin D deficiency has been associated with many diseases in recent years in addition to its well-known influence on bone disease. Low concentrations of vitamin D 25 OH in cross sectional studies have been implicated in overall mortality, heart disease, hypertension, diabetes, autoimmune diseases, and some cancers. Both polycystic ovary syndrome (PCOS) and vitamin D 25 OH deficiency are very common. PCOS affects more than 6% of women, and vitamin D deficiency is even more common. In PCOS women, androgen excess and insulin resistance with high serum insulin concentrations are characteristic features. Vitamin D deficiency has been associated with impaired glucose tolerance and insulin secretion in both humans and experimental animals. Kotsa investigated the effect of alphacalcidol (1-α-hydroxyvitamin D_3) on peripheral insulin resistance and effectiveness in women with documented PCOS. They observed that the first phase of insulin secretion and the lipid profile were significantly improved after treatment with the vitamin D_3 analog. Vitamin D deficiency is more common in obesity compared with normal weight persons. Additional studies in diabetics without PCOS would be informative about the influence of vitamin D on insulin secretion and action.

A. W. Meikle, MD

Bone Health in Men

Relation between Serum Testosterone, Serum Estradiol, Sex Hormone-Binding Globulin, and Geometrical Measures of Adult Male Proximal Femur Strength

Travison TG, Araujo AB, Beck TJ, et al (New England Res Insts, Watertown, MA; Johns Hopkins Univ School of Medicine, Baltimore, MD; et al)
J Clin Endocrinol Metab 94:853-860, 2009

Context.—Although previous studies have indicated associations between circulating testosterone (T) or estradiol (E2) concentrations and bone mineral density, the relationship between gonadal steroids and skeletal geometry is not well defined.

Objective.—Our objective was to uncover the relation between circulating T or E2 and proximal femur geometry in a diverse sample of men.

Design.—We used data on 808 men enrolled in the Boston Area Community Health/Bone Study. Serum concentrations of total and calculated free T and E2 were obtained via early-morning blood sampling. The geometry of the proximal femur at three sites (the narrow neck, intertrochanter, and shaft) was obtained using the Hip Structural Analysis technology. Analyses adjusted for subjects' age, height, total body lean mass and fat mass, and level of physical activity were performed.

Setting.—In-home interviews accompanied by subject visits to the General Clinical Research Center at Boston University School of Medicine were performed.

Study Participants.—A randomly selected cohort of men living in Boston, MA (ages 30–79 yr) was included in the study.

Interventions.—These were not applicable.

Main Outcome Measures.—Bone mineral density and bone outer diameter, cross-sectional area (measuring bone material), and section modulus (an index of bending strength) were calculated.

Results.—In age-adjusted models, E2 was positively associated with hip strength parameters, whereas T was not. Adjustment for age and other parameters resulted in substantial reductions in, but not complete elimination of, associations between E2 and hip strength parameters.

Conclusion.—Circulating E2 is strongly associated with proximal femur strength, an association that is partially mediated by body composition (Fig 2).

▶ Sex steroids are known to affect bone mineral density (BMD), and in men, aging is associated with alterations in sex steroid concentrations that might adversely affect BMD and predispose to fractures. Cross-sectional and longitudinal studies have shown a positive relationship between serum testosterone and estradiol concentrations and BMD with estradiol showing the stronger association. There are other factors besides sex steroids that affect bone fractures, and BMD is not directly associated with bone strength. In the study by Travison et al, 808 men were enrolled in a study to determine whether

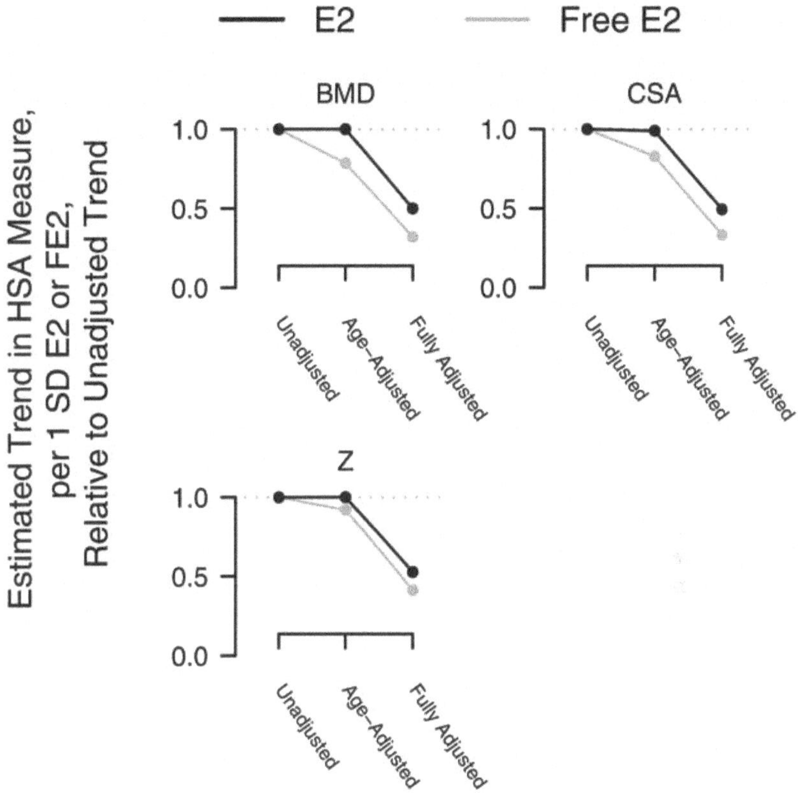

FIGURE 2.—Reduction in the magnitude of the association between E2 and NN hip geometry accompanying control for other parameters in a multivariate regression model. Points corresponding to "Age-adjusted" and "Fully Adjusted" models express the cross-sectional change in proximal femur strength indices accompanying a 1 SD increase in E2 or FE2, controlling for age and other parameters (LM, FM, PASE, and height). These differences are scaled to the crude difference observed when no other covariates are considered ("Unadjusted"). (Reprinted from Travison TG, Araujo AB, Beck TJ, et al. Relation between serum testosterone, serum estradiol, sex hormone-binding globulin, and geometrical measures of adult male proximal femur strength. *J Clin Endocrinol Metab.* 2009;94:853-860, with permission from The Endocrine Society.)

circulating sex steroids showed a relationship to proximal femur geometry in men aged 30 to 79 years. Results that estradiol but not testosterone was positively associated with hip strength parameters are consistent with other studies in elderly men that show stronger association serum estradiol concentrations than testosterone. Body composition also influences proximal femur strength. In studies of bone strength the measurement are imperfect, and longitudinal studies are needed rather than cross-sectional studies.

A. W. Meikle, MD

Hypogonadism and Aging

17β-Estradiol at Low Concentrations Acts through Distinct Pathways in Normal Versus Benign Prostatic Hyperplasia-Derived Prostate Stromal Cells

Park II, Zhang Q, Liu V, et al (Northwestern Univ Feinberg School of Medicine, Chicago, IL; Univ of Chicago, IL; et al)
Endocrinology 150:4594-4605, 2009

The aim of this study was to identify differential responses to low concentrations of 17β-estradiol (E2) in primary stromal cell cultures derived from either normal organ donors or benign prostatic hyperplasia or hypertrophy (BPH) specimens. Furthermore, we sought to identify the potential mechanism of E2 action in these cell types, through either a genomic or nongenomic mechanism. We initially treated stromal cells derived from five normal prostates or five BPH specimens with low concentrations of E2 (0.001–1.0 nM) and analyzed their growth response. To determine whether genomic or nongenomic pathways were involved, we performed studies using specific estrogen receptor antagonists to confirm transcriptional activity or MAPK inhibitors to confirm the involvement of rapid signaling. Results of these studies revealed a fundamental difference in the mechanism of the response to E2. In normal cells, we found that a nongenomic, rapid E2 signaling pathway is predominantly involved, mediated by G protein-coupled receptor-30 and the subsequent activation of ERK1/2. In BPH-derived prostate stromal cells, a genomic pathway is predominantly involved because the addition of ICI 182780 was sufficient to abrogate any estrogenic effects. In conclusion, prostate stromal cells respond to far lower concentrations of E2 than previously recognized or examined, and this response is mediated through two distinct mechanisms, depending on its origin. This may provide the basis for new insights into the causes of, and possible treatments for, BPH.

▶ Both benign prostatic hyperplasia (BPH) and prostate cancer occur frequently in men with age. By 50 years of age 50% of men will be diagnosed with BPH, and by 60 years of age 60% of men will be diagnosed with BPH. Both androgens and estrogens have been implicated in the occurrence of BPH, but the evidence for estradiol-17β in the development of BPH is less clear. In experimental animals estrogen has been shown to accelerate the development of BPH, possibly by increasing androgen receptor activity. Circulating estradiol-17β concentrations also increases with age. The investigation by Park and associates suggests that estradiol-17β genomic and nongenomic pathways are evidence in prostate tissue. They concluded that in normal prostate stromal cells the nongenomic pathway was predominate, while in BPH stroma the genomic pathway predominated. Low concentrations of estrogen produced these responses. Further study is needed to determine whether inhibition of estrogen action can prevent BPH or reduce prostate size in men with BPH.

A. W. Meikle, MD

Effects of Aromatase Inhibition on Bone Mineral Density and Bone Turnover in Older Men with Low Testosterone Levels

Burnett-Bowie S-AM, McKay EA, Lee H, et al (Massachusetts General Hosp, Boston, MA)

J Clin Endocrinol Metab 94:4785-4792, 2009

Context.—Aging is associated with declining gonadal steroid production, low bone mineral density (BMD), and fragility fractures. The efficacy and safety of testosterone replacement in older men remains uncertain.

Objective.—The objective of the study was to assess the effects of aromatase inhibition on BMD in older men with low testosterone levels.

Design and Setting.—This was a 1-yr, double-blind, randomized, placebo-controlled trial that was conducted at a tertiary care academic center in Boston, MA.

Participants.—Participants included 69 men aged 60+ yr with borderline or low testosterone levels and hypogonadal symptoms.

Intervention.—Intervention included 1 mg anastrozole daily or placebo.

Main Outcome Measures.—Changes in gonadal steroid hormone levels, BMD, and bone turnover markers were measured.

Results.—Mean serum testosterone increased from 319 ± 93 ng/dl at baseline to 524 ± 139 ng/dl at month 3 ($P < 0.0001$) and declined slightly to 474 ± 145 ng/dl by 1 yr. Estradiol levels decreased from 15 ± 4 pg/ml at baseline to 12 ± 4 pg/ml at month 3 and then remained stable ($P < 0.0001$). Posterior-anterior (PA) spine BMD decreased in the anastrozole group as compared with placebo ($P = 0.0014$). In the anastrozole group, PA spine BMD decreased from 1.121 ± 0.141 g/cm^2 to 1.102 ± 0.138 g/cm^2, whereas in the placebo group, PA spine BMD increased from 1.180 ± 0.145 g/cm^2 to 1.189 ± 0.146 g/cm^2. Qualitatively similar, but not statistically significant, changes occurred at the other sites. Bone turnover markers were not affected by anastrozole therapy.

Conclusions.—In older men, aromatase inhibition increases testosterone levels, decreases estradiol levels, and appears to decrease BMD. Aromatase inhibition does not improve skeletal health in aging men with low or low normal testosterone levels.

▶ Estrogen has feedback influence on gonadotropin secretion in men. In aging men, testosterone declines and the gonadotropin rise is insufficient to maintain normal serum testosterone concentrations in many men. Bone mineral density (BMD) also declines as men age. Blocking estrogen feedback by inhibitors of estrogen action or decreasing concentrations by agents that inhibit estrogen formation can increase gonadal function and increase serum concentrations of testosterone. In the current study, men 60 years and older were treated with an aromatase inhibitor, which increased serum concentrations of testosterone and dihydrotestosterone, but lowered serum estradiol concentrations. Treatment with an aromatase inhibitor also significantly decreased bone mineral density of the spine without affecting bone turnover markers. The decrease in BMD of the hip was not statistically significant, perhaps because of the small sample size, which was a limitation of the study. In addition, despite the rise in testosterone, concentrations to the mid-normal range body composition did not improve with aromatase inhibitor therapy. These agents are also used in younger men to normalize gonadal function for improvement of fertility status. The current study indicates that long-term therapy with aromatase inhibitors is not recommended.

A. W. Meikle, MD

Effects of Testosterone on Muscle Strength, Physical Function, Body Composition, and Quality of Life in Intermediate-Frail and Frail Elderly Men: A Randomized, Double-Blind, Placebo-Controlled Study

Srinivas-Shankar U, Roberts SA, Connolly MJ, et al (Univ of Manchester, UK; Univ of Auckland, New Zealand)

J Clin Endocrinol Metab 95:639-650, 2010

Context.—Physical frailty is associated with reduced muscle strength, impaired physical function, and quality of life. Testosterone (T) increases muscle mass and strength in hypogonadal patients. It is unclear whether T has similar effects in intermediate-frail and frail elderly men with low to borderline-low T.

Objective.—Our objective was to determine the effects of 6 months T treatment in intermediate-frail and frail elderly men, on muscle mass and strength, physical function, and quality of life.

Design and Setting.—We conducted a randomized, double-blind, placebo-controlled, parallel-group, single-center study.

Participants.—Participants were community-dwelling intermediate-frail and frail elderly men at least 65 yr of age with a total T at or below 12 nmol/liter or free T at or below 250 pmol/liter.

Methods.—Two hundred seventy-four participants were randomized to transdermal T (50 mg/d) or placebo gel for 6 months. Outcome measures included muscle strength, lean and fat mass, physical function, and self-reported quality of life.

Results.—Isometric knee extension peak torque improved in the T group (*vs.* placebo at 6 months), adjusted difference was 8.6 (95% confidence interval, 1.3–16.0; $P = 0.02$) Newton-meters. Lean body mass increased and fat mass decreased significantly in the T group by 1.08 ± 1.8 and 0.9 ± 1.6 kg, respectively. Physical function improved among older and frailer men. Somatic and sexual symptom scores decreased with T treatment; adjusted difference was −1.2 (−2.4 to −0.04) and −1.3 (−2.5 to −0.2), respectively.

Conclusions.—T treatment in intermediate-frail and frail elderly men with low to borderline-low T for 6 months may prevent age-associated loss of lower limb muscle strength and improve body composition, quality of life, and physical function. Further investigations are warranted to extend these results.

▶ Physical frailty affects many organ systems, and aging is associated with a decline in muscle mass and strength, which is then associated with falls, disability, hospitalizations, and death. Hypogonadism, with a decline particularly in free testosterone, increases as men age and is deemed related to frailty of aging men. Some investigators have demonstrated improvement in muscle function with testosterone treatment of aging men, but other studies have failed to confirm that finding. The strength of the study by Srinivas-Shanker et al was that it was a single-center study and was a double-blind placebo-controlled study of the effect of testosterone therapy on muscle strength, physical function, and quality of life in intermediate-frail and frail elderly men. Men qualified for the study if their total testosterone was below 12 nmol/L (345 ng/dL) or a free testosterone of <250 pg/L (72 pg/mL). Treatment was either placebo or transdermal testosterone gel of 50 mg/d. Compared with placebo, men treated with testosterone had improved isometric knee extension peak torque and were physically functional. Lean body mass improved and fat mass decreased, as did somatic and sexual symptoms scores. The study was only for 6 months, which was not long enough to answer questions of the long-term benefits and safety of testosterone therapy in aging frail men. Adverse event increases were restricted to some rise in prostate-specific antigen (PSA) and hematocrit in the treated group, and serious adverse events listed did not appear to be testosterone related.

A. W. Meikle, MD

Fatty Acid Metabolism in the Elderly: Effects of Dehydroepiandrosterone and Testosterone Replacement in Hormonally Deficient Men and Women

Koutsari C, Ali AH, Nair KS, et al (Mayo Clinic, Rochester, MN)

J Clin Endocrinol Metab 94:3414-3423, 2009

Context.—Aging, low dehydroepiandrosterone (DHEA), and testosterone are associated with increased adiposity and metabolic risk. Treatment with these hormones may improve these abnormalities.

Objective.—The objective of the study was to determine effects of aging, DHEA, or testosterone replacement on adiposity, meal fat partitioning, and postabsorptive lipolysis.

Design.—This was a cross-sectional, 2-yr, double-blind, randomized, placebo-controlled trial.

Setting.—The study was conducted in the general community.

Patients.—Elderly women and men (≥60 yr) with low DHEA sulfate (women and men) and bioavailable testosterone (men) concentrations and young adults.

Interventions.—Thirty elderly women each received 50 mg DHEA or placebo daily for 2 yr. Thirty elderly men received 75 mg DHEA, 29 received 5 mg testosterone (patch), and 32 received placebo daily for 2 yr. Thirty young women and 32 young men served as controls.

Main Outcome Measures.—*In vivo* measures of meal fat storage into sc fat, postabsorptive lipolysis, and regional adiposity at baseline and after treatment.

Results.—At baseline, the elderly had more body fat, greater systemic lipolysis (women, $P = 0.0003$; men, $P < 0.0001$) adjusted for resting energy expenditure, greater meal fat oxidation (women, $P = 0.026$; men, $P = 0.0025$), and less meal fat storage in sc fat (women, $P = 0.0139$; men, $P = 0.0006$). Although testosterone treatment increased meal fat storage into upper- *vs.* lower-body fat in elderly men, neither hormone affected regional adiposity, meal fat oxidation, or systemic lipolysis.

Conclusions.—Aging, in the context of low DHEA sulfate (women and men) and bioavailable testosterone (men) concentrations, is associated with changes in meal fat partitioning and postabsorptive lipolysis that are not corrected by DHEA and only partly corrected by testosterone replacement.

▶ Increased total body fat and visceral fat accumulation occur with aging in both men and women. Serum concentrations of adrenal androgens, dehydroepiandrosterone sulfate (DHEA-S), and DHEA, also decline in both sexes with aging and testosterone declines in men, which is associated with increase adiposity and lower lean body mass. DHEA administration to the elderly has been associated with a reduction in total body, visceral, and abdominal subcutaneous fat. Testosterone therapy of testosterone deficient men has also resulted in a reduction in adiposity of various sites. The study by Koutsari et al was designed to determine if DHEA in men and women and testosterone in the elderly affected meal fat use and systemic lipolysis pathways that modify total body or regional fat distribution. DHEA therapy failed to correct the changes associated with meal fat partitioning and postabsorptive lipolysis, but were partially corrected by testosterone. Whether differences between young and elderly are hormonally controlled by DHEA is not certain from the study and might be related to other factors, but testosterone may be a partial contributory to the changes associated with aging men.

A. W. Meikle, MD

Low circulating androgens and mortality risk in heart failure

Güder G, Frantz S, Bauersachs J, et al (Klinikum der Universität Würzburg, Germany)

Heart 96:504-509, 2010

Objective.—Deficiency of anabolic sex steroids is common in heart failure (HF). The pathophysiological implications of this phenomenon, however, have not been fully elucidated. This clinical study investigated the significance of low serum androgen levels in HF.

Design.—Prospective cohort study.

Patients and Methods.—In 191 consecutively recruited men with HF (mean age 64 years; New York Heart Association (NYHA) class I–IV 24%/35%/35%/6%) and reduced (ejection fraction (EF) ≤40%, n=96) or preserved (EF >40%, n=95) left ventricular function total and free serum testosterone, dehydroepiandrosterone sulfate (DHEAS) and sex hormone binding globulin (SHBG) were measured. The median observation period was 859 days.

Results.—During follow-up 53 patients (28%) died. Whereas total serum testosterone was normal in most patients (91%), free testosterone and DHEAS were reduced in 79% and 23%, respectively. DHEAS and free testosterone, but not total testosterone, were inversely associated with NYHA class (both $p<0.01$). Lower free testosterone and DHEAS and higher SHBG predicted all-cause mortality risk (hazard ratio (HR) 0.89, 95% CI 0.82 to 0.96 per 1 ng/dl free testosterone, $p=0.004$; HR 0.95, 95% CI 0.89 to 1.00 per 10 μg/dl DHEAS, $p=0.058$; and HR 1.18, 95% CI 1.05 to 1.33 per 10 nmol/l SHBG, $p=0.006$, respectively; adjusted for age and NYHA class). However, further adjustment for carefully selected confounding factors abolished these associations.

TABLE 4.—Association Between Androgens or SHBG and All-Cause Mortality Risk

	Model 1 HR (95% CI); p Value	Model 2 HR (95% CI); p Value	Model 3 HR (95% CI); p Value
Total testosterone, per 100 ng/dl	0.85 (0.69 to 1.04); 0.105	0.88 (0.73 to 1.07); 0.205	Not computed
Free testosterone, per 1 ng/dl	0.85 (0.76 to 0.94); 0.002	0.89 (0.82 to 0.96); 0.004	0.92 (0.84 to 1.02); 0.118
DHEAS, per 10 μg/dl	0.93 (0.87 to 0.98); 0.013	0.95 (0.89 to 1.00); 0.058	0.97 (0.91 to 1.03); 0.329
SHBG, per 10 nmol/l	1.13 (1.00 to 1.28); 0.050	1.19 (1.05 to 1.34); 0.006	1.06 (0.92 to 1.23); 0.411

Model 1: Adjustment for age. Model 2: Adjustment for age and New York Heart Association class. Model 3: Adjustment of model 2 extended by those variables that were associated with both mortality risk and the respective hormone level (ie, potential confounding factors). Confounders were: for free testosterone: renal function, atrial fibrillation, systolic blood pressure, C-reactive protein, N-terminal pro-brain natriuretic peptide (NT-proBNP), intake of diuretics, cortisol; for dehydroepiandrosterone sulphate (DHEAS): renal function, atrial fibrillation, total cholesterol, NTproBNP, intake of diuretics, intake of betablockers; for sex hormone binding globulin (SHBG): renal function, atrial fibrillation, NT-proBNP, intake of angiotensin-converting enzyme inhibitor, intake of statin, cortisol. HR, hazard ratio.

Conclusion.—In male HF patients, low serum levels of androgens are associated with adverse prognosis, but this relation is confounded by indicators of a poor health state. The results suggest that low serum androgens develop as a sequel of this progressive multifaceted systemic disorder (Table 4).

▶ There are reports of reduced longevity in aging men with low serum testosterone concentrations. It is uncertain if the reduction in serum testosterone is disease associated or causal to mortality. Anabolic hormones, such as testosterone and insulin-like growth factor 1 (IGF-1) decline with age, while catabolic hormones such as thyroid hormone and cortisol do not decline, which results in an imbalance between catabolic and anabolic hormones. Guder et al evaluated circulating serum testosterone and dehydroepiandrosterone sulfate (DHEAS) in older men with heart failure. In these men, total testosterone was deficient in only 9%, whereas free testosterone was subnormal in 79%. They concluded that neither total nor free testosterone, DHEAS, or sex hormone binding globulin (SHBG) were independent risk factors for mortality. Their findings did not indicate that androgens had a causal influence on progression of heart failure. The modest sample size limited the power of the analyses, and hormones were not measured serially. The results cannot be extrapolated to other chronic diseases in men with androgen alterations.

A. W. Meikle, MD

Non-competitive androgen receptor inhibition in vitro and in vivo

Jones JO, Bolton EC, Huang Y, et al (Univ of California San Francisco; et al)

Proc Natl Acad Sci USA 106:7233-7238, 2009

Androgen receptor (AR) inhibitors are used to treat multiple human diseases, including hirsutism, benign prostatic hypertrophy, and prostate cancer, but all available anti-androgens target only ligand binding, either by reduction of available hormone or by competitive antagonism. New strategies are needed, and could have an important impact on therapy. One approach could be to target other cellular mechanisms required for receptor activation. In prior work, we used a cell-based assay of AR conformation change to identify non-ligand inhibitors of AR activity. Here, we characterize 2 compounds identified in this screen: pyrvinium pamoate, a Food and Drug Administration-approved drug, and harmol hydrochloride, a natural product. Each compound functions by a unique, non-competitive mechanism and synergizes with competitive antagonists to disrupt AR activity. Harmol blocks DNA occupancy by AR, whereas pyrvinium does not. Pyrvinium inhibits AR-dependent gene expression

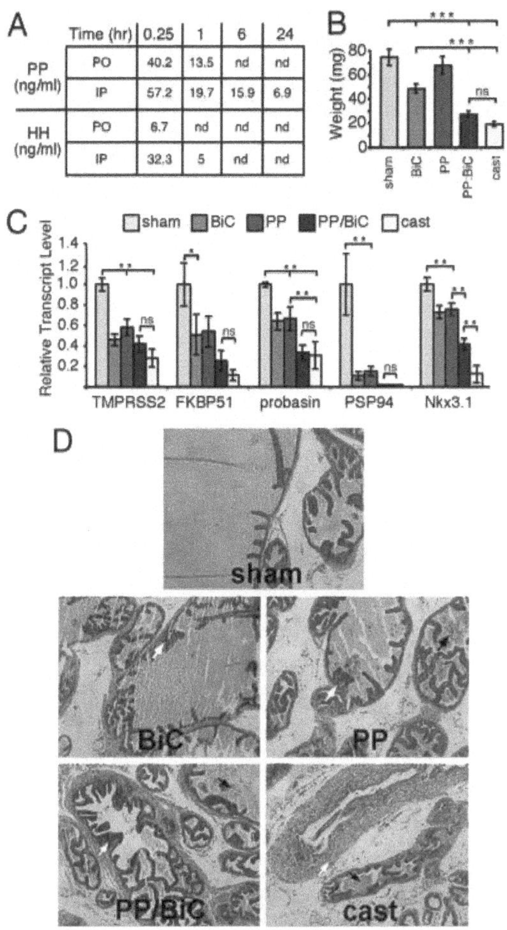

FIGURE 4.—Properties and efficacy of PP and HH in vivo. (*A*) Mice were administered 5 mg/kg PP or 2 mg/kg HH by the indicated methods. Plasma concentrations were determined by MS, and reported in ng/mL. (*nd*, compound not detected.) (*B and C*) Litter-mate-controlled FVB male mice were treated for 4 weeks with 100 mg/kg oral BiC ($n = 9$), an escalating dose of i.p. PP to 1 mg/kg ($n = 9$), or a combination of these treatments ($n = 9$). Cohorts of mice were castrated at the onset of the study ($n = 9$), or were sham-treated with i.p. and oral vehicles ($n = 10$). (*B*) Prostate wet weight was measured as a proximal marker of anti-androgen potency. (*C*) Quantitative PCR was performed on reverse-transcribed RNA isolated from mouse prostate tissues. Transcripts for each gene were normalized to RPL19, an androgen-unresponsive gene. (ANOVA, $^{*}P < 0.05$; $^{**}P < 0.01$; $^{***}P < 0.001$; *ns*, no significant difference between indicated populations; error bars indicate SEM.) (*D*) Representative sections of dorsal prostate from each treatment group were stained using hematoxylin and eosin. Substantial prostate atrophy is present in castrated and combination treatment samples. Signs of androgen deprivation are also visible in the samples of mice treated with BiC and PP alone. Note the loss of columnar epithelial architecture (white arrows), decreased secretory protein, increased nuclear staining, a relative thickening of the stromal layer, and dead cell accumulation in the lumen (black arrows). (Reprinted from Jones JO, Bolton EC, Huang Y, et al. Non-competitive androgen receptor inhibition in vitro and in vivo. *Proc Natl Acad Sci USA.* 2009;106:7233-7238.)

in the prostate gland in vivo, and induces prostate atrophy. These results highlight new therapeutic strategies to inhibit AR activity (Fig 1).

▶ Androgen receptor (AR) is a member of the nuclear hormone receptor family and is expressed in many tissues producing influences on physiological and pathological conditions. In women, androgens can cause hirsutism and virilization. While in males, androgens are necessary for sexual differentiation, cognition, muscle enlargement, bone health, prostate growth, and differentiation. In men, prostate disease and male pattern hair loss are undesirable consequences of androgen action. Commonly used current therapies for reducing unwanted androgen actions include reducing androgen concentrations or blocking androgen binding to the AR. Jones et al sought 2 noncompetitive androgen receptor inhibitors and observed that they block androgen action on growth of prostate tissue both in vitro and in vivo. Harmol hydrochloride blocked occupancy of by AR, and pyrvinium inhibited AR-dependent gene expression of prostate tissue. These are interesting findings and might provide new approaches to treatment of androgen-dependent diseases and disorders. Clinical trials will be needed to determine whether they have acceptable efficacy and toxicity and are superior in anyway to currently available inhibitors of androgen action.

A. W. Meikle, MD

Sex Hormones and Frailty in Older Men: The Osteoporotic Fractures in Men (MrOS) Study

Cawthon PM, for the Osteoporotic Fractures in Men (MrOS) Research Group (California Pacific Med Ctr, San Francisco; et al)

J Clin Endocrinol Metab 94:3806-3815, 2009

Context.—As men age, the prevalence of frailty increases whereas levels of androgens decline. Little is known about the relation between these factors.

Objective.—The aim of this study was to assess cross-sectional and longitudinal associations of estradiol, bioavailable estradiol, testosterone, bioavailable testosterone (bioT), and SHBG with frailty status.

Design and Setting.—The Osteoporotic Fractures in Men (MrOS) study was conducted at six U.S. clinical centers.

Participants.—A total of 1469 community-dwelling men at least 65 yr old with baseline data participated; 1245 men had frailty status reassessed 4.1 yr later.

Main Outcome Measure.—Proportional odds models estimated the likelihood of greater frailty status. Frail men had at least three of the following: weakness, slowness, low activity, exhaustion, and shrinking/sarcopenia; intermediate men had one or two criteria; and robust men had none. At follow-up, death was included as an additional ordinal

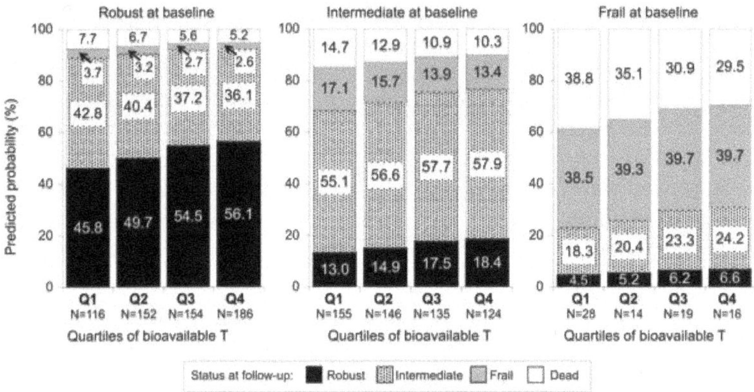

FIGURE 3.—Predicted probability of frailty status at follow-up, by quartile of bioavailable testosterone and frailty status at baseline for a 73.4-yr-old man. Cut-points for quartiles of bioavailable testosterone: Q1, ≤165.4 ng/dl; Q2, 165.4 to <201.5 ng/dl; Q3, 201.5 to <241.9 ng/dl; and Q4, ≥241.9 ng/dl. Probabilities derived from a partial proportional odds model, with age and bioavailable testosterone meeting the proportionality assumption, and frailty status at baseline not meeting the proportional odds assumption. The age assumed for the model (73.4 yr) is the mean age of the population at baseline. (Reprinted from Cawthon PM, for the Osteoporotic Fractures in Men (MrOS) Research Group. Sex hormones and frailty in older men: the osteoporotic fractures in men (MrOS) study. *J Clin Endocrinol Metab*. 2009;94:3806-3815, with permission from The Endocrine Society.)

outcome. Sex hormones were assayed by spectrometry/chromatographic methods.

Results.—In cross-sectional analyses, men in the lowest quartile of bioT had 1.39-fold (95% confidence interval, 1.02, 1.91) increased odds of greater frailty status compared to men in the highest quartile after adjustment for covariates including age, body size, health status, and medical conditions. In age-adjusted longitudinal analyses, men in the lowest quartile of bioT had 1.51-fold (95% confidence interval, 1.10, 2.07) increased odds of greater frailty status 4.1 yr later. This association was largely attenuated by adjustment for covariates. No other hormones were associated in a cross-sectional or longitudinal manner with frailty status after adjustment.

Conclusions.—Low levels of bioT were independently associated with worse baseline frailty status. Frailty status should be considered as an outcome in trials of testosterone supplementation (Fig 3).

▶ Frailty is associated with impaired function in older persons in response to external stressors. The characterization includes weakness (grip strength), shrinking/sarcopenia (weight loss), slowness (walking speed), self reported low activity level, and exhaustion. There is a parallel between decline in physical function and circulating androgen concentrations in men with aging, which may suggest an association between frailty and declining sex hormones. The study by Cawthon et al evaluated 1245 men over 65 years of age for association of frailty parameters and sex hormones. This was a cross-sectional study, but men within the lowest quartile for bioavailable testosterone (the presumed biologically active testosterone) had about 40% increased frailty compared with men in the highest quartile. Certainly, studies assessing the potential benefits of testosterone therapy of aging men with androgen deficiency must include parameters of frailty. A weakness of the current investigation is that it was cross-sectional rather than interventional. There are many factors besides a reduction in testosterone with aging that must be considered in assessing benefits of testosterone therapy to restore sex hormone levels, which will be components of future studies.

A. W. Meikle, MD

Testosterone and Growth Hormone Improve Body Composition and Muscle Performance in Older Men

Sattler FR, Castaneda-Sceppa C, Binder EF, et al (Univ of Southern California, Los Angeles; Tufts Univ, Boston, MA; Washington Univ, St. Louis, MO)
J Clin Endocrinol Metab 94:1991-2001, 2009

Context.—Impairments in the pituitary-gonadal axis with aging are associated with loss of muscle mass and function and accumulation of upper body fat.

Objectives.—We tested the hypothesis that physiological supplementation with testosterone and GH together improves body composition and muscle performance in older men.

Design, Setting, and Participants.—One hundred twenty-two community-dwelling men 70.8 ± 4.2 yr of age with body mass index of 27.4 ± 3.4 kg/m^2, testosterone of 550 ng/dl or less, and IGF-I in lower adult tertile (≤167 ng/dl) were randomized to receive transdermal testosterone (5 or 10 g/d) during a Leydig cell clamp plus GH (0, 3, or 5 μg/kg · d) for 16 wk.

Main Outcome Measures.—Body composition by dual-energy x-ray absorptiometry, muscle performance, and safety tests were conducted.

Results.—Total lean body mass increased (1.0 ± 1.7 to 3.0 ± 2.2 kg) as did appendicular lean tissue (0.4 ± 1.4 to 1.5 ± 1.3 kg), whereas total fat mass decreased by 0.4 ± 0.9 to 2.3 ± 1.7 kg as did trunk fat (0.5 ± 0.9 to 1.5 ± 1.0 kg) across the six treatment groups and by dose levels for each parameter ($P \leq 0.0004$ for linear trend). Composite maximum voluntary strength of upper and lower body muscles increased by 14 ± 34 to 35 ± 31% ($P < 0.003$ in the three highest dose groups) that correlated with changes in appendicular lean mass. Aerobic endurance increased in all six groups (average 96 ± 137 sec longer). Systolic and diastolic blood pressure increased similarly in each group with mean increases of 12 ± 14 and 8 ± 8 mm Hg, respectively. Other predictable adverse events were modest and reversible.

Conclusions.—Supplemental testosterone produced significant gains in total and appendicular lean mass, muscle strength, and aerobic endurance

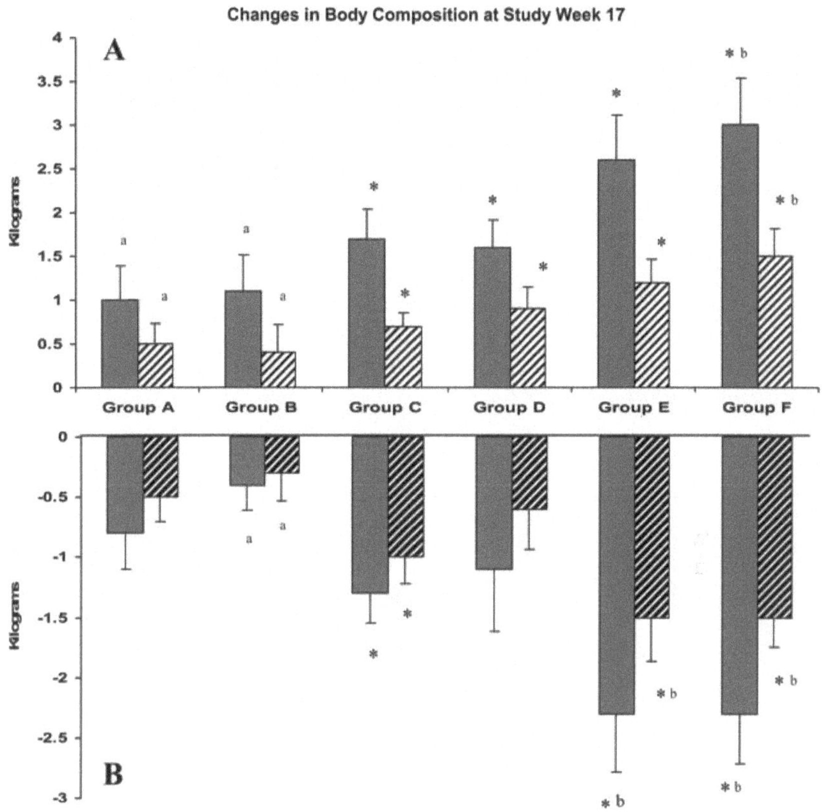

FIGURE 3.—DEXA-derived changes (mean ± 1 SE) in LBM and fat mass for each treatment group from baseline to wk 17. A, Increases in total LBM (*solid bars*) and appendicular lean mass (*hatched bars*). Changes across groups are significant for linear trend for total lean mass ($P = 0.0002$) and appendicular lean ($P = 0.0002$). B, Decreases in total body fat mass (*solid bars*) and trunk fat (*hatched bars*). Changes across groups are significant for linear trend for total fat mass ($P = 0.0004$) and trunk fat ($P = 0.0003$). *, Bonferoni adjusted within group changes ($P < 0.008$). Pairs of treatment groups with *different letters* (e.g. a *vs.* b) are significantly different by one-way ANCOVA with pairwise comparison (Tukey adjusted; $P < 0.05$). (Reprinted from Sattler FR, Castaneda-Sceppa C, Binder EF, et al. Testosterone and growth hormone improve body composition and muscle performance in older men. *J Clin Endocrinol Metab.* 2009;94:1991-2001, with permission from The Endocrine Society.)

with significant reductions in whole-body and trunk fat. Outcomes appeared to be further enhanced with GH supplementation (Fig 3).

▶ Aging men have impairment of gonadal function and a reduction in growth hormone secretion, which are associated with sarcopenia, decreased muscle strength, and increased body fat. The metabolic alterations have been shown to be reversible with testosterone therapy, and growth hormone has been shown to increase lean body mass and decrease body fat. The combination of therapy with testosterone and growth hormone has not been studied extensively in aging men. In the study by Sattler et al, the average age of the men was about 71 years and the men were randomized to receive various doses of testosterone with or without growth hormone. As might be expected, total and appendicular lean mass, muscle strength, and aerobic capacity improved significantly, and body fat and truck fat decreased. Growth hormone enhanced the response to testosterone. While these results are informative, this was a short-term study and long-term safety issues must be established for such intervention.

A. W. Meikle, MD

Male Hormone Replacement

A Novel Synthetic Androgen Receptor Ligand, S42, Works as a Selective Androgen Receptor Modulator and Possesses Metabolic Effects with Little Impact on the Prostate

Min L, Yanase T, Tanaka T, et al (Kyushu Univ, Fukuoka, Japan; et al)

Endocrinology 150:5606-5616, 2009

We identified a novel synthetic steroid, S42, as a promising candidate of selective androgen receptor (AR) modulator. Results of the whole-cell binding assay using COS-7 cells exogenously expressing various steroid receptors indicated that S42 specifically binds to AR and progesterone receptor. When orchiectomized Sprague Dawley rats were administered with S42 for 3 wk, the muscle weight of the levator ani was increased as markedly as that induced by 5α-dihydrotestosterone (DHT), but the weight of the prostate was not elevated at any doses in contrast to DHT. The plasma concentrations of gonadotropin and adiponectin, those down-regulated by DHT, were unaffected by S42. In addition, although the plasma triglyceride level was unaffected by DHT, it was significantly reduced by S42. This effect of S42 was associated with suppression of the SRBP-1c-mediated lipogenic and insulin-desensitizing pathway in the liver and visceral fat. Taken together, S42 works as an AR agonist in muscle and as an AR antagonist in the prostate, pituitary gland, and liver, accompanying beneficial potentials on lipid metabolism (Fig 4).

▶ Testosterone and dihydrotestosterone (DHT) are potent endogenous androgens and result in male sexual differentiation and characteristics. DHT is a more potent androgen than testosterone and is the main androgen promoting prostate growth. A search for an androgen that mediates desired anabolic effects without adversely affecting prostate growth has been sought. Min and associates report on a novel synthetic steroid, S42, that has promise as a selective androgen receptor modulator with limited affects on prostate growth. It is a prostate antagonist in prostate, pituitary, liver, and adipose tissue, and it is an agonist in muscle. It appears to have beneficial effects on insulin sensitivity in the liver, adipose tissue, and muscle without suppressing the gonadal axis. S42 also showed antagonistic effect on DHT-mediated androgen receptor transactivation. The explanation for the lowering of triglycerides by S42 is

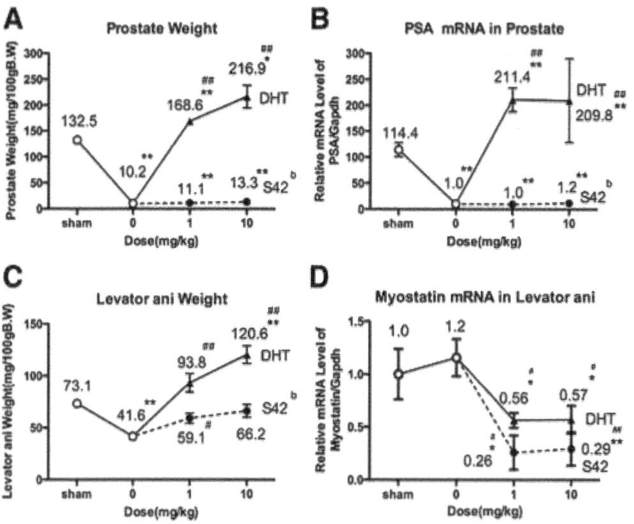

FIGURE 4.—S42 had no virilizing activity but had an anabolic action in orchiectomized rats over 3 wk of treatment. A, The prostate weight increased with DHT treatment but not with S42 treatment. B, PSA mRNA level was dramatically decreased by castration compared with the sham operation and was dose dependently increased by DHT treatment, and there was no change in PSA mRNA levels in the S42-treated groups. C, DHT and S42 increased the weight of levator ani (skeletal muscle). D, DHT reduced myostatin mRNA level by about 40%, whereas S42 more strongly reduced the level to about 70% as compared with the sham group. The assay procedure is described in *Materials and Methods. Points* show the sham and ORX groups, respectively. Each point and vertical bar represents the mean ± SE of three to five rats. *, $P < 0.05$, sham *vs.* ORX groups; **, $P < 0.01$ sham *vs.* ORX groups; #, $P < 0.05$, vehicle (DHT or S42, 0 mg) *vs.* treatment groups; ##, $P < 0.01$, vehicle (DHT or S42, 0 mg) *vs.* treatment groups. a, $P < 0.05$, S42 *vs.* DHT groups at the same dose; b, $P < 0.01$ S42 *vs.* DHT groups at the same dose; no designation indicates not significant. (Reprinted from Min L, Yanase T, Tanaka T, et al. A novel synthetic androgen receptor ligand, S42, works as a selective androgen receptor modulator and possesses metabolic effects with little impact on the prostate. *Endocrinology.* 2009;150:5606-5616.)

uncertain, but it could be related to its effect on up-regulation of peroxisome proliferator-activated receptor-δ (PPARδ). Further study in vivo is needed to fully develop the potential efficacy and safety on this new class of androgen.

A. W. Meikle, MD

N-Terminal Propeptide of Type III Procollagen as a Biomarker of Anabolic Response to Recombinant Human GH and Testosterone

Bhasin S, He EJ, Kawakubo M, et al (Boston Univ School of Medicine, MA; Univ of Southern California, Los Angeles; et al)

J Clin Endocrinol Metab 94:4224-4233, 2009

Context.—Biomarkers that predict musculoskeletal response to anabolic therapies should expedite drug development. During collagen synthesis in soft lean tissue, N-terminal propeptide of type III procollagen (P3NP) is released into circulation. We investigated P3NP as a biomarker

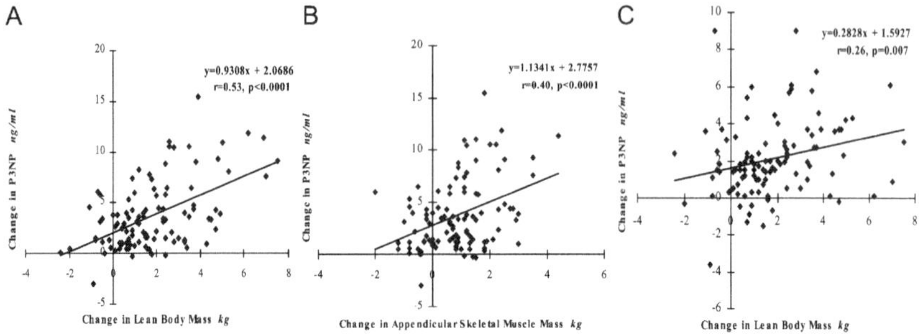

FIGURE 1.—A, Regression plot of change in total lean body mass (kilograms) from baseline to wk 16 relative to change in serum P3NP concentrations (nanograms per milliliter) from baseline to wk 16. B, Change in appendicular lean mass (kilograms) from baseline to wk 16 was plotted against change in serum P3NP concentrations (nanograms per milliliter) from baseline to wk 16. C, Change in lean body mass (kilograms) from baseline to wk 16 was plotted against change in serum P3NP concentrations (nanograms per milliliter) from baseline to wk 4 (n = 106 for all three panels). (Reprinted from Bhasin S, He EJ, Kawakubo M, et al. N-terminal propeptide of type III procollagen as a biomarker of anabolic response to recombinant human GH and testosterone. *J Clin Endocrinol Metab.* 2009;94:4224-4233, with permission from The Endocrine Society.)

of lean body mass (LBM) and muscle strength gains in response to testosterone and GH.

Design.—Community-dwelling older men received GnRH agonist plus 5 or 10 g testosterone gel plus 0, 3, or 5 μg recombinant human GH daily. P3NP levels were measured at baseline and wk 4, 8, 12, and 16. LBM and appendicular skeletal musclemass (ASM) were measured by dual-energy x-ray absorptiometry.

Results.—One hundred twelve men completed treatment; 106 underwent serum P3NP measurements. P3NP levels were higher at wk 4 than baseline (6.61 ± 2.14 *vs.* 4.51 ± 1.05, $P < 0.0001$) and reached plateau by wk 4 in men receiving testosterone alone. However, wk 8 P3NP levels were higher than wk 4 levels in men receiving testosterone plus recombinant human GH. Increases in P3NP from baseline to wk 4 and 16 were significantly associated with gains in LBM ($r = 0.26$, $P = 0.007$; $r = 0.53$, $P < 0.001$) and ASM ($r = 0.17$, $P = 0.07$; $r = 0.40$, $P < 0.0001$). Importantly, for participants receiving only testosterone, P3NP increases at wk 4 and 16 were related to muscle strength gains ($r = 0.20$, $P = 0.056$ and $r = 0.36$, $P = 0.04$). In stepwise regression, change in P3NP explained 28 and 30% of the change in ASM and LBM, respectively, whereas change in testosterone but not IGF-I and age provided only small improvements in the models.

Conclusion.—Early changes in serum P3NP levels are associated with subsequent changes in LBM and ASM during testosterone and GH administration. Serum P3NP maybe a useful early predictive biomarker of anabolic response to GH and testosterone (Fig 1).

▶ With an aging population, there is increasing interest in maintaining and improving physical function and preventing loss of bone and lean body and reducing body fat. Investigators have used androgens, myostatin inhibitors, growth hormone (GH), and selecting agents to increase physical function and increase muscle mass in an attempt to minimize frailty. Testosterone and GH alone or in combination have been increasingly evaluated in aging persons. In the study by Bhasin and associates, N-terminal propeptide of type III procollagen (P3NP) was used as a biomarker of the anabolic responses of testosterone and GH. They observed that testosterone alone increased P3NP and GH augmented the response to testosterone. P3NP may be an early marker of improvement in lean body mass and appendicular skeletal muscle mass. Other investigators have shown that recombinant human GH (rhGH) elevates P3NP and the effect persists for several days after discontinuing GH therapy. Exercise will also increase P3NP. Long-term studies are needed to determine the balance between efficacy and adverse effects of these potent anabolic agents in aging persons.

A. W. Meikle, MD

Metabolic Syndrome and Hypogonadism

Effect of Roux-en-Y Gastric Bypass Surgery on the Sex Steroids and Quality of Life in Obese Men

Hammoud A, Gibson M, Hunt SC, et al (Univ of Utah, Salt Lake City; et al)
J Clin Endocrinol Metab 94:1329-1332, 2009

Context.—The effect of bariatric surgery on the reproductive function of obese men is not entirely elucidated.

Objective.—The aim of the study was to define the effect of Roux-En-Y gastric bypass surgery on the reproductive hormones and sexual function in obese men.

Design and Setting.—The cohort was followed for 2 yr at a clinical research center.

Patients.—Sixty-four severely obese men (22 who had gastric bypass surgery and 42 controls) participated in the study.

Intervention(s).—Anthropometrics [weight, body mass index (BMI), and percentage body fat] and reproductive hormones were measured. The sexual quality of life was assessed using the Impact of Weight on the Quality Of Life-Lite questionnaire.

Main Outcome Measure(s).—Reproductive hormones and sexual quality of life were measured.

Results.—The mean age was 48.9 ± 1.2 yr. At baseline, mean weight was 333.0 ± 7.1 lb, BMI was 46.2 ± 0.9 kg/m^2, and total testosterone was 339.9 ± 21.32 ng/dl. BMI correlated positively with estradiol and negatively with total and free testosterone. Indices of dissatisfaction with sexual quality of life correlated positively with measures of obesity. Difficult sexual performance and low sexual desire correlated negatively with free and total testosterone ($r = -0.273$, $P = 0.038$; and $r = -0.267$, $P = 0.042$, respectively). After 2 yr, the gastric bypass surgery group had a significant decrease in BMI (−16.6 ± 1.2 *vs.* −0.46 ± 0.51 kg/m^2) and

TABLE 2.—The 2-yr Change in Anthropometric, Hormonal, and Sexual Quality of Life Measures in the Gastric Bypass Surgery and Control Groups

Mean 2-year Change (mean ± SE)	Roux-en-Y Gastric Bypass (n = 22)	Control Group (n = 42)	*P* Value for the Unpaired *t* test
BMI	−16.6 ± 1.2[a]	−0.46 ± 0.51	<0.001
Body fat (%)	11.1 ± 1.65[a]	0.89 ± 1.04	<0.001
Hormonal parameters			
Estradiol (pg/ml)	−8.1 ± 2.4[a]	1.6 ± 1.4	0.006
Total testosterone (ng/dl)	310.8 ± 47.6[a]	14.2 ± 15.3	<0.001
SHBG (nmol/liter)	21.6 ± 2.8[a]	2.3 ± 0.8[a]	<0.001
Free testosterone (pg/ml)	45.2 ± 5.1[a]	−0.4 ± 3.0	0.047
C-reactive protein (mg/dl)	−0.5 ± 0.1[a]	−0.0 ± 0.05	<0.001
LH (IU/liter)	0.9 ± 0.36[a]	1.0 ± 0.31[a]	0.385
FSH (IU/liter)	1.0 ± 0.36[a]	0.7 ± 0.20[a]	0.759
Sexual quality of life			
Avoid sexual encounters	−1.8 ± 0.3[a]	−0.0 ± 0.2	<0.001
Difficulty with sexual performance	−2.3 ± 0.3[a]	−0.1 ± 0.2	<0.001
Have little sexual desire	−1.9 ± 0.2[a]	0.05 ± 0.2	<0.001
Do not enjoy sex	−1.7 ± 0.3[a]	−0.05 ± 0.2	<0.001
Total score of dissatisfaction	−7.5 ± 1.2[a]	−0.1 ± 0.6	<0.001

[a]Significant difference of the two year value when compared to baseline.

estradiol (−8.1 ± 2.4 *vs.* 1.6 ± 1.4 pg/ml) and had an increase in total testosterone (310.8 ± 47.6 *vs.* 14.2 ± 15.3 ng/dl) and free testosterone (45.2 ± 5.1 *vs.* −0.4 ± 3.0 pg/ml). Sexual quality of life was improved after gastric bypass surgery.

Conclusion.—Hormonal alterations and diminished sexual quality of life among obese men are related to degree of obesity, and both are improved after gastric bypass surgery (Table 2).

▶ Obesity in men has been associated with decreased sexual quality of life, altered sperm parameters, and impaired fertility. It is also associated with hormone alterations, such as decreased total serum testosterone and sex hormone binding globulin (SHBG) concentrations and increased serum estradiol. This study was undertaken to determine the effect of weight loss from bariatric surgery on sex hormones and sexual quality of life in obese men. Weight loss associated with Roux-en-Y gastric bypass resulted in marked increase in free and total testosterone, and SHBG serum concentrations and a decrease in serum estradiol. All parameters of sexual quality of life improved compared with the control group that did not undergo bariatric surgery, which supports the association between improvement in sex hormone concentrations and sexual quality of life. A prospective study should be conducted to determine serial changes in these measurements. Strengths of the study are the large number of men studied and a follow-up interval of 2 years.

A. W. Meikle, MD

8 Neuroendocrinology

Introduction

Of the hundreds of articles published on various subtopics in neuroendocrinology in the past 12 months, 20 articles were selected for summary and review here. These articles were chosen for a variety of reasons, including their potential impact on the practice of medicine, the breadth of the audience to which they apply, and the strength of their investigational rigor. I believe these studies address fundamental issues in neuroendocrinology and are likely to have an important bearing on how we manage pituitary disease. Obviously, many outstanding and significant works were not discussed in this limited overview of the literature.

In the first section, 8 articles were selected in the area of growth hormone (GH) disorders. In the first article, Reid et al review the potentially changing characteristics of patients diagnosed with acromegaly over a 25-year period. Next, Karavitaki et al review the value of various tests in determining a cure of acromegaly after pituitary surgery. Four papers by Colao et al, Colao et al, Trainer et al, and Buhk et al characterize different pharmacologic approaches for the treatment of GH excess. The final 2 papers, by Miller et al and Colao et al, focus on GH deficiency and its effect in acromegalics as well as patients with other pituitary disorders.

The second section reviews 3 studies that focus on the treatment of hyperprolactinemia. In the first article, Dekkers et al look at recurrence of hyperprolactinemia after withdrawal from dopamine agonists. Second, Delgrange et al look at the role of cabergoline treatment in macroprolactinomas. And finally, Nachtigall et al retrospectively look at the effects of cabergoline treatment on cardiac valvular function.

Seven studies are reviewed in the third section on ACTH overproduction (Cushing's syndrome). The first 2 articles, by Valassi et el and Carroll et al, provide some insights into the complexity of the diagnostic work up of Cushing's syndrome using the Dex-CRH and late-night salivary cortisol tests. In the next 2 papers, Alexandraki et al shed some insight into the prevalence of the variable Cushing's disease, and Baid, et al evaluate the utility of screening the obese population for Cushing's syndrome. The final 3 studies by Valassi et al, Ben-shlomo et al, and Hoybye et al focus on various postsurgical management issues of the Cushing's patient, including discussions of delayed remission after pituitary surgery, ligand-mediated somatostatin signaling, and the role of GH replacement in Cushing's disease patients.

The fourth and final section on general pituitary disorders contains 2 papers. Fernandez et al address the prevalence of pituitary tumors in the general population, and McCormack et al look at effects of temozolomide in the treatment of aggressive pituitary tumors.

William H. Ludlam, MD, PhD

Growth Hormone

Features at diagnosis of 324 patients with acromegaly did not change from 1981 to 2006: acromegaly remains under-recognized and under-diagnosed

Reid TJ, Post KD, Bruce JN, et al (Columbia Univ, NY; Mt Sinai Med Ctr, NY)
Clin Endocrinol 72:203-208, 2010

Background.—Traditionally, acromegaly evaded diagnosis until in its clinically obvious later stages when treatment is more difficult. Over the last 25 years diagnostic tests have improved, but whether clinical disease detection also improved was unknown, so we tested if disease severity at diagnosis had changed from 1981 to 2006.

Methods.—Data on 324 consecutive acromegaly patients presenting from 1981 to 2006 at two New York City hospitals were collected by retrospective review ($n = 324$) and by interview ($n = 200$). The main complaint, acromegaly associated comorbidities, signs, symptoms, healthcare providers visited, preoperative GH and IGF-I levels and pituitary tumour size at diagnosis were compared in patients presenting in the earlier *vs.* later halves of the time period.

Results.—Times from symptom onset to diagnosis were 5·9 year (early) *vs.* 5·2 year (late; $P = \text{NS}$). At diagnosis, 96% of early and late groups had facial feature changes and/or hand/foot enlargement. Comorbidities included hypertension 37% (early) *vs.* 36% (late), carpal tunnel syndrome (24% *vs.* 24%), sleep apnoea (13% *vs.* 29%; $P < 0{\cdot}01$), osteoarthritis (25% *vs.* 23%) and diabetes mellitus (18% *vs.* 15%); each patient had 1·2 (early) *vs.* 1·3 (late; $P = 0{\cdot}53$) comorbidities. Groups were similar in signs, symptoms, tumour size, GH and IGF-I.

Conclusions.—Clinical, biochemical and tumour size characteristics at diagnosis of acromegaly patients were unchanged from 1981 to 2006. Most patients still have marked manifestations of acromegaly at diagnosis, suggesting that acromegaly remains clinically under-recognized. Healthcare professionals should more commonly consider acromegaly, which can lead to earlier diagnosis and better treatment outcome.

▶ The diagnosis of acromegaly is often delayed from 5 to 10 years (or longer) due to the nonspecific nature of the symptoms. With the development of improved assays and imaging techniques, it is unclear if earlier detection has resulted. Reid et al seek to address this question by retrospectively reviewing

324 cases of acromegaly over a 25-year period looking at presenting signs and symptoms in the earlier and later halves of that time interval. They noted that the time of symptom onset to diagnosis as well as the degree of progression of the signs and symptoms of disease and associated comorbidities were similar in the earlier and later halves of the time period studied. These authors conclude that the clinical, biochemical, and tumor size characteristics noted at the time of diagnosis had not changed, suggesting that despite improvement in testing and imaging, acromegaly remains under-recognized and underdiagnosed.

W. H. Ludlam, MD, PhD

The value of the oral glucose tolerance test, random serum growth hormone and mean growth hormone levels in assessing the postoperative outcome of patients with acromegaly

Karavitaki N, Fernandez A, Fazal-Sanderson V, et al (Churchill Hosp, Oxford, UK)

Clin Endocrinol 71:840-845, 2009

Background.—The nadir GH value following an oral glucose tolerance test (OGTT) and the mean GH levels obtained from a GH day curve (GHDC) are among the tools currently used for assessing therapeutic end-points in surgically treated acromegaly. The latter test, however, is cumbersome and costly.

Objectives.—To evaluate, by using a modern, two-site chemiluminescent immunometric GH assay, the degree of discordance between the nadir GH following an OGTT and the mean GH obtained from a GHDC after surgical treatment of acromegaly and to check whether the OGTT can replace reliably the GHDC for the assessment of the disease status postoperatively.

Patients and Methods.—Forty-nine patients [25 males/24 females, median age 52 years (range 18–70)] with a GH-secreting pituitary adenoma who had been surgically treated previously underwent hormonal evaluation of their disease status. The GHDC comprised of 9 × 30-min samples for GH collected in the morning after an overnight fast and rest.

Results.—Seven per cent of patients with mean GH <1·7 μg/l (5 mU/l) in the GHDC had nadir GH >0·7 μg/l (2 mU/l) in the OGTT, and 10% of those with mean GH >1·7 μg/l had nadir GH <0·7 μg/l in the OGTT (all cases with discrepancies had normal IGF-I). GH value at time 0 min <0·6 μg/l in the OGTT had positive predictive value 100% and negative predictive value 75% in predicting nadir GH <0·3 μg/l (1 mU/l) in the OGTT. Nadir GH <0·8 μg/l in the OGTT had positive predictive value 97% and negative predictive value 95% in predicting mean GH <1·7 μg/l in the GHDC. Mean GH in the OGTT <1·4 μg/l had a positive predictive value 90% and negative predictive value 95% in predicting mean GH <1·7 μg/l in the GHDC. Mean GH in the OGTT <2·5 μg/l had positive predictive value 100% and negative predictive value 81% in predicting normal IGF-I. GH at time 0 min in the GHDC <2·1 μg/l had positive predictive value 90% and negative predictive value 90% in predicting mean GH <1·7 μg/l in the GHDC.

Conclusions.—The hormonal data obtained from an OGTT (mean and nadir GH) can provide comprehensive information on the status of acromegaly following surgery and can replace the GHDC cost-effectively. Furthermore, a morning fasting GH sample has an excellent positive predictive value in predicting biochemical cure and an optimal prognostic profile in predicting "safe" mean GH levels.

▶ Although pituitary surgery remains the first-line treatment for treating acromegaly, accurately assessing postoperative cure can sometimes be difficult, particularly when there is discordance between biochemical markers such as insulin-like growth factor-1 (IGF-1) and random growth hormone (GH) spot measurements, average of serial GH measurements or nadir GH value after glucose suppression. To address this challenge, Karavitaki et al measured the degree of discordance between nadir GH value following oral glucose tolerance test and GH mean from GH day curve. Forty-nine patients with acromegaly who had undergone surgical resection of their pituitary adenoma were evaluated for disease status. They found that nadir GH level during a glucose suppression test and mean GH levels were very similar in their positive and negative predictive capacity to determine disease control. These authors conclude that measuring nadir GH as part of a glucose suppression test is as reliable as the more costly and cumbersome mean GH day curve.

W. H. Ludlam, MD, PhD

Significant tumour shrinkage after 12 months of lanreotide Autogel-120 mg treatment given first-line in acromegaly

Colao A, Auriemma RS, Rebora A, et al (Univ 'Federico II' of Naples, Italy; Univ of Genova, Italy)

Clin Endocrinol 71:237-245, 2009

Objective.—To evaluate GH and IGF-I control and tumour shrinkage in newly diagnosed patients with acromegaly treated first-line with lanreotide-Autogel (ATG) 120 mg.

Design.—Open, prospective.

Patients.—Twenty-six patients (17 women, aged 31–70 years): eight enclosed and 12 extrasellar (eight invasive) macroadenomas and six microadenomas (one invasive). ATG 120 mg initially given every 4 weeks for 12 weeks; then intervals between injections increased to every 6 or 8 weeks if GH levels were ≤ 2·5 or < 1 μg/l (equal to 6·5 and 2·6 mU/l), respectively.

Results.—Final dosage was ATG 120 mg every 4 weeks in nine patients (34·6%), every 6 weeks in eight patients (30·8%) and every 8 weeks in the remaining nine patients (34·6%). After 12 months, both GH and IGF-I were controlled in 14 patients (53·8%). The mean tumour volume decreased from 1405 ± 1827 mm^3 at study entry to 960 ± 1381 mm^3 after 6 months, and 799 ± 1161 mm^3 after 12 months ($P < 0{\cdot}0001$). Overall tumour shrinkage was 35·8 ± 28·1% after 6 months and 48·4 ± 27·6% after 12 months. After 12 months, 20 patients (76·9%) achieved > 25% tumour shrinkage: 12 of 14 with controlled disease (85·7%) and 8 of 12 with noncontrolled disease (66·7%; $P = 0{\cdot}49$). Hyperhydrosis, paresthesiae and arthralgias significantly reduced after treatment. No patient withdrew from the study because of adverse events.

Conclusion.—ATG 120 mg in newly diagnosed patients with acromegaly controls GH and IGF-I secretion in 53·8% and induces ≥ 25% tumour shrinkage in 76·9% during a 12-month period. The treatment was associated with improvement of clinical symptoms and with a good safety profile.

▶ Pituitary surgery remains the first-line treatment for acromegaly. When surgery is not successful at completely removing the GH-producing pituitary tumor or when surgery in contraindicated, somatostatin analogs are typically the second-line choice of treatment. Two somatostatin analogs are commonly used for this purpose: octreotide LAR and lanreotide-Autogel. Although octreotide LAR has been previously shown to have tumor shrinkage properties, not as much data is available to show whether lanreotide-Autogel has similar effects on tumor size. This open, prospective study investigates the long-term treatment (12 months) effects of lanreotide-Autogel on normalization of GH hypersecretion and on pituitary tumor shrinkage. Twenty-six patients with denovo acromegaly were treated with lanreotide-Autogel. Mean tumor shrinkage was 35.8% after 6 months of treatment and 53.8% after 12 months of treatment. Fourteen patients were biochemically well controlled based on GH and IGF-1 levels during this same time interval. This data supports the use of lanreotide-Autogel in patients where tumor shrinkage is an important clinical goal.

W. H. Ludlam, PhD, MD

Effects of Initial Therapy for Five Years with Somatostatin Analogs for Acromegaly on Growth Hormone and Insulin-Like Growth Factor-I Levels, Tumor Shrinkage, and Cardiovascular Disease: A Prospective Study

Colao A, Auriemma RS, Galdiero M, et al (Univ of Naples "Federico II", Italy)
J Clin Endocrinol Metab 94:3746-3756, 2009

Objective.—The objective of the study was to evaluate the efficacy of 5 yr of depot somatostatin analogs (SSAs) as first-line therapy in acromegaly.

Outcome Measures.—Primary measures were fasting GH 2.5 μg/liter or less and IGF-I normalized for age and tumor shrinkage. Secondary measures were control of hypertension, arrhythmias, left ventricular hypertrophy, diastolic and systolic dysfunction, and change in lipid and glucose profile.

Patients.—Patients included 45 *de novo* patients (18 women and 27 men, aged 20–82 yr); 28 were treated with octreotide-long-acting release and 17 with lanreotide.

Results.—GH was controlled in 100% and IGF-I levels in 97.8%, tumor shrinkage was 74.9 ± 22.1 and 78.2 ± 14.5%, in the octreotide-long-acting release and lanreotide groups, respectively. There was a significant improvement in the prevalence of hypertension (from 46.7 to 22.2%, $P = 0.027$), arrhythmias (from 17.8% to zero, $P = 0.01$), left ventricular hypertrophy (from 82.2 to 42.2%, $P < 0.0001$), diastolic dysfunction (from 60.0 to 15.6%, $P < 0.0001$), systolic dysfunction (from 40.0 to 4.4%, $P < 0.0001$), and hypertriglyceridemia (from 40.0 to 4.4%, $P < 0.0001$). The prevalence of impaired glucose tolerance (IGT; from 28.9 to 20.0%. $P = 0.46$) and diabetes mellitus (from 22.4 to 31.1%, $P = 0.64$) did not change.

Conclusions.—In patients with severe comorbidities and those who refuse surgery, 5 yr of exclusive SSA therapy induce successful control of GH and IGF-I; tumor shrinkage (by median 80%), and improvement of hypertension, cardiac performance; and dyslipidemia. No patient was withdrawn from treatment because of side effects, and glucose tolerance was stable. We suggest that first-line SSA treatment may be safely continued in patients with acromegaly, according to an individual patient's indications and preferences.

▶ Pituitary surgery is typically considered the first-line treatment for patients with acromegaly. However, with the availability of several medical options that are safe and effective at normalizing the acromegaly-related biochemistry, and in many cases lead to tumor shrinkage, the option of using medical therapy for the treatment of de novo acromegaly is being considered on a more frequent basis. However, relatively little data are available to support that decision. To address this issue, Colao et al look at the efficacy of somatostatin analog treatment (octreotide LAR or lanreotide) in 45 de novo acromegalics over a 5-year period. They note that nearly all patients treated in the study achieved biochemical control of their acromegaly, that there was tumor shrinkage in 75% and 78% of the patients treated with octreotide LAR and lanreotide, respectively, and that other markers such as hypertension, cardiac function, and lipid profile improved significantly. They conclude that for patients who are not surgical candidates or who refuse pituitary surgery, the first-line medical treatment of their acromegaly with somatostatin analogs is a viable option.

W. H. Ludlam, PhD, MD

A randomized, controlled, multicentre trial comparing pegvisomant alone with combination therapy of pegvisomant and long-acting octreotide in patients with acromegaly

Trainer PJ, Ezzat S, D'Souza GA, et al (Christie Hosp, Manchester, UK; Mount Sinai Hosp and Univ of Toronto, Ontario, Canada; Pfizer Global Res and Development, Sandwich, Kent, UK; et al)

Clin Endocrinol 71:549-557, 2009

Objective.—For patients with acromegaly who are suboptimally controlled on long-acting octreotide (LAR), treatment options are to switch to pegvisomant monotherapy (PM) or add pegvisomant to LAR (P-LAR). Our objective was to evaluate if the safety and efficacy of these regimens differ.

Design.—This was an open-label, multicentre, randomized, 40-week outpatient study. The control arm consisted of patients controlled on LAR ($n = 28$).

Patients.—A total of 27 patients with suboptimally controlled acromegaly [as indicated by a serum IGF-I level ≥ 1·3 × upper limit of normal (ULN) of the age-related reference range] were randomized to PM (10 mg once daily initially, then adjusted in 5-mg increments every 8 weeks based on IGF-I levels) and 29 to P-LAR (LAR dosing remained fixed).

Measurements.—The primary end-point was adverse events (AEs). The secondary end-point was biochemical IGF-I-based efficacy. The RIA for IGF-I was discontinued by the manufacturer during the study and a chemiluminescent assay was subsequently used. Previously obtained IGF-I levels were re-analysed.

Results.—PM and P-LAR were well tolerated and there were no differences in the number of AEs. Patients receiving P-LAR tended to be more likely to have clinically significant increases in hepatic transaminase levels, especially those receiving high-dose LAR. Normalization of IGF-I was similar with both regimens (56% and 62% of patients for PM and P-LAR respectively). The change in IGF-I assay resulted in lower rates of IGF-I normalization than expected. Reductions in fasting glucose levels were greater with PM than with P-LAR (−0·8 mmol/l; 95% confidence interval −1·16, −0·53 mmol/l).

Conclusions.—In patients suboptimally controlled on LAR, PM and P-LAR were equally well tolerated and effective in normalizing IGF-I, and overall clinical improvement was observed with both regimens. Thus, pegvisomant monotherapy and adjunctive therapy are equally viable options for the treatment of LAR-resistant acromegaly.

▶ The primary treatment for acromegaly is surgical resection of the causative pituitary somatotroph adenoma. But when pituitary surgery does not completely remove the GH-producing pituitary tumor or when surgery is contraindicated, somatostatin analogs are often used as a therapeutic alternative. If the adjunct therapy with a somatostatin analog does not normalize the GH hypersecretion, therapy with a GH receptor blocker can be effective when used as either a single agent or in combination with a somatostatin analog. However, it is not known whether these agents used in combination is superior to the treatment with GH receptor blocker alone. To address this issue, Trainer et al performed an open-label, multicenter, randomized trial comparing pegvisomant monotherapy (GH receptor blocker alone) with combination therapy with pegvisomant and octreotide LAR (combination of somatostatin analog with GH receptor blocker). Twenty-seven patients with inadequately controlled acromegaly were randomized to the 2 groups. They noted that both the monotherapy group (pegvisomant alone) and the combination therapy group (pegvisomant and octreotide LAR) had similar adverse event profiles. Furthermore, the percentage of patients normalizing their IGF-1 was similar for the 2 groups (56% and 62% for the pegvisomant monotherapy group and the combination group, respectively). These authors conclude that both GH receptor blocker monotherapy and GH receptor blocker plus somatostatin analog combination therapy are viable treatment options for somatostatin analog-resistant acromegaly.

W. H. Ludlam, PhD, MD

Tumor Volume of Growth Hormone-Secreting Pituitary Adenomas during Treatment with Pegvisomant: A Prospective Multicenter Study

Buhk J-H, Jung S, Psychogios MN, et al (Univ of Goettingen, Germany; et al)
J Clin Endocrinol Metab 95:552-558, 2010

Context.—Clinical and biochemical remission in acromegaly can frequently be achieved with the recombinant GH receptor antagonist pegvisomant, even when other treatments fail. However, increases in tumor volume have been reported.

Objective.—Because previous studies suffer from inhomogenous magnetic resonance imaging (MRI) protocols, this prospective study examined the long-term course of adenoma volume during pegvisomant therapy by standardized MRI.

Design.—Five centers in Germany participated. High-resolution MRI was performed at baseline and 6, 12, and 24 months after enrollment.

Setting/Patients.—Patients were outpatients, and pegvisomant is third-line therapy in most of the cases.

Main Outcome Measures.—The primary end point was tumor volume at 24 month follow-up, measured by a single, double-blinded rater.

Results.—Forty-five of 61 patients completed 24 months' follow-up (73.8%). Tumor volume increase greater than 25%during the study was observed in three of 61 patients (4.9%), all during the first year of enrollment. All three patients had had octreotide treatment before initiation of pegvisomant; none of them had had radiotherapy. All volumetric findings were comparable with clinical radiological interpretations. ANOVA revealed no significant change in tumor volume after 24 months ($n = 45$).

Conclusions.—This study shows that pegvisomant therapy infrequently coincides with tumor growth during long-term treatment of acromegaly.

Because all significant tumor volume increases occurred during the first year, these changes might correlate to the change of medication and thus be the result of a rebound from somatostatin-induced shrinkage.

▶ Medical therapy is often effective at controlling the biochemical aspects of acromegaly when pituitary surgery is not successful or is contraindicated. Somatostatin analogs are typically the first line of medical therapy because of their relatively good efficacy and tolerability. Somatostatin analogs have also been shown to reduce tumor size in many patients. When somatostatin analog treatment is not effective at normalizing growth hormone (GH) and insulin-like growth factor 1 (IGF-1) or when side effects (primarily gastrointestinal complaints) limit use, a GH receptor blocker (pegvisomant) can be used. Although the use of a GH receptor blocker can be extremely effective at blocking the effects of excess GH and normalizing IGF-1 and are generally very well tolerated, their tumor shrinkage or maintenance properties are not well characterized. To address this issue, Buhk et al studied 61 patients initially treated with somatostatin analogs and then transitioned to pegvisomant. Forty-five of the 61 patients (73.8%) continued treatment for the 24-month duration of the study. These authors found that tumor volume increased more than 25% in 3 of 61 patients (4.9%). Since all significant tumor growth occurred in the first year of transition from somatostatin analog treatment to GH receptor blocker treatment, these authors feel this may be due to a rebound effect of transitioning treatment. This study shows that GH receptor treatment is safe in terms of tumor growth in the majority (> 95%) of patients.

W. H. Ludlam, MD, PhD

Growth Hormone Deficiency after Treatment of Acromegaly: A Randomized, Placebo-Controlled Study of Growth Hormone Replacement

Miller KK, Wexler T, Fazeli P, et al (Massachusetts General Hosp and Harvard Med School, Boston)

J Clin Endocrinol Metab 95:567-577, 2010

Context.—The effects of GH replacement therapy in patients who develop GH deficiency (GHD) after cure of acromegaly have not been established in a placebo-controlled study.

Objective.—The objective of the study was to determine whether GH replacement improves body composition, cardiovascular risk markers and quality of life in patients with GHD and prior acromegaly.

Design.—This was a 6-month, randomized, placebo-controlled study.

Setting.—The study was conducted at a clinical translational science center.

Study Participants.—Participants included 30 subjects with prior acromegaly and current GHD.

Intervention.—Interventions included GH or placebo.

Main Outcome Measures.—Body composition (dual-energy x-ray absorptiometry and cross-sectional computed tomography at L4), cardiovascular risk markers (high-sensitivity C-reactive protein (hsCRP), total, high-density lipoprotein and low-density lipoprotein cholesterol, fibrinogen, and carotid intimal-medial thickness), and quality of life were measured.

Results.—The mean GH dose at 6 months was 0.58 ± 0.26 mg/d. Total fat mass, visceral adipose tissue (−15.3 ± 18.6 *vs.* 1.3 ± 12.5%, $P = 0.01$), and total abdominal fat decreased, and fat-free mass increased, in the GH *vs.* placebo group. Mean hsCRP levels decreased, but there was no GH effect on other cardiovascular risk markers. There was no change in glycosylated hemoglobin or homeostasis model assessment insulin resistance index. Quality of life improved with GH. Side effects were minimal.

Conclusions.—This is the first randomized, placebo-controlled study of the effects of GH replacement therapy on body composition and cardiovascular end points in patients who have developed GH deficiency after treatment for acromegaly, a disease complicated by metabolic and body composition alterations and increased cardiovascular risk. GH replacement decreased visceral adipose tissue, increased fat-free mass, decreased hsCRP, and improved quality of life in patients with GHD after cure of acromegaly, with minimal side effects and without an increase in insulin resistance.

▶ Growth hormone deficiency (GHD) can sometimes occur in patients with a history of acromegaly, either as a result of the destructive mass effects of the somatotroph tumor crushing the pituitary gland or as a consequence of pituitary damage from surgery or irradiation to the pituitary tumor. These patients can develop severe symptoms of GHD. The effects of GH replacement in this patient population have not been established. To address this issue, Miller et al performed a 6-month, randomized, placebo-controlled study to access body composition, cardiovascular risk markers, and quality of life. These authors noted an improvement in each of these areas in the GH-treated group and noted very little adverse effects of GH treatment. They conclude that acromegalic patients that subsequently develop GHD may benefit from a trial of GH replacement. These data suggest that patients with GHD who once had a history of acromegaly may benefit from GH treatment and that there are no risks of treatment specific to the acromegaly population.

W. H. Ludlam, MD, PhD

A Reappraisal of Diagnosing GH Deficiency in Adults: Role of Gender, Age, Waist Circumference, and Body Mass Index

Colao A, Di Somma C, Savastano S, et al (Univ of Naples "Federico II," Italy; et al)

J Clin Endocrinol Metab 94:4414-4422, 2009

Objective.—The objective of the study was to reevaluate the diagnostic accuracy of GH peak after GHRH plus arginine test (GHRH + ARG) according to patients' age, body mass index (BMI), and waist circumference to diagnose GH deficiency (GHD).

Outcome Measures.—GH peak after GHRH + ARG and IGF-I levels reported as SD score.

Subjects.—Subjects included 408 controls (218 women, 190 men, aged 15–80 yr) and 374 patients with hypopituitarism (167 women, 207 men, aged 16–83 yr).

Results.—In the healthy subjects 15–25 yr old (young), 26–65 yr old (adults) and older than 65 yr (elderly), GH cutoffs were 15.6, 11.7, and 8.5 μg/liter, 11.8, 8.1, and 5.5 μg/liter, and 9.2, 6.1, and 4.0 μg/liter, respectively, in the lean, overweight, and obese subjects. Waist circumference was the best predictor of GH peak ($t = -7.6$, $P < 0.0001$) followed by BMI ($t = -6.7$, $P < 0.0001$) and age ($t = -5.7$, $P < 0.0001$). Based on the old (<9.1 μg/liter) and new GH cutoff, 286 (76.5%) and 276 (73.8%) of 374 hypopituitary patients had severe GHD. The receiving-operator characteristic analysis showed GH cutoffs in line with the third percentile or slightly higher results so that the prevalence of GHD increased to 90.1%.

Conclusions.—The results of the current study show that waist circumference and BMI are the strongest predictors of GH peak after GHRH + ARG followed by age. However, the old cutoff value of 9.0 μg/liter was in line with the new cutoffs in 95% of patients.

▶ There are a variety of biochemical stimuli commonly used as a part of growth hormone (GH) stimulation tests, which are conducted to assess for GH deficiency in adults. These stimuli include insulin tolerance test-induced hypoglycemia, glucagon, GH releasing hormone (GHRH) plus arginine, L-DOPA, etc. The optimal cutoff of GH peak during the GHRH plus arginine GH stimulation test has been debated. The purpose of this study was to reassess the diagnostic accuracy of the GH peak after the GHRH plus arginine GH stimulation test relative to several objective markers, including patients' age, body mass index (BMI), and waist circumference. To do this, these authors performed a GHRH plus arginine GH stimulation test in 408 controls and 374 patients with hypopituitarism. They noted that waist circumference and BMI best correlated with GH peak after GHRH plus arginine GH stimulation test. They conclude that there is need to improve the diagnostic accuracy of GH deficiency tests to optimize the cost and effectiveness of the treatment.

W. H. Ludlam, MD, PhD

Prolactin

Recurrence of Hyperprolactinemia after Withdrawal of Dopamine Agonists: Systemic Review and Meta-Analysis

Dekkers OM, Lagro J, Burman P, et al (Leiden Univ Med Ctr, The Netherlands; Univ Hosp, Malmö, Sweden; et al)
J Clin Endocrinol Metab 95:43-51, 2010

Context.—Dopamine agonists are the treatment of choice for prolactinomas and symptomatic idiopathic hyperprolactinemia. However, the optimal treatment strategy and treatment duration is not clear in all details.

Objective.—The aim of the study was to assess the effect of dopamine agonist withdrawal in patients with idiopathic hyperprolactinemia and prolactinomas.

Data Sources.—PubMed, the Cochrane Library, the Web of Science, and EMBASE were searched electronically. No restriction was made with respect to language.

Study Selection.—Studies reporting the proportion of normoprolactinemic patients after withdrawal of dopamine agonist or studies in which this proportion could be calculated were eligible. Both observational studies and clinical trials were eligible. Nineteen studies were included in the meta-analysis, with a total of 743 patients.

Data Extraction.—Data extraction was performed by two reviewers independently.

Data Synthesis.—The pooled proportion of patients with persisting normoprolactinemia after dopamine agonist withdrawal was 21% in a random effects model [95% confidence interval (CI), 14–30%; I^2 81%). Stratified analysis showed higher proportions of treatment success in idiopathic hyperprolactinemia (32%; 95% CI, 5–80%), compared with both microprolactinomas (21%; 95% CI, 10–37%), and macroprolactinomas (16%; 95% CI, 6–36%). In a random effects meta-regression adjusting for cause of hyperprolactinemia, a longer treatment duration was associated with treatment success ($P = 0.015$), whereas the use of cabergoline showed a trend of effect ($P = 0.07$).

Conclusions.—This meta-analysis showed that hyperprolactinemia will recur after dopamine agonist withdrawal in a considerable proportion of patients. The probability of treatment success was highest when cabergoline was used for at least 2 yr.

▶ Dopamine agonists (DA) are typically very effective at treating prolactin-producing pituitary tumors and idiopathic hyperprolactinemia. Markers of effective treatment include normalization of elevated prolactin levels and tumor shrinkage (in the case of prolactinomas). How long treatment of hyperprolactinemia with DA should be is not clear. Dekkers et al performed a meta-analysis of 19 articles (including 743 patients), which addressed this subject. They found that 21% of the patients had continued normalization of their prolactin levels after withdrawal of cabergoline. Specifically, 32% of patients with idiopathic hyperprolactinemia had continued normalization of prolactin levels after DA withdrawal, whereas only 21% of microadenomas and 16% of macroprolactinomas had continued normalization of prolactin. These authors conclude that hyperprolactinemia will recur in a substantial proportion of patients with history of hyperprolactinemia (either due to a prolactinoma or idiopathic cause) after withdrawal of DA treatment. They further note that the likelihood of long-term success with DA treatment was highest when the duration of DA treatment exceeded 2 years.

W. H. Ludlam, MD, PhD

Characterization of resistance to the prolactin-lowering effects of cabergoline in macroprolactinomas: a study in 122 patients

Delgrange E, Daems T, Verhelst J (Université Catholique de Louvain, Belgium; Univ of Antwerp, Belgium; et al)

Eur J Endocrinol 160:747-752, 2009

Context.—Macroprolactinomas poorly responsive to dopamine-agonists are often more aggressive and are usually termed 'resistant' but this clinical concept has always been defined empirically.

Objective.—To define resistance to cabergoline (CAB) on the basis of a dose–response relationship established in a large series of macroprolactinoma patients and to assess the influence of gender and tumor invasiveness on the response to treatment.

Design.—Retrospective study.

Methods.—One hundred and twenty-two patients (72 women and 50 men) primarily treated with CAB for at least 1 year were included. Main outcome measures were serum prolactin (PRL) and tumor size.

Results.—Normalization of PRL was obtained in 115 out of the 122 patients (94%). The majority of patients (96/115, 83%) were controlled with a CAB dose ≤1.5 mg/week. Most of the other patients (19/26) had only a partial resistance, responding to a further increase of the CAB dose. Beyond the dose of 3.5 mg/week, there was no clear advantage in further increasing the dose instead of continuing the treatment at the same dose. Most tumors (98/119 assessable cases, 82%) showed a significant shrinkage during CAB treatment. It was more likely to occur in cases of PRL normalization. Both cavernous sinus invasion and male gender were significantly and independently associated with partial or complete resistance to treatment.

Conclusions.—Most macroprolactinomas primarily treated with CAB are adequately controlled with doses ≤ 1.5 mg/week. About 20% of patients, mainly men and/or those with invasive tumors will require a higher dose of CAB. We suggest defining such patients as resistant to CAB.

▶ Prolactin-producing pituitary adenomas (prolactinomas) are typically very sensitive to dopamine agonist (DA) treatment in terms of its ability to normalize hyperprolactinemia and shrink tumor size. However, some prolactinomas, particularly macroprolactinomas, are DA resistant. The objective of this study is to determine whether certain characteristics in patients with macroprolactinomas correlate with DA resistance. To do this, case reports for 121 patients with macroprolactinomas who were treated with cabergoline for at least 1 year were retrospectively analyzed. These authors found that 83% of these patients were well controlled with cabergoline (doses at or below 1.5 mg per week) as determined by normalization of prolactin and associated tumor shrinkage. They found that male gender and cavernous sinus invasion were predisposing risk factors for DA resistance in this patient population and that doses of cabergoline greater than 3.5 mg per week had no greater likelihood of shrinking tumor size in DA resistant prolactin-producing tumors.

W. H. Ludlam, MD, PhD

Gender effects on cardiac valvular function in hyperprolactinaemic patients receiving cabergoline: a retrospective study

Nachtigall LB, Valassi E, Lo J, et al (Massachusetts General Hosp and Harvard Med School, Boston)

Clin Endocrinol 72:53-58, 2010

Background.—Ergot-derived dopamine agonists are associated with increased risk of valvular dysfunction in Parkinson's disease. The risk of valvular disease associated with lower doses of cabergoline used to treat prolactinomas remains controversial.

Objective.—To determine whether there is an association of cabergoline and valvular function in patients with hyperprolactinaemia according to gender.

Design.—Case-record retrospective study.

Setting.—Outpatient neuroendocrine clinical centre at a tertiary care hospital.

Study Participants.—One hundred patients (48 men and 52 women) with hyperprolactinaemia who had an echocardiogram while receiving cabergoline for at least 6 months.

Controls.—One hundred controls (48 men and 52 women) selected from Massachusetts general hospital (MGH) database of echocardiograms without clinically significant findings, matched to patients for age, gender, body mass index (BMI) and hypertension.

Main Outcome Measure.—Echocardiogram.

Results.—There were no significant differences in valvular function in patients compared with controls. However, women patients had a higher prevalence of mild tricuspid regurgitation (TR) than female controls (15·4% *vs.* 1·9%, $P = 0.03$). Among men only, patients had more trace TR than controls (68·8% *vs.* 45·8%, $P = 0.02$). The mild valvular regurgitation in patients was not clinically significant and did not correlate with dose, duration or cumulative dose.

Conclusions.—Overall cabergoline was not associated with valvulopathy. However, subdivided by gender, hyperprolactinaemic men and women had higher prevalence of trace or mild TR, respectively, compared with gender matched controls. There may be gender differences in valvular dysfunction associated with cabergoline. Longer term, larger studies are necessary to evaluate definitively an effect of cabergoline on valvular function in hyperprolactinaemic patients.

▶ Patients with prolactin-producing pituitary tumors are typically treated with dopamine agonists, with the therapeutic goal of normalizing prolactin levels and shrinking the tumor. In most cases, medical treatment of hyperprolactinemia is very effective in helping the patients to avoid surgery and/or irradiation to the pituitary tumor. However, since the majority of these patients will require dopamine agonist treatment indefinitely to maintain tumor control, potential long-term side effects of dopamine agonists are a concern. This concern has been heightened in recent years, with the discovery that the incidence of valvular heart disease increases in Parkinson's disease patients treated with relatively high doses of cabergoline over a prolonged period of time. However, it remains controversial whether the lower doses of cabergoline used to treat prolactinomas also induce valvular heart disease. To address this question, Nachtigall et al performed a case-record retrospective study. One hundred patients who had a baseline echocardiogram and who were treated with cabergoline over a 6-month period were evaluated. Overall, there was no significant difference in terms of incidence of valvulopathy between the cabergoline treated and untreated groups. Interestingly, when the data were subdivided by gender, there was a slight increased incidence of trace or mild tricuspid regurgitation when compared with their gender-matched controls.

W. H. Ludlam, MD, PhD

ACTH

Concomitant Medication Use Can Confound Interpretation of the Combined Dexamethasone-Corticotropin Releasing Hormone Test in Cushing's Syndrome

Valassi E, Swearingen B, Lee H, et al (Massachusetts General Hosp and Harvard Med School Boston)

J Clin Endocrinol Metab 94:4851-4859, 2009

Context.—The ability of combined dexamethasone-corticotropin releasing hormone (Dex-CRH) testing to distinguish pseudo-Cushing's syndrome (PCS) from Cushing's syndrome is controversial. One factor potentially impairing diagnostic efficacy is the concomitant use of commonly prescribed medications that may alter dexamethasone metabolism.

Objective.—Our objective was to assess the diagnostic accuracy of the Dex-CRH test and evaluate the potential impact of concomitant drugs.

Design.—The study was a retrospective one.

Participants.—Participants included 101 patients [60 Cushing's disease (CD); 41 PCS] who underwent 112 Dex-CRH tests. Patients were divided into two groups, depending on use of medications potentially interfering with dexamethasone metabolism: 58 tests were classified as No Meds (32 CD; 26 PCS) and 54 as Meds (34 CD; 20 PCS). The latter group was further subdivided into patients taking one medication *vs.* those taking multiple medications.

Main Outcome Measures.—Diagnostic accuracy of different serum cortisol and ACTH thresholds at baseline and 15 min after CRH injection was assessed.

Results.—The specificity of a baseline post-low-dose-dexamethasone-suppressed test cortisol lower than 1.4 μg/dl (38 nmol/liter) was significantly higher in the No Meds *vs.* the Meds group ($P = 0.014$). Sensitivity and specificity using a post-CRH cortisol cutoff of 1.4 μg/dl (38 nmol/liter) were 93.1% (95% confidence interval = 88.4–97.8) and 92.3% (95% confidence interval = 87–97.6) in the No Meds group. The specificity of a cortisol lower than 1.4 μg/dl (38 nmol/l) at 15 min after CRH was significantly higher in patients taking only one medication *vs.* those on multidrug treatment ($P < 0.05$).

Conclusions.—Medications commonly prescribed in hypercortisolemic patients undergoing Dex-CRH testing may contribute to the variable diagnostic accuracy of this test. Prospective studies to address this issue are needed.

▶ Distinguishing Cushing's syndrome from pseudo-Cushing's syndrome can be diagnostically challenging. The dexamethasone-corticotropin releasing hormone (Dex-CRH) test has been proposed to be a highly specific and sensitive test for this purpose, but its utility in this setting is not clear. For example, the use of concomitant medications during the test may alter the dexamethasone level in the blood, thus affecting the accuracy of the test. To address the question of whether concomitant medications may alter the accuracy of the Dex-CRH test, Valassi et al performed a retrospective study of 101 patients (60 patients with Cushing's syndrome and 41 patients with pseudo-Cushing's syndrome) who had Dex-CRH tests performed and divided the patients into Meds versus No Meds groups. They then looked at the diagnostic accuracy of the test in patients concomitantly treated with medications versus those not treated with medications. They noted that the Dex-CRH test had a lower diagnostic accuracy in those patients that had concomitant medication use. Therefore, care should be used when interpreting the Dex-CRH test under these circumstances.

W. H. Ludlam, MD, PhD

Late-night salivary cortisol for the diagnosis of Cushing syndrome: a meta-analysis

Carroll T, Raff H, Findling JW (Med College of Wisconsin, Milwaukee)

Endocr Pract 15:335-342, 2009

Objective.—To report a meta-analysis of late-night salivary cortisol testing for the diagnosis of Cushing syndrome.

Methods.—MEDLINE and EMBASE computer databases were searched to identify relevant articles published between January 1950 and December 2007. The search strategy used the following medical subject headings and keywords: cortisol, Cushing or Cushing's, saliva, salivary, late-night, nocturnal, and nighttime. The results were limited to studies in humans older than 18 years. Titles and abstracts of all articles, as well as full text of relevant articles, were reviewed. Sensitivity, specificity, likelihood ratio positive, likelihood ratio negative, and diagnostic odds ratio were extracted by 2 authors. Discrepancies were resolved by mediation and discussion with a third author.

Results.—Seven articles contained sufficient information to be included in the analysis. A total of 947 patients (339 with Cushing syndrome) were identified. Pooled data from the 7 studies revealed a sensitivity of 92% (95% confidence interval [CI], 88%-94%), specificity of 96% (95% CI, 94%-97%), and diagnostic odds ratio of 311 (95% CI, 92-1059). Likelihood ratio positive was 21 (95% CI, 10-43), with a likelihood ratio negative of 0.08 (95% CI, 0.02-0.32). Inconsistencies for each of these results measured by the I^2 statistic ranged from moderate to high.

Conclusion.—This analysis demonstrates that late-night salivary cortisol has excellent diagnostic characteristics and as such, is a robust, convenient test for screening and diagnosis of Cushing syndrome.

▶ Correctly diagnosing mild Cushing syndrome often can be clinically difficult. Late-night salivary cortisol measurement is a simple and relatively inexpensive screening tool to detect hypercortisolemia and is potentially a very powerful test to diagnose diagnostically challenging cases of Cushing syndrome. Because of this, in the last several years, the use of late-night salivary cortisol measurements has become commonplace in the work up of Cushing syndrome. To address the question of whether late-night salivary cortisol measurements accurately diagnose Cushing syndrome and appropriately differentiate it from other ailments, such as generalized obesity, hypertension, diabetes, etc, Carroll et al performed a meta-analysis of articles published over a 57-year period (1950–2007) and selected those articles that contained data describing the diagnostic accuracy of late-night salivary cortisol measurements. Nine hundred forty-seven patients (339 with Cushing syndrome) in 7 articles were identified. The authors determined that late-night salivary cortisol measurements have a sensitivity of 92% and a specificity of 96% and is therefore a powerful screening tool for the work-up of Cushing syndrome and has excellent diagnostic characteristics.

W. H. Ludlam, MD, PhD

The prevalence and characteristic features of cyclicity and variability in Cushing's disease

Alexandraki KI, Kaltsas GA, Isidori AM, et al (St Bartholomew's Hosp, London, UK)

Eur J Endocrinol 160:1011-1018, 2009

Objective.—Cyclical Cushing's syndrome may render the diagnosis and management of Cushing's disease difficult. The aim of the present study was to investigate the prevalence of cyclicity and variability in patients with Cushing's disease, and to identify putative distinctive features.

Design.—Retrospective case-note study.

Methods.—We analysed the case-records of 201 patients with Cushing's disease in a retrospective case-note study. Cyclicity was considered as the presence of at least one cycle, defined as a clinical and/or biochemical hypercortisolaemic peak followed by clinical and biochemical remission, and by a new clinical and/or biochemical hypercortisolaemic peak. The fluctuations of mean serum cortisol levels, as assessed by a 5-point cortisol day curve, defined the variability.

Results.—Thirty (14.9%; 26 females) patients had evidence of cyclicity/variability. 'Cycling' patients were older but no difference in sex or paediatric distribution was revealed between 'cycling' and 'non-cycling' patients. The median number of cycles was 2 for each patient, and 4 years was the median intercyclic period. A trend to lower cure rate post-neurosurgery and lower adenoma identification was observed in 'cycling' compared to 'non-cycling' patients. In multivariate analysis, older patients, longer follow-up, female sex, and no histological identification of the adenoma were associated with an increased risk of cyclic disease.

Conclusions.—This large population study reveals that cyclicity/variability is not an infrequent phenomenon in patients with Cushing's disease, with a minimum prevalence of 15%. Physicians should be alert since it can lead to frequent problems in diagnosis and management, and no specific features can be used as markers.

▶ Cushing's disease can at times be a very difficult disease to diagnose, partly because of the discordance between biochemical markers and the signs and symptoms of the disease. This can sometimes be accounted for by variability in corticotroph tumor activity leading to inconsistent states of hypercortisolemia. The incidence of cyclic or variable Cushing's disease is thought to be rare (only a few small series and case reports have been reported), but determining the incidence of an entity that is difficult to biochemically identify is problematic. These authors set out to determine the incidence of cyclic or variable Cushing's disease in the Cushing's disease population. To do this, they reviewed case reports of 201 patients with the diagnosis of Cushing's disease and looked for patients with 2 hypercortisolemic peaks and an intervening period of clinical and biochemical remission. They found that 15% of the patients reviewed had cyclicity/variability as defined. These data suggest that cyclicity/variability in Cushing's disease is not a rare phenomenon and that the diagnosis should be considered in difficult cases of inconsistently hypercortisolemic patients or those with discordant biochemical test results.

W. H. Ludlam, MD, PhD

Specificity of Screening Tests for Cushing's Syndrome in an Overweight and Obese Population

Baid SK, Rubino D, Sinaii N, et al (Natl Insts of Health, Bethesda, MD; The George Washington Univ Weight Management Program, DC)

J Clin Endocrinol Metab 94:3857-3864, 2009

Context.—Recent reports suggest a higher prevalence (1–5%) of Cushing's syndrome in certain patient populations with features of the disorder (*e.g.*, diabetes), but the prevalence in the over-weight and obese population is not known.

Objective.—The aim of the study was to evaluate the diagnostic performance of screening tests for Cushing's syndrome in overweight and obese subjects with at least two other features of the disorder.

Design and Setting.—We conducted a cross-sectional prospective study.

Subjects and Methods.—A total of 369 subjects (73% female) completed two or three tests: a 24-h urine cortisol, and/or late-night salivary cortisol, and/or 1 mg dexamethasone suppression test (DST). If any result was abnormal [based on laboratory reference range or cortisol after DST $\geq$1.8 μg/dl (50 nmol/liter)], tests were repeated and/or a dexamethasone-CRH test was performed. Subjects with abnormal DST results and a low dexamethasone level were asked to repeat the test with 2 mg of dexamethasone.

Results.—In addition to obesity, subjects had a mean of five to six features of Cushing's syndrome. None was found to have Cushing's syndrome. Test specificities to exclude Cushing's syndrome for subjects who completed three tests were: urine cortisol, 96% [95% confidence interval (CI), 93–98%]; DST, 90% (95% CI, 87–93%); salivary cortisol, 84% by RIA (95% CI, 79–89%) and 92% by liquid chromatography-tandem mass spectrometry (95% CI, 88–95%). The combined specificity (both tests normal) for all combinations of two tests was 84 to 90%, with overlapping CIs.

Conclusion.—These data do not support widespread screening of overweight and obese subjects for Cushing's syndrome; test results for such patients may be falsely abnormal.

▶ The incidence of Cushing's syndrome in the general population is estimated to be about 3.5 cases per million people. However, the incidence is much higher (1%-5%) in specific subpopulations such as poorly controlled diabetics. Distinguishing Cushing's syndrome from generalized obesity is very important clinically, but the incidence of Cushing's syndrome in this subpopulation is not known. To address this question, Baid et al performed a cross-sectional prospective study looking at 369 patients who were screened for Cushing syndrome using 24-hour urinary free cortisol, late-night salivary cortisol, or low-dose (1 mg) overnight dexamethasone suppression tests. Although they found that the screened patients had between 5 and 6 clinical features (in addition to obesity) consistent with Cushing's syndrome, they found none of the patients screened actually had Cushing's syndrome. They conclude that widespread screening for Cushing's syndrome in the obese population is not appropriate and that such screening may lead to false-positive results and unnecessary treatment.

W. H. Ludlam, MD, PhD

Delayed Remission after Transsphenoidal Surgery in Patients with Cushing's Disease

Valassi E, Biller BMK, Swearingen B, et al (Massachusetts General Hosp and Harvard Med School, Boston; et al)

J Clin Endocrinol Metab 95:601-610, 2010

Background.—Transsphenoidal surgery (TSS) is the treatment of choice for Cushing's disease (CD). Postoperative hypercortisolemia mandates further therapy.

Objective.—The aim of the study was to characterize patients without immediate postoperative remission who have a delayed decrease to normal or low cortisol levels without further therapy.

Design and Setting.—A retrospective case series was conducted at three tertiary care centers.

Patients and Intervention.—We reviewed the records of 620 patients (512 females, 108 males; mean age, 38 ± 13 yr) who underwent transsphenoidal pituitary surgery for CD between 1982 and 2007.

Results.—Outcomes were classified into the following three groups based upon the postoperative pattern of cortisol testing: group IC (immediate control) included 437 of the 620 patients (70.5%) with hypocortisolism and/or cortisol normalization throughout the postoperative follow-up; group NC (no control) included 148 of 620 patients (23.9%) with persistent hypercortisolism; and group DC (delayed control) included 35 of 620 patients (5.6%)who had early elevated or normal UFC levels and developed a delayed and persistent cortisol decrease after an average of 38 ± 50 postoperative days. The total rate of recurrence was 13% at a median follow-up time of 66 months after TSS; the cumulative rate of recurrence at 4.5 yr was significantly higher in group DC *vs.* group IC (43 *vs.* 14%; $P = 0.02$).

Conclusions.—Hormonal assessment in the immediate postoperative period after TSS for CD may be misleading because delayed remission can occur in a subset of patients. Expectant management and retesting may spare some patients from unnecessary further treatment. Optimal timing to determine the need for further therapy after TSS remains to be determined.

▶ Pituitary surgery is the first-line treatment for Cushing's disease but is successful in only 80% to 90% of cases in the hands of an experienced surgeon. Interestingly, because of the typically small size of the pituitary lesions and the difficulty of accurately assessing the biochemical and pathologic outcomes, it can be difficult at times to determine if a patient has undergone complete resection of their corticotroph pituitary lesion. When surgery is not successful, other often invasive or toxic treatment options include bilateral adrenalectomy, pituitary radiation, or medications. Therefore, correctly determining whether a patient is cured is critical when developing long-term follow-up treatment plans. To address this issue, Valassi et al performed a retrospective case series of 620 patients in 3 tertiary centers to determine the incidence of delayed biochemical remission after pituitary surgery. They found that 70.5% of the patients had immediate control of their hypercortisolism, 23.9% never obtained control, and 5.6% had delayed control after an average of 38 postoperative days. They noted a 13% recurrence of Cushing's disease at 5.5 years. They conclude that caution should be used when interpreting postoperative biochemical analysis and careful reassessment of cortisol status may save patients unnecessary additional procedures.

W. H. Ludlam, MD, PhD

Differential Ligand-Mediated Pituitary Somatostatin Receptor Subtype Signaling: Implications for Corticotroph Tumor Therapy

Ben-Shlomo A, Schmid H, Wawrowsky K, et al (Cedars Sinai Med Ctr, Los Angeles, CA; Novartis Pharmaceuticals, Basel, Switzerland; et al)

J Clin Endocrinol Metab 94:4342-4350, 2009

Objective.—Pituitary targeted pharmacotherapy for Cushing's disease is challenging and ineffective. Unlike octreotide and lanreotide, the multisomatostatin receptor (SST) analog pasireotide that exhibits SST5 greater than SST2 binding affinity offers potential for treating Cushing's disease. Because corticotroph cells express SST5 more abundantly than SST2, pasireotide likely exerts superior corticotroph action mainly through SST5. However, there is no direct evidence for this assumption, and moreover, the ligand effect on corticotroph SST2 is not known.

Results.—We used AtT20 mouse pituitary corticotroph tumor cells stably overexpressing SST2 or SST5 and TtT/GF mouse pituitary folliculostellate cells stably or transiently expressing SST receptors to examine ligand-receptor activation by SST2- and SST5-selective agonists. We show that pasireotide was more potent than either octreotide or somatostatin-14 in mouse corticotroph cells. Pasireotide potency is not affected by SST2 abundance, SST2 antagonist treatment, or octreotide cotreatment in SST2-overexpressing cells. Pasireotide also does not induce SST2 internalization and attenuates octreotide or SRIF14-induced SST2 internalization only at superphysiological dose ranges. In contrast, octreotide attenuates pasireotide potency in SST5-overexpressing cells. Moreover, short exposure to pasireotide causes prolonged inhibition of forskolin or CRH-induced cAMP accumulation, in contrast to somatostatin-14- and SST2-selective agonists that induced postwithdrawal cAMP rebound. Long-term pasireotide signaling effects are enhanced by SST5 overexpression.

Conclusion.—The results indicate that SST5 determines short- and long-term enhanced pasireotide action in corticotroph cells, whereas the ligand action on SST2 is negligible.

▶ There is currently no effective pituitary targeted treatment for Cushing's disease. Although the 2 commercially available somatostatin receptor analogs (octreotide and lanreotide) predominantly affect somatostatin 2 (SST2) receptors, corticotroph tumors predominantly express the SST5 receptor. Although the novel SST receptor analog SOM230 (pasireotide) has high affinity for the SST5 receptor, there is little evidence to date that pasireotide exerts a superior corticotroph action at the SST5 receptor. To correlate potential biologic activity induced by the binding of pasireotide to the SST5 receptor, these authors used AtT20 mouse pituitary corticotroph tumor cells, which stably overexpress SST2 and SST5 receptors, as well as cells that transiently express these receptors and examined ligand-specific activity. They found that pasireotide was more potent than octreotide or lanreotide in mouse pituitary corticotroph cells and that this activity is specific to the SST5 receptor. These authors conclude that the presence of SST5 receptors effects the action of pasireotide in corticotroph cells and gives biochemical rational to the premise that pasireotide has effectiveness in treating patients with Cushing's disease due to the affinity that it has for the ST5 receptor.

W. H. Ludlam, MD, PhD

Clinical features of growth hormone (GH) deficiency and effects of 3 years of GH replacement in adults with controlled Cushing's disease

Höybye C, Ragnarsson O, Jönsson PJ, et al (Karolinska Univ Hosp, Stockholm, Sweden; Sahlgrenska Univ Hosp, Gothenburg, Sweden; KIMS Med Outcomes, Sollentuna, Sweden; et al)

Eur J Endocrinol 162:677-684, 2010

Objective.—Patients in remission from Cushing's disease (CD) have many clinical features that are difficult to distinguish from concomitant GHD. In this study, we evaluated the features of GHD in a large cohort of controlled CD and assessed the effect of GH treatment.

Design and Methods.—Data were obtained from KIMS, the Pfizer International Metabolic Database. A retrospective cross-sectional comparison of background characteristics in unmatched cohorts of patients with CD (n=684, 74% women) and non-functioning pituitary adenomas (NFPA) (n=2990, 39% women) was conducted. In addition, a longitudinal evaluation of 3-years of GH replacement in a subset of patients with controlled CD (n=322) and NFPA (n=748) matched for age and gender was performed.

Results.—The cross-sectional study showed a significant delay to GHD diagnosis in the CD group, who had a higher prevalence of hypertension, fractures and diabetes mellitus. In the longitudinal, matched study, the CD group had a better metabolic profile but a poorer quality of life (QoL) at baseline, **assessed with the disease specific questionnaire QoL-AGHDA.** After 3 years of GH treatment (mean dose at 3 years 0.39 mg/day in CD and 0.37 mg/day in NFPA), total and LDL-cholesterol decreased, while glucose and HbA1C increased. Improvement in QoL was observed, greater in the CD group (−6 CD group vs. −5 NFPA group, p<0.01).

Conclusion.—In untreated GHD, co-morbidities, including impairment of QoL, were more prevalent in controlled CD. Overall, both groups responded similarly to GH replacement, suggesting that patients with GHD due to CD benefit from GH to the same extent as those with GHD due to NFPA.

▶ Treating Cushing's disease with pituitary surgery or irradiation may cause damage to the pituitary gland in some cases. Distinguishing the clinical signs and symptoms of growth hormone deficiency (GHD) from the persistent sequelae of previously treated Cushing's disease can be difficult. Hoybye et al obtained data from the kinetic interaction of microparticles in a solution (KIMS) database (Pfizer) and performed a retrospective analysis of cross-matched cohorts with Cushing's disease and nonfunctioning pituitary adenomas. In those patients with 3 or more years of GH treatment, markers such as lipid profile, glucose control, and quality of life were improved similarly in both the Cushing's disease group and the nonfunctioning pituitary tumor group. These authors also noted that there was a significant delay in the diagnosis of GHD in patients with history of Cushing's disease. They conclude that GH treatment is as beneficial in GHD patients with a history of Cushing's disease as those patients with a history of nonfunctioning pituitary tumors and that GHD should be considered in patients treated for Cushing's disease despite the potentially persistent sequelae of prior longstanding hypercortisolemia.

W. H. Ludlam, PhD, MD

Pituitary-General

Prevalence of pituitary adenomas: a community-based, cross-sectional study in Banbury (Oxfordshire, UK)

Fernandez A, Karavitaki N, Wass JAH (Churchill Hosp, Oxford, UK)

Clin Endocrinol 72:377-382, 2010

Background.—Pituitary adenomas (PAs) are associated with increased morbidity and mortality. The optimal delivery of services and the provision of care for patients with PAs require distribution of the resources proportionate to the impact of these conditions on the community. Currently, the resource allocation for PAs in the health care system is lacking a reliable and an up-to-date epidemiological background that would reflect the recent advances in the diagnostic technologies, leading to the earlier recognition of these tumours.

Objectives.—To determine the prevalence, the diagnostic delay and the characteristics of patients with PA in a well-defined geographical area of the UK (Banbury, Oxfordshire).

Patients and Methods.—Sixteen general practitioner (GP) surgeries covering the area of Banbury and a total population of 89 334 inhabitants were asked to participate in the study (data confirmed on 31 July 2006). Fourteen surgeries with a total of 81,449 inhabitants (91% of the study population) agreed to take part. All cases of PAs were found following an exhaustive computer database search of agreed terms by the staff of each Practice and data on age, gender, presenting manifestations and their duration, imaging features at diagnosis, history of multiple endocrine neoplasia type 1 and family history of PA were collected.

Results.—A total of 63 patients with PA were identified amongst the study population of 81,149, with a prevalence of 77·6 PA cases/100,000 inhabitants (prolactinomas; PRLoma: 44·4, nonfunctioning PAs: 22·2, acromegaly; ACRO: 8·6, corticotroph adenoma: 1·2 and unknown functional status; UFS: 1·2/100,000 inhabitants). The distribution of each PA subtype was for PRLoma 57%, nonfunctioning PAs 28%, ACRO 11%, corticotroph adenoma 2% and UFS 2%. The median age at diagnosis and the duration of symptoms until diagnosis (in years) were for PRLoma 32·0 and 1·5, nonfunctioning PAs 51·5 and 0·8, ACRO 47 and 4·5 and corticotroph adenoma 57 and 7, respectively. PRLoma was the most frequent PA diagnosed up to the age of 60 years (0–20 years: 75% and 20–60 years: 61% of PAs) and nonfunctioning PA after the age of 60 years (60% of PAs). Nonfunctioning PAs dominated in men (57% of all men with PA) and PRLoma in women (76% of all women with PA). Five patients (7·9%) presented with classical pituitary apoplexy, with a prevalence of 6·2 cases/100,000 inhabitants.

Conclusions.—Based on a well-defined population in Banbury (Oxfordshire, UK), we have shown that PAs have a fourfold increased prevalence than previously thought; our data confirm that PAs have a higher burden on the Health Care System and optimal resource distribution for both clinical care and research activities aiming to improve the outcome of these patients are needed.

▶ The estimated prevalence of pituitary adenomas in the general population has been reported to be as low as 25 cases per 100 000 people. There can be significant morbidity and mortality associated with undiagnosed pituitary tumors, and once identified, these patients often require substantial medical resources to manage their disease. For this reason, it is important to obtain an accurate assessment of the true incidence and diagnostic characteristics of pituitary tumors in the general population. To address this need, Fernandez et al performed a review of patients with pituitary adenomas in a well-defined region of nearly 90 000 inhabitants in the United Kingdom. Ninety-one percent of this population was successfully analyzed in the study. These authors identified 63 patients (of the final study population of just over 80 000 people), which resulted in a prevalence of 77.6 cases per 100 000 people. The proportion of pituitary tumor types identified was as follows: 57% prolactinomas, 28% nonfunctional, 11% somatotroph, 2% corticotroph, and 2% other. These authors conclude that the prevalence of pituitary tumors is significantly higher than previously thought and that there needs to be optimization of medical resources to better manage this patient population.

W. H. Ludlam, MD, PhD

Low O^6-methylguanine-DNA methyltransferase (MGMT) expression and response to temozolomide in aggressive pituitary tumours

McCormack AI, McDonald KL, Gill AJ, et al (Royal North Shore Hosp, Sydney, New South Wales, Australia; et al)
Clin Endocrinol 71:226-233, 2009

Context.—Recent case reports detail the successful use of temozolomide in the management of aggressive pituitary tumours. O^6-methylguanine-DNA methyltransferase (MGMT) is a DNA repair protein that counteracts the effect of temozolomide.

Objective.—To study MGMT expression in pituitary tumours and consider whether MGMT expression is associated with response to temozolomide therapy in aggressive pituitary tumours.

Patients.—We report two patients with aggressive pituitary tumours treated with temozolomide, one who responded to temozolomide and the other who did not. MGMT expression was assessed in a further 88 archived pituitary tumour samples.

Design.—MGMT expression was assessed by immunohistochemistry. *MGMT* promoter methylation was studied by methylation-specific polymerase chain reaction (MSP), sequencing of *MGMT* was performed and loss of heterozygosity (LOH) analysis undertaken.

Results.—Low MGMT expression and *MGMT* promoter methylation were found in the pituitary tumour of the patient who responded to temozolomide. Conversely, high MGMT expression was seen in the patient demonstrating a poor response to temozolomide. Eleven out of 88 archived tumour samples (13%) had low MGMT expression. Prolactinomas were more likely to have low MGMT expression compared with other pituitary tumour subtypes ($P < 0{\cdot}001$). There was no significant difference in MGMT expression between invasive and noninvasive tumours, or between recurrent and nonrecurrent tumours. A significant inverse correlation was found between MGMT expression and promoter methylation ($P = 0{\cdot}012$).

Conclusion.—MGMT expression as assessed by immunohistochemistry may predict response to temozolomide therapy in patients with aggressive pituitary tumours. *MGMT* promoter methylation is likely to explain low MGMT expression in some, but not all, pituitary tumours.

▶ Temozolomide, an alkylating chemotherapeutic drug, has been shown to effectively manage aggressive pituitary tumors in some cases. O^6-methylguanine-DNA methyltransferase (MGMT) is a DNA repair protein that potentially blocks the effect of temozolomide treatment. These authors studied MGMT expression in 2 patients with aggressive pituitary tumors (1 patient responded to temozolomide treatment and 1 did not) to determine if there is a correlation between MGMT expression and temozolomide effectiveness. They found that MGMT expression and MGMT promoter methylation was low in the patient who responded to temozolomide. By contrast, these 2 markers were high in the patient who did not respond to temozolomide treatment. They also noted that 11 of 88 archived tumor samples from other patients had low MGMT expression, and there was a higher proportion of low MGMT expression in patients with prolactinomas. There was no difference in MGMT expression in patients with aggressive versus nonaggressive pituitary tumors. They conclude that MGMT expression may predict response to temozolomide treatment in patients with aggressive pituitary tumors.

W. H. Ludlam, MD, PhD

9 Pediatric Endocrinology

Introduction

The selections chosen for this edition of the YEAR BOOK represent a broad array of topics of interest in pediatric endocrinology. These include rare conditions as well as common ones, along with new discoveries in the varied realms of clinical management, molecular genetics, quality of life, and long-term outcomes. Taken together, they touch on many of the questions and issues frequently encountered while taking care of patients, formulating ideas for research, and teaching trainees.

Leading off the chapter is the first study to demonstrate a direct relationship between maternal vitamin D status and fetal bone development. While the precise postnatal variables affecting skeletal programming have not been elucidated, this study is yet another example of how our disease risk profile truly begins during prenatal life! The second selection also deals with bone, but in an entirely different context. This selection reviews the BoneXpert system, a promising automated method for bone age determination. As bone ages are the single most frequently ordered test in the pediatric endocrine clinic, adoption of such a system would have a profound impact on this aspect of routine care.

Selections 3 and 4 both address the topic of short stature from a broad-based perspective; one is a meta-analysis and the other is a population-based study. The first of these examines the impact of the exon-3 deleted growth hormone (GH) receptor polymorphism on growth response in GH-deficient children; the second provides reassurance about the absence of psychological problems in a cohort of healthy short children during the middle school years. Selection 5 illuminates valuable prognostic information pertaining to a rare problem in a rare condition, namely hypercortisolism in McCune-Albright syndrome. In contrast, the next selection deals with Turner syndrome, which is relatively common, occurring in approximately 1 in 2500 liveborn females. Despite the existence of comprehensive consensus guidelines for the care of affected women, the revelation that only a tiny fraction are receiving it highlights the lack of effective transition so ubiquitous in the pediatric setting.

Selections 7-9 all report novel mutations resulting in drastically different phenotypic consequences. The first report of a loss of function mutation in the GnRH gene was a long-awaited but predictable cause of hypogonadotropic hypogonadism, while the activating mutation in KISS1 joins one other example of a genetic basis for central precocious puberty in the GPR54/Kisspeptin system. In contrast, the novel homozygous mutation in the ligand-binding domain of the glucocorticoid receptor in an infant with profound hypoglycemia due to generalized glucocorticoid resistance was completely unexpected and importantly expands the differential diagnosis of neonatal hypoglycemia.

Finally, the last 2 selections this year deal with pediatric thyroid disease. Selection 10 examines the role of fine-needle aspiration in the evaluation of thyroid nodules in children, whereas selection 11 challenges the assumption that a normal newborn screen for congenital hypothyroidism (using both T_4 and TSH tests) makes the presence of hypopituitarism unlikely.

In conclusion, I hope that these YEAR BOOK selections will serve to educate as well as stimulate novel ideas and challenge existing assumptions. Ultimately, may the incorporation of new knowledge continually enhance our efforts as physicians and scientists!

Erica Eugster, MD

Bone/Calcium

Genetic Variations in Sex Steroid-Related Genes as Predictors of Serum Estrogen Levels in Men

Eriksson AL, Lorentzon M, Vandenput L, et al (Gothenburg Univ, Sweden; et al)

J Clin Endocrinol Metab 94:1033-1041, 2009

Context.—The risk of many conditions, including prostate cancer, breast cancer, and osteoporosis, is associated with serum levels of sex steroids.

Objective.—The aim of the study was to identify genetic variations in sex steroid-related genes that are associated with serum levels of estradiol (E2) and/or testosterone in men.

Design.—Genotyping of 604 single nucleotide polymorphisms in 50 sex steroid-related candidate genes was performed in the Gothenburg Osteoporosis and Obesity Determinants (GOOD) study (n = 1041 men; age, 18.9 ± 0.6 yr). Replications of significant associations were performed in the Osteoporotic Fractures in Men (MrOS) Sweden study (n = 2568 men; age, 75.5 ± 3.2 yr) and in the MrOS US study (n = 1922 men; age, 73.5 ± 5.8 yr). Serum E2, testosterone, and estrone (E1) levels were analyzed using gas chromatography/mass spectrometry.

Results.—The screening in the GOOD cohort identified the single nucleotide polymorphism rs2470152 in intron 1 of the CYP19 gene, which codes for aromatase, responsible for the final step of the biosynthesis of E2 and E1, to be most significantly associated with serum E2 levels ($P = 2 \times 10^{-6}$). This association was confirmed both in the MrOS Sweden

TABLE 4.—Serum Levels of Sex Steroids According to CYP19 rs2470152 Genotype

	AA	AG	GG	*P*	GG *vs.* AA[a]
GOOD	n = 241	n = 514	n = 286		
E2 (pg/ml)	17.5 ± 6.2[b,c]	18.8 ± 6.1[b]	19.8 ± 6.2[c]	1×10^{-5}	+13%
E1 (pg/ml)	21.8 ± 7.4[b]	22.5 ± 7.5[b]	24.0 ± 8.2[c]	3×10^{-3}	+10%
T (ng/ml)	4.5 ± 1.6	4.6 ± 1.5	4.7 ± 1.4	NS	
SHBG (nmol/liter)	20.4 ± 7.6	20.7 ± 7.1	20.1 ± 6.9	NS	
MrOS Sweden	n = 551	n = 1249	n = 768		
E2 (pg/ml)	19.7 ± 7.5[b,c]	21.1 ± 8.0	21.9 ± 8.1	4×10^{-6}	+11%
E1 (pg/ml)	31.8 ± 12.8[b,c]	33.8 ± 14.2[b]	36.8 ± 17.2[c]	1×10^{-9}	+16%
T (ng/ml)	4.4 ± 1.8	4.4 ± 1.7	4.7 ± 1.8	NS	
SHBG (nmol/liter)	43.2 ± 22.7	44.4 ± 21.3	43.9 ± 21.0	NS	
MrOS US	n = 484	n = 944	n = 494		
E2 (pg/ml)	21.6 ± 7.9[b,c]	22.8 ± 8.6	23.4 ± 8.2	4×10^{-4}	+8%
E1 (pg/ml)	31.3 ± 13.4[b,c]	34.1 ± 15.7[b]	35.8 ± 15.8[c]	1×10^{-6}	+14%
T (ng/ml)	3.9 ± 1.5	4.0 ± 3.9	3.9 ± 1.7	NS	
SHBG (nmol/liter)	48.3 ± 16.7	49.7 ± 19.1	49.2 ± 19.9	NS	

Values are adjusted for race (in the MrOS US cohort), age, and BMI and are given as mean ± SD. *P* values are for comparison of the three genotypes (ANOVA with Tukey's *post hoc* test). NS, Nonsignificant.
[a]Difference between GG and AA genotype given in percent for significant differences.
[b]$P < 0.05$ *vs.* GG.
[c]$P < 0.05$ *vs.* AG.

study ($P = 9 \times 10^{-7}$) and in the MrOS US study ($P = 1 \times 10^{-4}$). When analyzed in all subjects (n = 5531), rs2470152 was clearly associated with both E2($P = 2 \times 10^{-14}$) and E1 ($P = 8 \times 10^{-19}$) levels. In addition, this polymorphism was modestly associated with lumbar spine BMD ($P < 0.01$) and prevalent self-reported fractures ($P < 0.05$).

Conclusions.—rs2470152 of the CYP19 gene is clearly associated with serum E2 and E1 levels in men (Table 4).

▶ It is known that hereditary and environmental factors influence serum sex steroid concentrations, and sex steroids are associated with clinical disorders, such as breast and prostate cancer and osteoporosis. In his study, genetic variation in sex-steroid related genes associated with serum estrogens, sex hormone binding globulin (SHBG), and testosterone were investigated. They observed that the rs2470152 of the CYP19 gene, which codes the aromatase, was associated with serum estradiol and estrone in men, but not SHBG and testosterone. This gene polymorphism was also associated with lumbar spine bond mineral density. The limitations of the study include single measurements of sex steroids and associations of parameters. It might be expected that higher estradiol concentrations might cause an elevation of serum SHBG and a reduction in serum testosterone, but this was not observed. This might imply that there is an associated alteration of estrogen responsiveness. Additional studies are needed to clarify the gene interaction of sex steroid synthesis, serum concentration, and action.

A. W. Meikle, MD

Maternal Vitamin D Status Determines Bone Variables in the Newborn

Viljakainen HT, Saarnio E, Hytinantti T, et al (Univ of Helsinki, Finland; Helsinki Univ Central Hosp, Finland; et al)

J Clin Endocrinol Metab 95:Epub ahead of print, 2010

Context.—Vitamin D regulates 3% of the human genome, including effects on bone health throughout life. Maternal vitamin D status may program neonatal skeletal development. The objective here was to determine the association of mothers' vitamin D status with bone variables of their newborns.

Subjects and Methods.—In a birth hospital, pregnant women (n = 125) participated in a cross-sectional study with a longitudinal follow-up of the pregnancy. The mean (SD) values for age, body mass index before pregnancy, pregnancy weight gain, and total vitamin D intake in mothers were 31 (4) yr, 23.5 (3.7) kg/m^2, 13.1 (4.3) kg, and 14.3 (5.8) μg, respectively. All newborns were full-term, 99% were appropriate for gestational age, and 53% were boys. Blood samples were collected from mothers during the first trimester and 2 d postpartum and from umbilical cords at birth for analysis of serum 25-hydroxyvitamin D (S-25-OHD), PTH, and bone remodeling markers. Bone variables were measured by pQCT at the 20% site of the newborn tibia on an average of 10 (11) d postpartum. Bone contour was analyzed with a single threshold of 180 mg/mm^3 for the detection of total bone mineral density (BMD), bone mineral content (BMC), and cross-sectional area (CSA).

Results.—Mean S-25-OHD was 41.0 (13.6), 45.1 (11.9), and 50.7 (14.9) nmol/liter during the first trimester, postpartum, and in the umbilical cord, respectively. The median value of the individual means for first trimester and the 2-d postpartum S-25-OHD was 42.6 nmol/liter, which was used as cutoff to define two equal-sized groups. Groups are called below median and above median in the text. Newborns below median were heavier ($P = 0.05$), and 60% were boys. Tibia bone mineral content was 0.047 (95% confidence interval, 0.011–0.082) g/cm higher ($P = 0.01$), and cross-sectional area was 12.3 (95% confidence interval, 2.0–22.6) mm^2 larger ($P = 0.02$), but no difference in bone mineral density was observed, above median compared with below median group. These results were adjusted for newborn Z-score birth weight, maternal height, and newborn age at the measurement. A positive, significant correlation was observed between remodeling markers in mothers at different time points and above median group in the cord.

Conclusions.—Although the mean total intake of vitamin D among mothers met current Nordic recommendations, 71% of women and 15% of newborns were vitamin D deficient during the pregnancy. Our results suggest that maternal vitamin D status affects bone mineral accrual during the intrauterine period and influences bone size. More efforts should be made to revise current nutrition recommendations for pregnant women that may have permanent effects on the well-being of children.

▶ This interesting study is a useful reminder that the establishment of an individual's risk and resilience factors for human disease begins not at birth, but during prenatal life. As the first investigation of the relationship between maternal vitamin D status and fetal bone development, this study represents a significant contribution to current understanding of intrauterine bone biology and growth. As seen in Fig 2 in the original article, infants born to mothers with above median 25-hydroxyvitamin D levels had higher tibial bone mineral content and cross-sectional area than those with maternal below mean 25, OHD concentrations, although no differences in bone mineral density were seen. Importantly, these results persisted after adjustment for Z-score birth weight. One of the most striking findings of the study was that > 95% of the mothers were deemed vitamin D deficient or insufficient during the first trimester as well as in the postpartum period, despite the fact that 80% were getting the recommended daily supplement of vitamin D for pregnant women. Since a linear relationship between maternal and cord blood vitamin D concentration was seen, this suggests that the recommended daily intake of vitamin D for Nordic women during pregnancy should be drastically revised. While maternal vitamin D status appears to directly impact fetal bone variables, to what extent it influences skeletal programming is less clear. Similarly, how postnatal factors might modulate the effect of intrauterine vitamin D exposure remains to be elucidated.

E. Eugster, MD

Growth/Growth Hormone

An Automated Method for Determination of Bone Age

Thodberg HH (Visiana, Holte, Denmark)

J Clin Endocrinol Metab 94:2239-2244, 2009

Context.—Bone age rating is associated with a considerable rater variability, which limits its usefulness in modern pediatric endocrinology. An automated computerized method would theoretically solve this problem but has been surprisingly difficult to establish.

Evidence Acquisition.—We review the development of automated bone age assessment and describe how the conceptual understanding of bone age rating shifted from a rule-based theory to a more intuitive and experience-based approach. The role of the CASAS system from 1992 is described. The BoneXpert system from 2008 employs deformable models of each bone to locate the bones and extracts the component of the bone appearance related to maturity in a holistic, statistical manner. Two clinical studies have been published on its accuracy, defined as the root mean square deviation from manual rating. Other studies addressed the precision of the method, defined as its ability to give the same result on a repeated x-ray, expressed as the SD on a single measurement.

Evidence Synthesis.—The accuracy of the automated bone age determination was 0.71–0.72 yr, and the precision was 0.17–0.18 yr. More than 98.6% of the images could be analyzed. The system was validated on children with various diagnoses of short stature in the bone age range 2.5–17 yr for boys and 2–15 yr for girls.

Conclusion.—The reviewed validation studies suggest that this automated bone age determination system has adequate accuracy, precision, and efficiency to be clinically useful.

▶ Ask anyone in Pediatrics what the pediatric endocrinologists' favorite test is and they will quickly reply "A bone age X-ray!" Not only is this due to the frequency with which this test is ordered, but it is also related to our insistence that we review the actual radiographs ourselves rather than rely on the (less qualified) radiologist's interpretation. Despite our fondness for bone ages, the fact that they provide an imprecise measure is undisputed. One reason is that the system is inherently subjective, often yielding quite discrepant results from several independent but equally experienced readers, as well as varying interpretations of the same film by the same examiner on different days. Added to that is a certain mystique to bone age interpretation that many of us learned in fellowship and incorporate to this day. For example, I (as well as some, but not all, of my colleagues) was taught that the pages depicting the 11- and 12-year-old radiographs for girls were reversed in the Greulich and Pyle Atlas, creating extra uncertainty about accuracy when reading an X-ray near this level of maturation. Finally, our results are subject to multiple sources of bias, ranging from knowledge of the chronological age to our own personal prejudices regarding stature, gender, growth, and puberty. Given that treatment decisions often rest heavily on our imperfect assessments, the concept of an automated and highly accurate method for bone age interpretation is attractive indeed. This review, and an additional abstract from the United States,[1] highlight the cumulative evidence that such a method exists in the form of the BoneXpert system. Whether this system is ready for clinical prime time depends in part on the willingness of pediatric endocrinologists to adopt it in their practices. Only if it is also proven to be reliable for making accurate height predictions in a longitudinal fashion in both the clinical and research arenas could it ever be postulated to truly supplant the old-fashioned way.

E. Eugster, MD

Reference

1. Lee PA, Thodberg HH. Evaluation of automated bone age determination in American children with precocious puberty. (poster), Endo Soc Annual Meeting P1-342, June 2009; Washington DC

Impact of the exon 3-deleted GH receptor polymorphism on baseline height and the growth response to recombinant human growth hormone therapy in growth hormone deficient (GHD) and non-GHD children with short stature: a systematic review and meta-analysis

Wassenaar MJE, Dekkers OM, Pereira AM, et al (Leiden Univ Med Ctr, The Netherlands)

J Clin Endocrinol Metab 94:3721-3730, 2009

Context.—The exon-3 deleted growth hormone receptor (GHR_{d3}) polymorphism is associated with an increased growth response to recombinant human GH (rhGH) therapy in some, but not all, studies in growth hormone deficient (GHD) and non-GHD children with short stature.

Objective.—To assess the effects of GHR_{d3} on baseline height and the 1st year's growth response to rhGH treatment in pre-pubertal GHD and non-GHD children with short stature.

Design.—Systematic review and meta-analysis.

Methods.—Fifteen studies reporting the effect of GHR_{d3} on growth parameters were included. Principal outcomes were baseline height SDS, and the weighted average of change in growth velocity (delta cm/yr) and height gain (delta height SDS) after 1 year of rhGH.

Results.—In GHD, not in non-GHD, baseline height SDS was 0.159 SD higher (95%CI 0.020,0.298) in GHR_{d3} compared with $GHR_{wt\text{-}wt}$. In GHR_{d3} rhGH therapy resulted in a higher increase in growth velocity (0.521 cm/yr, 95%CI 0.196,1.015) and height gain (0.075 SD; 95%CI 0.007, 0.143) compared with $GHR_{wt\text{-}wt}$. Meta-regression demonstrated a larger difference between GHR_{d3} and $GHR_{wt\text{-}wt}$ in studies using lower rhGH doses and carried out at a higher age, independently of the cause of short stature.

Conclusions.—This meta-analysis in prepubertal children with short stature indicates that GHR_{d3} is associated with increased baseline height in GHD, but not in non-GHD. Furthermore, GHR_{d3} stimulates growth velocity by an additional effect of ~0.5 cm during the first year of rhGH treatment and this effect is more pronounced at lower doses of rhGH and higher age.

▶ Many attempts have been made to identify physiological factors that are related to individual differences in sensitivity to human recombinant growth hormone (GH) therapy. One of the more intriguing of these has been the suggestion that a common polymorphism of the GH receptor, the exon 3-deleted version, confers a higher degree of responsiveness to exogenous GH than the wild type. However, studies published to date that have examined this possibility have yielded conflicting results. Therefore, the authors of this article are to be commended for amassing what appears to be the world's extant literature on this subject. As with all meta-analyses, only a fraction of the originally identified articles, 11% in this case, met inclusion criteria. Of the 15 articles that were included, significant heterogeneity of sample size, clinical characteristics, and GH dose existed. Despite those inherent problems, collectively the data present good evidence for a positive, albeit very modest, effect of the exon 3-deleted GH receptor polymorphism on baseline height and 1-year growth velocity in prepubertal GH deficient children. Although this is clearly the take-home message, inconsistencies remain. Of the 11 articles reporting the effect of heterozygosity versus homozygosity of the exon 3-deleted GH receptor, 4 report differences in growth velocity between these 2 groups (although not necessarily in the same direction), while 7 do not. Although this meta-analysis does not represent the final word on the question at hand, it is an important contribution that provides a modicum of clarity to an otherwise murky topic.

E. Eugster, MD

Short Stature in a Population-Based Cohort: Social, Emotional, and Behavioral Functioning

Lee JM, Appugliese D, Coleman SM, et al (Univ of Michigan, Ann Arbor; Boston Univ, MA; et al)

Pediatrics 124:903-910, 2009

Objective.—The goal was to determine whether there were significant differences between children of normative versus short stature in behavioral functioning and peer relationships, according to teacher and child reports.

Methods.—The study included 712 boys and girls in the sixth grade, from the National Institute of Child Health and Human Development Study of Early Child Care and Youth Development. Main outcome measures included Achenbach Teacher's Report Form internalizing, externalizing, and total scores; Children's Depression Inventory scores (child report); Life Orientation Test-Revised scores (child report); Child Behavior with Peers questionnaire asocial with peers, excluded by peers, and peer victimization subscale scores (teacher report); peer social support and victimization scores (child report); and relationships with peers score (teacher report). In bivariate comparisons, these outcomes were compared for children of relatively short (height of <10th percentile) versus nonshort (height of ≥10th percentile) stature, and effect sizes were calculated. Multivariate linear regression models adjusted for maternal education, income/needs ratio, race, and gender.

Results.—Effect sizes ranged from 0.00 to 0.35. Short children reported marginally higher levels of self-perceived peer victimization, compared with their nonshort peers. There were no significant differences in the rest of the outcomes for children of short versus nonshort stature, in either unadjusted or adjusted models.

Conclusion.—Although short children from a population-based sample reported marginally higher levels of self-perceived peer victimization, they did not differ from their nonshort peers in a range of social, emotional, and behavioral outcomes.

▶ Approximately 40% of new patient referrals to the pediatric endocrine clinic are due to concerns about short stature. Not only is small size perceived as a physical disadvantage, but also the fact that it is also psychologically debilitating is a frequent assumption made by parents and primary care providers. Therefore, a study such as this one, which emphasizes the importance of a community based, rather than a clinic referred sample, serves as a useful reality check when addressing these concerns. Particularly informative is that children were assessed at ~age 11, which often coincides with Middle School angst regarding real or imagined differences from one's peers. An additional strength of the study is that it included assessments from teachers, parents, and children themselves. That findings were consistent across these different sources is reassuring. The trend toward higher self-perceived peer victimization among short children is undoubtedly related to increased rates of teasing. The lack of any other effect of stature on overall functioning is in line with previous assertions that teasing in and of itself does not result in psychopathology. Although parents who are certain that their short child is suffering will be skeptical, results from this article should be included in conversations about the importance of height in children's quality of life. Future similar analyses targeted at the very shortest children (those with heights < 5th percentile) are needed.

E. Eugster, MD

Miscellaneous

Cushing Syndrome in the McCune-Albright Syndrome

Brown RJ, Kelly MH, Collins MT (Natl Insts of Health, Bethesda, MD)
J Clin Endocrinol Metab 95:1508-1515, 2010

Context.—Cushing syndrome (CS) is a rare but potentially fatal feature of McCune-Albright syndrome (MAS). Optimal management, prognostic features, and long-term follow-up of this disorder have not been described.

Setting.—The study was conducted at an academic tertiary care center.

Patients.—A total of 112 patients participating in a natural history study at the National Institutes of Health (NIH) were evaluated, and 21 published cases were reviewed.

Interventions.—Subjects received observation, medical management, or bilateral adrenalectomy.

Main Outcome Measures.—We measured prevalence, prognostic factors, and natural history.

Results.—The prevalence of CS among NIH patients was 7.1%. The median age at diagnosis was 3 months. Clinical features included "Cushingoid facies" (66.7%), failure to thrive (60.0%), low birth weight (50.0%), liver disease (36.7%), and heart disease (26.7%). Six patients (20.0%) died, four after adrenalectomy. Death was more likely in patients with comorbid heart disease (odds ratio, 13.3; $P < 0.05$). Of 23 survivors,

13 underwent adrenalectomy, and 10 exhibited spontaneous resolution. Two patients with spontaneous resolution who were tested later in life (3 and 15 yr after resolution) continued to have low-level, autonomous adrenal function with biochemical adrenal insufficiency. Compared to MAS patients without CS, patients with CS were more likely to have a cognitive/developmental disorder (44.4 *vs.* 4.8%; $P < 0.001$; odds ratio, 8.8).

Conclusions.—Comorbid heart and liver disease were poor prognostic markers and may indicate the need for prompt adrenalectomy. The high incidence of cognitive disorders indicates a need for close developmental follow-up and parental counseling. Patients with spontaneous resolution of CS may develop adrenal insufficiency, and they require long-term monitoring.

▶ The extreme rarity of McCune-Albright syndrome (MAS) has made it difficult to determine the incidence rates of specific manifestations of the condition. In addition, prognostic features and information about the natural history of the various endocrinopathies associated with this complex disorder have been lacking. Thus, the major contribution of this retrospective review is that the authors were able to amass an impressive number ($n = 112$) of subjects with MAS, of whom 30 had Cushing syndrome (CS), with the last follow-up occurring at up to ~16 years of age. A few of the findings are particularly noteworthy: One of these is the extremely young age at diagnosis of CS, which often occurred before any of the other features associated with MAS were recognized. This emphasizes the importance of maintaining a high index of suspicion for the disorder in a multitude of potential clinical scenarios. Another interesting feature of CS in these patients was the high rate of spontaneous resolution, believed to be due to involution of the fetal zone of the adrenals in the postnatal period. Lastly, the observation that cognitive problems were more prevalent in the group with cortisol excess than in those without is intriguing. However, information regarding whether standardized assessments of cognitive function were performed in all subjects is lacking. Given that most of these data regarding those with CS were extracted from previously published reports, it seems safe to assume that there were no standardized assessments of cognitive function performed. Regardless, this study provides valuable information regarding the incidence, associated clinical features, and natural history of CS in patients with MAS.

E. Eugster, MD

Determinants of Medical Care for Young Women with Turner Syndrome

Devernay M, Ecosse E, Coste J, et al (Robert Debré Hosp and Univ Paris 7 Denis Diderot, France; Groupe hospitalier Cochin-Saint Vincent de Paul and Univ Paris Descartes, France)

J Clin Endocrinol Metab 94:3408-3413, 2009

Context.—Turner syndrome is associated with reduced life expectancy. Lifelong follow-up is strongly recommended, but follow-up during the transition between pediatric and adult care has been little evaluated.

Objective.—Our objective was to evaluate the medical follow-up of a population-based cohort of young adult patients.

Design, Setting, and Patients.—A questionnaire study was conducted with a national cohort of 568 women, aged 22.6 ± 2.6 yr (range, 18.3–31.2), a mean of 6 yr after stopping GH treatment (StaTur cohort).

Main Outcome Measures.—We assessed the proportion of patients with adequate follow-up at seven medical assessments over 4 yr and its determinants.

Results.—Most participants were followed by gynecologists or general practitioners. Medical assessments were performed in 16%(audiometry) to 68%(lipid level determinations) of participants, with little consistency in individual patients. Only 20 of 568 patients (3.5%) underwent all assessments in the 4-yr period. Multivariate analysis identified the type of physician as the only factor consistently associated with follow-up, which was more adequate with endocrinologists than with other physicians. Other variables associated with at least one adequate follow-up assessment were paternal socioeconomic class, education level, number of Turner syndrome disease components, size of the medical center following the patient in childhood, and physical health dimensions of Short Form 36 questionnaire.

Conclusions.—By contrast with the intensive medical follow-up in childhood, follow-up was grossly inadequate during the transition phase. During this phase, patients should be sent to physicians specializing in Turner syndrome and particular attention should be paid to patients with lower levels of education and from families of low socioeconomic status.

▶ Although it occurs as often as 1 in ~2500 live female births, the medical homeland for girls with Turner syndrome (TS) has always been the pediatric endocrinology, rather than the primary care, setting. Not only do we prescribe growth hormone and sex steroid replacement, but we also coordinate ongoing surveillance for other problems that girls with TS are at risk for, and typically take the lead on, referring to other subspecialty clinics when needed. One reason for this sense of ownership is that the diagnosis is often made by a pediatric endocrinologist, and is followed by the establishment of a long-standing relationship built on mutual trust and appreciation. In addition, we are the ones who educate trainees and primary care colleagues about the syndrome, and are integral to the process of formulating consensus guidelines, and to promoting the TS research and advocacy agendas. The significant investment made in our young patients during childhood and adolescence is in stark contrast to the findings of this study, which are disheartening to say the least. The revelation that only 3.5% of this large cohort of young women had undergone all recommended assessments in the previous 4-year period is simply stunning. No matter how careful and comprehensive the medical care is that we provide to our pediatric patients, it appears that we are ultimately failing them through a system that has no safeguards to ensure safe passage to adult providers. Where to lay the blame? One illuminating finding from this study is that care tended to be most acceptable in the hands of an endocrinologist, emphasizing the importance of identifying one of our adult counterparts for each patient discharged from our clinic. A greater emphasis must also be placed on educating and empowering patients to be their own health care advocates, and on providing personalized medical histories and written guidelines regarding ongoing care. Finally, training more Med-Peds endocrinologists is an obvious solution because they are able to provide knowledgeable care from childhood and beyond. Sadly, this breakdown in transition is ubiquitous in the pediatric realm. Only a concerted and collaborative endeavor on the part of us, our patients and our adult colleagues will eventually improve the quality of this critical development juncture for graduates of the pediatric setting.

E. Eugster, MD

Isolated Familial Hypogonadotropic Hypogonadism and a *GNRH1* Mutation

Bouligand J, Ghervan C, Tello JA, et al (Hôpital de Bicêtre, Paris; Univ of Medicine and Pharmacy Iuliu Hatieganu, Cluj-Napoca, Romania; The Queen's Med Research Inst, Edinburgh; et al)
N Engl J Med 360:2742-2748, 2009

We investigated whether mutations in the gene encoding gonadotropin-releasing hormone 1 (*GNRH1*) might be responsible for idiopathic hypogonadotropic hypogonadism (IHH) in humans. We identified a homozygous *GNRH1* frameshift mutation, an insertion of an adenine at nucleotide position 18 (c.18-19insA), in the sequence encoding the N-terminal region of the signal peptide–containing protein precursor of gonadotropin-releasing hormone (prepro-GnRH) in a teenage brother and sister, who had normosmic IHH. Their unaffected parents and a sibling who was tested were heterozygous. This mutation results in an aberrant peptide lacking the conserved GnRH decapeptide sequence, as shown by the absence of immunoreactive GnRH when expressed in vitro. This isolated autosomal recessive GnRH deficiency, reversed by pulsatile GnRH administration, shows the pivotal role of GnRH in human reproduction.

▶ Every textbook chapter and review article devoted to the topic of Delayed Puberty includes a section detailing the molecular genetic causes of hypogonadotropic hypogonadism (HH). Invariably, the discussion also contains an acknowledgment that a mutation in the gene encoding Gonadotropin-Releasing Hormone (GnRH) has never been identified. This fact has been deserving of attention because it has seemed a rather glaring absence in the growing list of human molecular mutations in genes involved in GnRH neuronal migration, signaling, and release. Implicit in this observation has likewise been the assumption that "It's only a matter of time" before such an abnormality is found. Thus, the discovery of a homozygous mutation in GNRH1, which encodes prepro-GnRH, in a pair of normosmic siblings with complete obliteration of GnRH secretion, is noteworthy indeed. There are several strengths of this report. These include the in-vitro functional studies as well as administration of exogenous GnRH to the affected female sibling, which underscored the physiologic role of GnRH by stimulating pulsatile LH release and recruitment of a dominant ovarian follicle. Finally, the screening of 445 controls for the mutation, including 145 with idiopathic HH and 200 who were ancestrally matched with the index family, was critical for providing insight into the likely origin and incidence of this genetic defect in similarly affected patients. Identification of a single ancestrally related control harboring a heterozygous form of the same mutation indicates a founder effect, while its complete absence in the other HH subjects and controls confirms the extreme rarity of the GNRH1 mutation. Therefore, while this mutation will not allow investigators to make significant headway in delineating the pathogenesis of HH in the sizable percentage of patients in whom the etiology remains unknown, it is nonetheless a landmark discovery in the field of human reproductive biology.

E. Eugster, MD

Mutations of the *KISS1* Gene in Disorders of Puberty

Silveira LG, Noel SD, Silveira-Neto AP, et al (Faculdade de Medicina da Universidade de São Paulo, Brasil; Brigham and Women's Hosp, Boston, MA; et al)

J Clin Endocrinol Metab 95:2276-2280, 2010

Context.—Kisspeptin, encoded by the *KISS1* gene, is a key stimulatory factor of GnRH secretion and puberty onset. Inactivating mutations of its receptor (*KISS1R*) cause isolated hypogonadotropic hypogonadism (IHH). A unique *KISS1R*-activating mutation was described in central precocious puberty (CPP).

Objective.—Our objective was to investigate *KISS1* mutations in patients with idiopathic CPP and normosmic IHH.

Patients.—Eighty-three children with CPP (77 girls) and 61 patients with IHH (40 men) were studied. The control group consisted of 200 individuals with normal pubertal development.

Methods.—The promoter region and the three exons of *KISS1* were amplified and sequenced. Cells expressing *KISS1R* were stimulated with synthetic human wild-type or mutant kisspeptin-54 (kp54), and inositol phosphate accumulation was measured. In a second set of experiments, kp54 was preincubated in human serum before stimulation of the cells.

Results.—Two novel *KISS1* missense mutations, p.P74S and p.H90D, were identified in three unrelated children with idiopathic CPP. Both mutations were absent in 400 control alleles. The p.P74S mutation was identified in the heterozygous state in a boy who developed CPP at 1 yr of age. The p.H90D mutation was identified in the homozygous state in two unrelated girls with CPP. *In vitro* studies revealed that the capacity of the P74S and H90D mutants to stimulate IP production was similar to the wild type. After preincubation of wild-type and mutant kp54 in human serum, the capacity to stimulate signal transduction was significantly greater for P74S compared with the wild type, suggesting that the p.P74S variant is more stable. Only polymorphisms were found in the IHH group.

Conclusion.—Two *KISS1* mutations were identified in unrelated patients with idiopathic CPP.Thep.P74S variant was associated with higher kisspeptin resistance to degradation in comparison with the wild type, suggesting a role for this mutation in the precocious puberty phenotype.

▶ The exciting discovery of the role of kisspeptin in human reproductive physiology has paved the way for the identification of novel molecular genetic abnormalities in this system as the basis for pubertal disorders in children. This is the second such report, following on the heels of the 2008 publication describing a GPR54 activating mutation in a girl with central precocious puberty (CPP).[1] In this study, 3 mutations in the *KISS1* gene were identified, accounting for 3.6% of cases of CPP in this cohort of 83 subjects. Functional studies of the heterozygous P74S mutation, discovered in a boy with the onset of idiopathic CPP at 12 months of age, indicated enhanced resistance to degradation as the basis for increased signaling by the mutant protein. This is a similar mechanism to that postulated in the case of the GPR54 mutation in which a reduced rate of receptor desensitization was observed in in vitro studies. The pathogenesis of CPP in the 2 girls harboring the homozygous H90D mutation could not be elucidated from the studies performed, however, and the investigators are appropriately cautious about attributing the early puberty to this genetic variant. Regardless, it is fascinating that the mother of one of these girls had menarche at age 10, and additional studies are clearly needed. While the vast majority of cases of CPP remain idiopathic, further exploration of genetic determinants of pubertal timing will surely lead to a progressive unraveling of the biological basis for both atypical and on-time activation of the hypothalamic-pituitary-gonadal (HPG) axis.

E. Eugster, MD

Reference

1. Teles MG, Bianco SD, Brito VN, et al. A GPR54-activating mutation in a patient with central precocious puberty. *N Engl J Med.* 2008;358:709-715.

Neonatal Complete Generalized Glucocorticoid Resistance and Growth Hormone Deficiency Caused by a Novel Homozygous Mutation in Helix 12 of the Ligand Binding Domain of the Glucocorticoid Receptor Gene (NR3C1)

McMahon SK, Pretorius CJ, Ungerer JPJ, et al (Royal Children's Hosp, Queensland, Australia; Dept of Chemical Pathology, Queensland, Australia; et al)

J Clin Endocrinol Metab 95:297-302, 2010

Context.—Glucocorticoid resistance is a rare genetic condition characterized by reduced sensitivity to cortisol signaling and subsequent hyperactivation of the hypothalamic-pituitary-adrenal axis.

Objective.—The objective was to confirm the diagnosis of glucocorticoid resistance in the patient, to determine the degree of suppression of cortisol and ACTH levels in response to dexamethasone, and to determine the underlying genetic abnormality and functional consequences of the mutation.

Patient and Methods.—The patient presented on the first day of life with profound hypoglycemia. Initial cortisol levels were appropriately elevated; however, the patient was found to have persistently elevated levels of both cortisol and ACTH. The baby developed a tanned appearance and severe hypertension and fatigued easily with feeding. Serial oral dexamethasone suppression tests were performed with doses escalating from 0.125 mg to 12 mg dexamethasone given at 2300 h. Sequencing of the glucocorticoid receptor gene was performed along with functional studies of the glucocorticoid receptor. GH secretion was assessed with an arginine glucagon stimulation test.

Results.—Cortisol and ACTH levels did not suppress with doses of up to 12 mg dexamethasone. A 2-bp deletion was found at amino acid position 773 of the glucocorticoid receptor ligand binding domain. A complete lack of dexamethasone binding and *in vitro* biological effect was demonstrated. GH stimulation testing was consistent with GH deficiency.

Conclusion.—The homozygous mutation in the ligand-binding domain of the glucocorticoid receptor gene resulted in a functionally inactive glucocorticoid receptor and apparent complete glucocorticoid resistance with biochemical GH deficiency.

▶ This fascinating report serves to remind us that the differential diagnosis of commonly encountered scenarios, such as neonatal hypoglycemia, must continually expand to accommodate new discoveries in human molecular biology. As was definitively demonstrated by a full panel of functional studies, the novel homozygous mutation in the ligand binding domain of the glucocorticoid receptor identified in this patient effectively obliterated all response to both endogenous and exogenous glucocorticoids. This case also demonstrates the importance of natural history in the diagnostic process. Although the finding of a normal cortisol in the setting of hypoglycemia was initially reassuring, the baby's progressive hyperpigmentation and hypertension eventually led to a presumptive diagnosis of generalized glucocorticoid resistance at 5 weeks of age. Another interesting aspect of the case is the concurrent growth hormone resistance, which the authors attribute to 2 possible and equally plausible mechanisms, and which also contributed to the infants' hypoglycemic state. Finally, it is obviously significant that the same homozygous mutation was identified in paraffin-embedded tissue from the deceased sibling. Whether this infant will survive, and what the phenotypic consequences of this previously unidentified defect will be going forward, remains to be seen.

E. Eugster, MD

Pediatric thyroid fine-needle aspiration cytology: a meta-analysis

Stevens C, Lee JKP, Sadatsafavi M, et al (Univ of British Columbia, Vancouver, Canada)

J Pediatr Surg 44:2184-2191, 2009

Background.—There is conflicting evidence in the current literature regarding the use of fine-needle aspiration (FNA) biopsy in the diagnosis of a thyroid nodule in the pediatric population. There are numerous studies that look at the sensitivity and specificity of this test with varying results. A meta-analysis will provide further insight into this topic.

Purpose.—Our objective was to investigate the diagnostic parameters of FNA biopsy in the diagnosis of a thyroid nodule in the pediatric population, specifically, to determine the sensitivity, specificity, accuracy, positive predictive value (PPV), and negative predictive value (NPV) of the test in differentiating malignant vs benign tumors.

Material and Methods.—We performed a literature search of Medline, Embase, and evidence based medicine (EBM) reviews for English studies that looked at FNA biopsy in thyroid nodules in the pediatric population, in which diagnostic values were present or could be calculated and where FNA results were compared to an acceptable reference standard. Two reviewers independently selected all abstracts, and from these, studies to review. Two reviewers also independently checked diagnostic values in the studies or calculated them from data available. A meta-analysis was performed, and pooled diagnostic test values were calculated using a random-effects, bivariate meta-regression model. Studies were also assessed for quality using the quality assessment for diagnostic accuracy studies tool.

Results.—Twelve studies were included for review. The quality of the studies in general was good. The pooled estimate of sensitivity and specificity were 94% (95% confidence interval [CI], 86%-100%) and 81% (95% CI, 72%-91%), respectively. Assuming 20% of nodules are malignant, the accuracy, PPV, and NPV were 83.6%, 55.3%, and 98.2%, respectively.

Conclusion.—This meta-analysis provides good evidence that FNA biopsy of thyroid nodules is a sensitive test in the pediatric population and may be a useful tool for excluding malignancy in young patients. Future prospective studies are needed to evaluate this further.

▶ Unlike in adults, thyroid nodules in children and adolescents are rare. Due to the established higher incidence of thyroid cancer in isolated pediatric versus adult thyroid nodules, these lesions are also considered to be far more worrisome than in the adult population. Therefore, many pediatric endocrinologists have traditionally followed the practice of routinely referring such patients to an ENT specialist or pediatric surgeon to have a hemithyroidectomy or thyroidectomy performed. However, thyroid surgery is not without risks, which include laryngeal nerve damage and hypoparathyroidism, which may be permanent. Thus, the ability to accurately differentiate benign nodules from thyroid cancer would prevent unnecessary thyroid surgeries and enhance clinical care. A major strength of this meta-analysis is the stringent criteria used for including studies. Given the scarcity of reports of using fine-needle aspiration (FNA) in the diagnostic evaluation of pediatric thyroid nodules, combining the results of existing studies to derive the sensitivity and specificity of this tool in children makes intuitive sense. Nonetheless, it should be noted that all studies were retrospective and not all of them used ultrasound-guided FNA, which would be considered standard of care at most institutions. The take-home message of the authors' findings is that FNA of thyroid nodules in children does appear to be quite sensitive in excluding malignancy, and is undoubtedly underused as a diagnostic tool. It would behoove pediatric endocrinologists to identify the appropriate personnel to perform this procedure in their own institution, and to consider it in the evaluation of select patients. Additional guidelines regarding whether and when to repeat FNA, the significance of nodule size in predicting pathology, and how to deal with equivocal results are also needed.

E. Eugster, MD

Pituitary

Newborn Screening Results in Children with Central Hypothyroidism

Nebesio TD, McKenna MP, Nabhan ZM, et al (Indiana Univ School of Medicine, Indianapolis)
J Pediatr 156:990-993, 2010

Objective.—To investigate newborn screening results in children with congenital hypopituitarism, including central hypothyroidism, and to determine whether there were differences between children who had abnormal results and children with normal newborn screening results.

Study Design.—Medical records of children with central hypothyroidism observed in our pediatric endocrinology clinics from 1990 to 2006 were reviewed.

Results.—Forty-two subjects (22 boys) were identified. Eight children (19%) had a low total thyroxine level (<5.0 mcg/dL) on the newborn screening test. The average total thyroxine level in the remaining 34 subjects was 9.8 ± 3.4 mcg/dL. Thyrotropin levels were within the reference range in all children. No differences were found in the 2 groups for birth history, jaundice (53% overall), hypoglycemia (36% overall), or micropenis (43% of boys). Fifty-seven percent of children had septo-optic dysplasia, and 98% had multiple pituitary hormone deficiencies. Children with an abnormal newborn screening results were initially examined by a pediatric endocrinologist at an average age of 4.6 ± 5.0 months, and children with normal newborn screening results were initially examined at an average age of 16.9 ± 26.7 months (P =.037).

Conclusions.—Most children with congenital central hypothyroidism have normal thyroid function at birth. Normal newborn screening results can be falsely reassuring and may contribute to a delay in diagnosis of hypopituitarism despite classic clinical features.

▶ Hallmarks of congenital hypopituitarism include hypoglycemia, micropenis (in boys), and jaundice. While the combination of all 3 is compelling, none of these clinical features are pathognomonic and can obviously result from a number of different etiologies. Additional evaluation of neonates with suspected hypopituitarism involves biochemical assessment of pituitary function, including results of the newborn screen for congenital hypothyroidism. There is a tacit assumption that if this test comes back normal, the presence of hypopituitarism is less likely. This article turns that notion on its head. After being burned by a delayed diagnosis of panhypopituitarism in a 3-month-old baby with septo-optic dysplasia, the authors took advantage of the fact that their state was fortuitously 1 of only 2 that measured both T4 and thyroid-stimulating hormone (TSH) on all newborns. What they found was quite unexpected. Of a cohort of children with congenital central hypothyroidism, fully 81% had normal thyroid function at birth and developed a low thyroxine only in the subsequent weeks and months that followed. Although no difference in clinical signs consistent with hypopituitarism was seen in infants with a normal versus abnormal newborn screen, the subjects with a normal initial T4 were first evaluated by a pediatric endocrinologist at a significantly older age than those in whom it was initially low. This suggests that the normal newborn screen in these infants led to a false sense of security that ultimately contributed to a delayed diagnosis of hypopituitarism. The take-home messages of this novel study are straightforward. One is that congenital hypothyroidism screening programs that use a TSH-only protocol are unlikely to miss cases of central hypothyroidism that would otherwise be detected by measuring T4 because most affected infants will have normal thyroid function at birth. Even more important is that while thyroid levels absolutely should be obtained, normal results should not decrease our index of suspicion for hypopituitarism in a neonate one iota!

E. Eugster, MD

Article Index

Chapter 1: Diabetes

Chapter 2: Lipoproteins and Atherosclerosis

Chapter 3: Obesity

Chapter 4: Thyroid

Chapter 5: Calcium and Bone Metabolism

Chapter 6: Adrenal Cortex

Chapter 7: Reproductive Endocrinology

Chapter 8: Neuroendocrinology

Chapter 9: Pediatric Endocrinology

Author Index

F

G

H

I

J

K

L

FSC
www.fsc.org
MIX
Papier | Fördert gute Waldnutzung
FSC® C083411

Kolibri 360 GmbH
Ferdinand-Jühlke-Straße 7
99095 Erfurt, Deutschland
produktsicherheit@kolibri360.de